*Changing Addictive Behavior*

D1279959

# Changing Addictive Behavior

## Bridging Clinical and Public Health Strategies

Edited by

Jalie A. Tucker
Dennis M. Donovan
G. Alan Marlatt

*Foreword by Frederick B. Glaser*

THE GUILFORD PRESS
New York    London

© 1999 The Guilford Press
A Division of Guilford Publications, Inc.
72 Spring Street, New York, NY 10012
www.guilford.com

Printed in the United States of America

This book is printed on acid-free paper.

Last digit is print number:   9   8   7   6   5   4

**Library of Congress Cataloging-in-Publication Data**

Changing addictive behavior : bridging clinical and public health
    strategies / edited by Jalie A. Tucker, Dennis M. Donovan, G. Alan
    Marlatt : foreword by Frederick B. Glaser.
        p.   cm.
    Includes bibliographical references.
    ISBN 1-57230-439-1 (hc.)   ISBN 1-57230-677-7 (pbk.)
    1. Substance abuse—Treatment.   2. Addicts—Rehabilitation.
I. Tucker, Jalie A. (Jalie Ann), 1954–       .   II. Donovan, Dennis M.
(Dennis Michael)   III. Marlatt, G. Alan.
RC564.C468     1999
616.86′06—dc21                                              99-22744
                                                              CIP

*To those seeking to come to terms with addictive behaviors and to gain balance and harmony in their lives*

# About the Editors

**Jalie A. Tucker, PhD, MPH,** is Alumni Professor of Psychology at Auburn University, Alabama. Originally educated as a clinical psychologist, Dr. Tucker has variously worked as a faculty researcher, educator, therapist, and administrator in medical school and psychology department settings. Her research on help-seeking and addictive behavior change patterns is supported by the National Institute on Alcohol Abuse and Alcoholism. Dr. Tucker recently completed a masters of public health degree in health care organization and policy, an endeavor made possible by a Research Scientist Development Award from the NIAAA. A consistent contributor to the scientific literature on substance abuse, she is a past president of the Division on Addictions (50) of the American Psychological Association and a past leader of the Addictive Behaviors Special Interest Group of the Association for Advancement of Behavior Therapy.

**Dennis M. Donovan, PhD,** is Director of the University of Washington's Alcohol and Drug Abuse Institute and is a Professor in the Department of Psychiatry and Behavioral Sciences and Adjunct Professor in the Department of Psychology at the University of Washington. Dr. Donovan was affiliated with the Addictions Treatment Center at the Seattle Department of Veterans Affairs Medical Center for 17 years, where he was involved in clinical, administrative, training, and research activities. During that time he was instrumental in the development of, and served as Associate Director of, the first Center of Excellence in Substance Abuse Treatment and Education (CESATE). He has over 120 publications in the area of alcoholism and addictive behaviors, and has served as Associate Editor and as a member of the editorial boards of the *Journal of Studies on Alcohol* and *Psychology of Addictive Behaviors*. His research has been funded by the National Institute on Alcohol Abuse and Alcoholism, the National Institute on Drug Abuse, and the Center for Substance Abuse Treatment.

**G. Alan Marlatt, PhD,** is Professor of Psychology and Director of the Addictive Behaviors Research Center at the University of Washington, Seattle. In 1996, Dr. Marlatt was appointed as a member of the National Advisory Council on Drug Abuse for the National Institute on Drug Abuse. His research is supported by a Senior Scientist Award and a MERIT Award from the National Institute on Alcohol Abuse and Alcoholism. In 1990, he received the Jellinek Memorial Award for outstanding contributions to knowledge in the field of alcohol studies. Widely published, he is the coeditor of *Assessment of Addictive Behaviors* (with Dennis M. Donovan) and *Relapse Prevention* (with Judith R. Gordon), and a coauthor of *Brief Alcohol Screening and Intervention for College Students (BASICS)* (with Linda A. Dimeff, John S. Baer, and Daniel R. Kivlahan).

# Contributors

**David B. Abrams, PhD,** Center for Behavioral and Preventive Medicine, and Department of Psychiatry and Human Behavior, Brown University School of Medicine, Providence, Rhode Island; The Miriam Hospital, Providence, Rhode Island

**Curtis Breslin, PhD,** Addiction Research Foundation of Ontario, University of Toronto, Toronto, Ontario, Canada

**Matthew M. Clark, PhD,** Center for Behavioral and Preventive Medicine, and Department of Psychiatry and Human Behavior, Brown University School of Medicine, Providence, Rhode Island

**Susan J. Curry, PhD,** Center for Health Studies, Group Health Cooperative of Puget Sound, Seattle, Washington; Department of Health Services, University of Washington at Seattle, Seattle, Washington

**Dennis M. Donovan, PhD,** Department of Psychiatry and Behavioral Sciences, Alcohol and Drug Abuse Institute, University of Washington at Seattle, Seattle, Washington

**Michael F. Fleming, MD, MPH,** Department of Family Medicine, University of Wisconsin at Madison Medical School, Madison, Wisconsin; Director, Center for Addiction Research and Education, Madison, Wisconsin

**John G. Heilman, PhD,** College of Liberal Arts, Auburn University, Auburn, Alabama

**Stephen T. Higgins, PhD,** Department of Psychiatry, University of Vermont, Burlington, Vermont

**Jay Joseph, MSc,** Addiction Research Foundation of Ontario, University of Toronto, Toronto, Ontario, Canada

**Eleanor L. Kim, MS,** Department of Psychology, University of Washington at Seattle, Seattle, Washington

**Teresa K. King, PhD,** Center for Behavioral and Preventive Medicine, and Department of Psychiatry and Human Behavior, Brown University School of Medicine, Providence, Rhode Island

**Michele Pukish King, PhD,** Addictive Behavior and Health Studies, Department of Psychology, Auburn University, Auburn, Alabama; Montgomery Psychiatry and Associates, Montgomery, Alabama

**G. Alan Marlatt, PhD,** Department of Psychology; and Addictive Behaviors Research Center, University of Washington at Seattle, Seattle, Washington

**René P. McEldowney, PhD,** Department of Political Science, Auburn University, Auburn, Alabama

**David B. Rosengren, PhD,** Alcohol and Drug Abuse Institute, University of Washington at Seattle, Seattle, Washington

**Laura A. Schmidt, MSW, MPH,** Alcohol Research Group, Public Health Institute, Berkeley, California

**Harvey Skinner, PhD,** Department of Public Health Sciences, University of Toronto, Toronto, Ontario, Canada

**Linda C. Sobell, PhD, ABPP,** Center for Psychological Studies, Nova Southeastern University, Fort Lauderdale, Florida

**Mark B. Sobell, PhD, ABPP,** Center for Psychological Studies, Nova Southeastern University, Fort Lauderdale, Florida

**Jalie A. Tucker, PhD, MPH,** Department of Psychology, Auburn University, Auburn, Alabama

**Rudy E. Vuchinich, PhD,** Department of Psychology, Auburn University, Auburn, Alabama

**Constance M. Weisner, DrPH, MSW,** Alcohol Research Group, Public Health Institute, Berkeley, California; School of Public Health, University of California at Berkeley, Berkeley, California

**Allen Zweben, DSW,** School of Social Welfare, University of Wisconsin at Milwaukee, Milwaukee, Wisconsin; Center for Addiction and Behavioral Health Research, Milwaukee, Wisconsin

# Foreword

The squirming facts exceed the squamous mind,
If one may say so. And yet relation appears,
A small relation expanding like the shade
Of a cloud on sand, a shape on the side of a hill.
— WALLACE STEVENS, *Connoisseur of Chaos*

Relation of the kind celebrated by the poet certainly appears in this book. It contains a creative synthesis of many individual research studies, most of them conducted within the last decade, brought together into a coherent whole with important implications for the future of the field. Thereby the individual research studies are endowed with a much greater level of meaning and significance.

All who were involved in the Institute of Medicine report of 1990, *Broadening the Base of Treatment for Alcohol Problems,* will read the current volume with a sense of deep satisfaction. The work of a decade ago has been a primary point of departure for this new synthesis. Erik H. Erikson, the painter turned psychoanalyst who developed a theory of the stages of human development (Erikson, 1950), saw generativity as a pinnacle of the life cycle. To the extent that the IOM Committee has contributed to the development of this volume, we have scaled that exalted height.

Yet this detracts in no way from the magnitude of the present achievement. Its relationship to the prior report resembles the relationship of a rocket to a launching platform. A solid base has been provided to send the space probe on its way, but the new exploration ultimately finds itself far from the customary skies of the former effort. And so it should. In the intervening period much has been learned, and much has changed. New charts are required for guidance into the future. This book provides them.

The IOM report and the present work are more similar in form than in content. They are the products of scholarship rather than research. They represent an attempt to find meaning in existing data more than an attempt to create new data.

Research and scholarship are closely related, but are not identical. Their relationship resembles that between building materials and an architect's design for a structure. The architect certainly works with specific building materials and their characteristics firmly in mind. But what he or she produces is not necessarily predictable from the characteristics of the materials. The whole that the architect strives for may be greater than the sum of its parts. He or she can create a novel synthesis that makes use of the materials and their properties but at the same time transcends them.

In academia, research tends to be more prevalent and is richly rewarded, while scholarship tends to be less prevalent and is not rewarded in an equivalent manner. Promotions committees, for example, place the highest value on articles published in peer-reviewed journals, and characteristically assign much less value to books or book chapters. Yet it is precisely these longer and freer forms that are most conducive to a scholarly synthesis.

In its thoroughgoing detail, *Changing Addictive Behavior* is an exceptional example of the fruits of collaborative scholarly creativity. Utilizing the building blocks of a vast array of research studies, it proposes a vision of the future in which the individual therapeutic encounter is extended and complemented by a broad spectrum of additional approaches, ranging from modifications of standard treatment practices through interventions that have a preventive more than a reparative orientation and on to novel policy initiatives. It proposes pushing the envelope of our current efforts to help persons with addictive behavior problems by making them both more comprehensive and more effective for a much broader target population—the entire population, indeed, rather than only those who have the most serious problems.

While this is a novel approach to the proposed future development of the addictions field, similar trajectories to the one urged here have been proposed for other of the healing arts. Medicine is an example. Historically, it has tended to place an almost exclusive emphasis upon the encounter between the physician and the patient. The effectiveness of medical care, for example, has been offered as an explanation of the astonishing growth in world population in the postindustrial era. To evaluate this hypothesis, Thomas McKeown examined the earliest available mortality records, the English parish registers (McKeown, 1976). He found that mortality had declined in a linear fashion long before medical treatment was effective enough to result in a significant difference in the survival of individuals. His conclusions echo those of the present volume:

In the classical tradition there were two ideas concerning man's health: one, associated with the goddess Hygieia, that it could be achieved by a rational way of life; the other, personified by the god Asclepius, that it depended largely on the role of the physician as healer of the sick. Both concepts are to be found in Hippocractic writings, and they have survived in medical thought and practice down to the present day. However, since the seventeenth century at least, the Asclepian approach has been dominant. Philosophically, it derived support from Descartes' concept of the living organism as a machine which might be taken apart and reassembled if its structure and function were understood; practically, it seemed to find confirmation in the work of Kepler and Harvey and in the success of the physical sciences in manipulating inanimate matter. It is only in the past few decades that it has become evident that this interpretation is quite inaccurate, that the health of man is determined essentially by his behaviour, his food and the nature of the world around him, and is only marginally influenced by personal medical care. Intuitively we believe that *we are ill and are made well;* it is nearer the truth to say that *we are well and are made ill.* (McKeown, 1976, p. 162; emphasis in the original)

The valuable and consistent view of the implications of current research for the future of the substance abuse field that is the gift of this volume can appropriately be termed a vision. The vision embodied herein has not been implemented—not yet, in any case. Visions, however, do not require implementation to be of value. They constitute potential alternative futures that allow us to exercise our imaginations, and ultimately permit us the luxury of making a better informed choice in shaping the actual future. Without the guidance that visions can provide we would simply blunder into whatever happened to evolve. With that guidance we become the connoisseurs of chaos of Wallace Stevens' poem. Through the exercise of creative scholarship, we begin to put things together and to advance with a greater measure of confidence into what would otherwise be a shapeless void. Again in the words of the poet, we benefit from the vision of

> The pensive man . . . He sees that eagle float
> For whom the intricate Alps are a single nest.

FREDERICK B. GLASER, MD, FRCP(C)
*Professor of Psychiatric Medicine*
*Director, Division of Substance Abuse*
*East Carolina University School of Medicine*
*Greenville, North Carolina*

# REFERENCES

Erikson, E. H. (1950). *Childhood and society.* New York: Norton.

Institute of Medicine. (1990). *Broadening the base of treatment for alcohol problems.* Washington, DC: National Academy Press.

McKeown, T. (1976). *The modern rise of population.* London: Edward Arnold.

Stevens, W. (1993). *Poems* (Selected by H. Vendler). New York: Knopf.

# Preface

This edited volume reflects a collective journey that is ongoing for us and others who share an interest in helping individuals with addictive behavior problems. During the 20th century, popular and professional opinion shifted somewhat away from viewing addictive behaviors as character flaws deserving of stigmatization and punishment in favor of viewing them as a disease deserving of treatment. This shift, while generally positive, is incomplete and falls short of responding to addictive behaviors as the prevalent public health problem that they represent. Adopting a public health perspective makes salient the need to move beyond now dominant clinical approaches to care and to develop a continuum of interventions that spans clinical, preventive, and policy initiatives and that better matches the heterogeneous problems that result from addictive behaviors.

The need for further evolution in approaches to reducing addictive behaviors was articulated a decade ago in the Institute of Medicine's (1990) visionary report, *Broadening the Base of Treatment for Alcohol Problems*. The Study Director of the committee that produced the report was Frederick Glaser (see Foreword), and one of us (G.A.M.) was a committee member. The present volume extends the IOM's major thesis as formulated in the context of alcohol problems to other addictive behaviors and incorporates developments during the past decade that have advanced a broadened approach to behavior change. Using clinical interventions as a point of departure, the volume describes clinical and public health approaches to changing addictive behavior and seeks to empower practitioners in both communities with the knowledge needed to extend the reach and effectiveness of interventions, including coordinated, interdisciplinary initiatives.

The book is divided into two main parts. The first part reviews previous intervention approaches, summarizes recent scientific advances in understanding addictive behavior change, and offers a reformulated perspective that views problem resolution as a dynamic, temporally extended

process that is heavily influenced by motivational and environmental variables, in addition to effects of time-limited interventions. Recognition of
the importance of these extratherapeutic variables is a recent development because addictive behavior change has long been viewed as dependent upon participation in intensive treatment or mutual help groups
guided by 12-step principles. The second part discusses interventions
needed in an expanded perspective on addictive behavior change and begins to lay the groundwork for necessary evolutions in the roles of behavior change specialists in the era of managed care and in the age of AIDS.
Applications are discussed that span the formal health care system and
community settings and include chapters on brief interventions, the Community Reinforcement Approach, and stepped-care approaches to triaging and coordinating service delivery across the continuum of care. The
book concludes with a chapter on cost–benefit analysis of intervention
programs.

The book will be of interest to the diverse audience who shares an interest in promoting addictive behavior change and in designing and evaluating interventions to facilitate it. The book includes contributions from
authors who represent many fields, including psychology, psychiatry, social
work, public health, political science, and health administration. Collectively, they illustrate the interdisciplinary approach that is essential to developing the range of interventions needed to address the diversity of addictive behavior problems.

While the book should have relevance to several disciplines, it remains the case that it was conceived and largely written by clinical psychologists, including the three of us and several chapter authors. It thus
heavily reflects the experiences, struggles, and breakthroughs of mental
health professionals who were educated and who practiced within the clinical model to broaden their vista to include public health and public policy
perspectives, rather than the other way around. During a series of discussions in 1994 when the three of us were in Seattle (thanks to a leave for
J.A.T. sponsored by G.A.M.), we discovered that, in each of our respective
programs of research and scholarship, developments were occurring that
required us to move beyond the familiar clinical model and to consider
public health approaches to addictive behavior change. The IOM report,
while not predating our initiatives, had been influential in moving our
thinking forward and had provided a vital framework for combining clinical and public health perspectives.

The present book is the spontaneous outgrowth of our discussions
and one whose conception and implementation emerged easily because
the forces that had been acting upon us also were influencing and energiz-
ing many of our colleagues. We continue to learn about and to be en-
riched by this expanded worldview that subsumes, but does not replace,

the clinical perspective. It is a viewpoint that we believe will bring help to the underserved majority of persons with addictive behavior problems who find conventional clinical treatment unappealing and who could benefit from alternative interventions that span community and health care settings and that offer a range of behavior change goals.

JALIE A. TUCKER
DENNIS M. DONOVAN
G. ALAN MARLATT

# Contents

## II  EXPANDING THE RANGE OF
## BEHAVIOR CHANGE INITIATIVES

# I

## REFORMULATING THE ADDICTIVE BEHAVIOR CHANGE PROCESS

# 1

# Changing Addictive Behavior: Historical and Contemporary Perspectives

## JALIE A. TUCKER

As the 20th century comes to a close, most Americans would probably agree that the widespread use of licit and illicit drugs has shaped our collective social fabric. Drug preferences and availability have changed over time, but the demand for psychoactive substances has been a constant of American life, and we have developed a distinctive American approach to dealing with drugs and the drug problem. On the one hand, we are a culture saturated with access to drugs and other hedonic pursuits, and their use is often encouraged and glamorized. On the other hand, when individuals indulge themselves beyond normative limits, we bring severe social controls to bear on their alcohol or other drug use and insist that they abstain, often permanently, in an environment that remains rich with temptation. There is no middle ground in contemporary American views of drug use and other pleasurable activities that carry a risk of harm to self or society, and we cycle between excess and punishment at high social and economic cost. This book is aimed at articulating the middle ground and at developing a continuum of behavior change goals and interventions that better match the continuum along which addictive behavior problems lie.

The two major government-sponsored initiatives in this century to reduce drug use have both been punitive in nature, and both have failed. In the first, Prohibition (1920–1933) was instituted by the 18th Amendment to the U.S. Constitution, which made the production, sale, and transport of alcoholic beverages illegal, but not drinking itself. Prohibition

3

resulted in modest, short-lived reductions in per capita alcohol consumption, but failed to curtail alcohol use and abuse significantly and produced untoward social effects that contributed to its repeal (Boardman, 1989; Wiebe, 1967). Criminal activity related to the production, transport, and sale of alcohol greatly increased (the "Gangster" era of the 1920s and 1930s), and nearby countries such as Canada, Bermuda, and the Bahamas substantially increased their manufacture or importation of liquor, with a substantial portion of it finding its way into the United States. Stills became commonplace, and private drinking clubs proliferated as America kept drinking but attempted to hide it from the law. The repeal of Prohibition by the 21st Amendment did not result in rapid and sustained increases in alcohol consumption as some feared it would.

In a second, similar development initiated in the 1980s with Congressional, but not with constitutional support, the U.S. government launched the War on Drugs against all illicit drug use. Like Prohibition, the War on Drugs is a "supply side" approach to the drug problem that seeks to eliminate drug use by eliminating sources of drug availability through expensive interdiction efforts. Unlike Prohibition, it includes criminal penalties for individual drug use, in addition to penalties for the production, transport, and sale of drugs (Nadelmann, 1998). Similar to Prohibition, the War on Drugs has been accompanied by increased drug production in neighboring countries in Central and South America, and by increased drug-related crimes. U.S. incarceration rates have soared and have disproportionately involved minorities, especially African Americans and Hispanics (Courtland, 1996/1997; Marlatt, 1996; Szasz, 1992).[1] Like Prohibition, the War on Drugs has had little positive impact on drug use and drug-related problems, while producing a range of negative effects, including the loss of property rights and civil liberties (Heather, Wodak, Nadelmann, & O'Hare, 1993; Nadelmann, 1998; Szasz, 1992).

In a related development made possible by laboratory testing technologies, the War on Drugs has promoted widespread testing for illicit drug use in work-site, school, and other institutional settings, and home-test kits are available for parents to use to monitor their children's drug use. Drug testing is generally accepted in occupations where drug use would risk the public safety, but testing when public safety is not an issue and when there is no probable cause for suspecting drug use conflicts with rights to privacy and protection against unfair search and seizure. The deterrence value of drug testing is not well established (Britt, Gottfredson, & Goldkamp, 1992; Coombs & Ryan, 1990), and the practice probably has contributed to the growing use of certain over-the-counter (OTC) medications and herbal food supplements as "legal highs" because they escape detection or identification as recreational drugs during routine drug tests. For example, mixtures of caffeine, ephedrine (a common decongestant), and phenylpropanolamine (the active ingredient in OTC diet pills) mimic cocaine and amphetamine in drug discrimination studies using animals (e.g., Gavin, Harland, Michaelis, & Holloway, 1989; Gavin, Moore, Youngblood, & Holloway, 1993). Companies that sell such products appear to be doing a brisk business, including sales over the Internet.

These highlights of the U.S. drug experience and approach to the drug problem during the past century are instructive in several ways. First, like it or not, drug use and abuse clearly are enduring features of American life, and anthropological research suggests that we are not unique in this respect. Across time and geography, history yields one example after another of human drug taking, and the extent of drug-related social problems in a given culture typically varies inversely with the extent to which drug use is incorporated into normative social rules and rituals (Bennett, 1988; DeRios & Smith, 1977; Heath; 1987; MacAndrew & Edgerton, 1969; Maloff, Becker, Fonaroff, & Rodin, 1979; Zinberg & Harding, 1979; Zinberg, Harding, & Winkeller, 1977). These findings suggest that a zero tolerance approach to drug use will almost certainly fail to eliminate use and also will retard the development and social transmission of sumptuary rules for alcohol or other drug use that minimize harm to individuals and to society. Such rules often are developed within drug-defined communities, even if they are not accepted by the larger society (Harding, Zinberg, Stelmark, & Berry, 1980; Maloff et al., 1979; Zinberg et al., 1977).

Second, U.S. policies and laws designed to eliminate drug availability and to punish drug use have not only failed to solve the problem, but also have produced negative effects ranging from increased drug-related crime and incarceration rates to underfunded treatment programs to failing to slow the spread of HIV among intravenous (IV) drug users who share infected syringes (Marlatt, 1996; Heather et al., 1993; Nadelmann, 1998; Szasz, 1992). The zero tolerance approach of the War on Drugs heavily stigmatizes drug use and abuse, and the stigma extends to drug treatment and to drug treatment providers (Fink & Tasman, 1992). It thus should be no surprise that treatment-seeking samples are skewed in the direction of individuals with more severe problems (Jordan & Oei, 1989; Marlatt, Tucker, Donovan, & Vuchinich, 1997) and that the vast majority of substance abusers do not seek help (Narrow, Regier, Rae, Manderscheid, & Locke, 1993; Regier, Narrow, Rae, Manderscheid, Locke, & Goodwin, 1993). The stigma and risks of entering treatment are further compounded when the substance abuser is HIV positive.

Conspicuously absent in American drug control policies are adequate efforts to help those with drug problems. This reflects the punitive stance of policies and laws that favor interdiction and criminal penalties over treatment and prevention. The federal drug control budget reflects this bias; for example, the 1994 allocation of over $12.5 billion included

$8.2 billion for international and domestic law enforcement, and $2.5 billion for treatment and prevention (Robert Wood Johnson Foundation, 1993). Sadly, many individuals with drug-related problems have had to rely on one another for help because the "help" offered by mainstream institutions carries risks of legal action, fines, and aversive social controls, especially if the drug of abuse is illegal (Pringle, 1982; Szasz, 1992). In the aftermath of Prohibition, Alcoholics Anonymous (AA) emerged in 1935 at the grassroots level as a social movement designed to help alcoholics recover (AA World Services, 1985). In the safe haven provided by AA, members accepted the social stigma of alcoholism and vowed to give up alcohol for life, to make amends for alcohol-related transgressions, and to help other alcoholics. In return, they received an opportunity to regain a productive role in mainstream society, while receiving support from the AA community (Makela et al., 1996).

The 12-step principles of AA and similar medical notions about the disease of alcoholism (Jellinek, 1960) have since been disseminated and generalized on such a scale that they have become a cultural metaphor for all impulse control problems (e.g., alcohol and drug abuse, gambling, overeating, sex and computer addiction), at least in the United States (Peele, 1991). During the 1970s and 1980s, these principles were incorporated into for-profit "chemical dependency" treatment programs and assured that the perspective remained the dominant American view of addiction and its treatment. Although the latter development helped move addiction treatment into the health care system, it remains a marginal member of the system and continues to be delivered in segregated programs.

Three recent developments have questioned the U.S. emphasis on interdiction and favor an expansion of interventions to reduce the demand for drugs and the harm drug use creates. The first, most important influence is the AIDS epidemic (early 1980s to the present). A major route for HIV transmission into heterosexual (including pediatric) populations occurs when heterosexuals have unprotected sex with HIV-infected IV drug users, who can contract and spread HIV by sharing unclean needles (Glasner & Kaslow, 1990; Leigh & Stall, 1993). This has forced greater consideration of demand-side interventions to reduce personal preferences for drug use and the risks associated with it (e.g., through clean needle exchanges, condom distribution, and drug treatment). Such interventions have been relatively neglected during the War on Drugs, as epitomized by the simple-minded "Just Say No" campaign of the 1980s.

Second, scientific knowledge about substance abuse has grown rapidly during the last quarter century, following the establishment in the early 1970s of the National Institute on Alcohol Abuse and Alcoholism (NIAAA) and the National Institute on Drug Abuse (NIDA). Research clearly supports the need for expanded intervention approaches to meet the heterogeneous needs of substance abusers. In contrast to the stereo-type of the alcoholic or addict as an end-stage, out-of-control drug fiend who is impervious to the negative consequences of drug use, research has consistently shown that (1) drug use is sensitive to environmental contingencies, even among physically dependent users; and (2) substance use patterns and problems are heterogeneous in nature and lie along a continuum of severity. Most persons have less severe problems that do not prevent them from working (albeit with diminished capacity in some cases) and from fulfilling at least some of their family and social responsibilities. This strongly suggests that intensive treatment, which removes individuals from their usual environment for extended periods, is excessively costly, disruptive, and sweeping in scope for those with mild to moderate problems, although it may be necessary for those with severe problems. Intervention alternatives that are less intensive and more problem focused are needed to meet the needs of substance abusers with more circumscribed problems.

Third, recent efforts to contain health care costs have begun to exert pressure to move substance abuse treatment into the health care system. Research has shown that substance abuse treatment tends to more than pay for itself by reducing substance abusers' utilization of more expensive medical services, which otherwise is higher compared to persons without such problems (e.g., Fuller, 1995; Hoffman & Miller, 1992; Holder & Blose, 1992; Putnam, 1982). This pattern also holds for their family members (e.g., Sax, Dougherty, Esty, & Fine, 1983), who tend to be above-average utilizers of medical services as long as the substance abuser is drinking or using drugs abusively. The negative impact of substance abuse on health services utilization and costs has helped increase coverage of substance abuse treatment in health care plans, although those services remain poorly integrated into primary health care. In another development that will advance the inclusion of substance use disorders in health care practice and research, in 1992 NIDA and NIAAA (along with the National Institute of Mental Health) were reorganized as institutes within the National Institutes of Health (NIH).

These developments, coupled with the enduring nature of the U.S. drug problem despite repeated, massive supply-side interventions, have led many scientists and drug policy analysts (e.g., Heather et al., 1993; Marlatt, 1996; Nadelmann, 1998; Reuter & Caulkins, 1995) to recommend pursuing a more balanced policy—that is, one that abandons a near-exclusive emphasis on drug supply reduction in favor of shifting some resources toward demand reduction strategies and by reducing criminal penalties for drug use, but not necessarily for drug trafficking. The high economic costs and limited effectiveness of the War on Drugs have contributed to this recommendation, in addition to the social, legal, and health care access problems discussed earlier. For example, a recent Rand Corporation research brief (1995) summarized cost-effectiveness evaluations of different cocaine control strategies. Drug treatment, even with its known limited effects on behavior change, was far more cost-effective in reducing cocaine consumption compared to domestic law enforcement, interdiction at U.S. borders, and source-country control of coca production. Based on these findings, a partial, but not total, shift in monetary resources toward treatment was recommended, in part because of barriers that impede help-seeking and behavior change even when treatment is freely available (see Chapters 3–5, this volume).

Although not widely pursued in the United States, a more balanced approach between supply and demand reduction strategies is emerging in other industrialized nations under the rubric of harm reduction programs (Heather et al., 1993; Marlatt, 1996, 1998). Harm reduction is a public health approach aimed at reducing the harmful consequences of substance use for both the user and the community, and any change that reduces harm or the risk of harm is encouraged and accepted, even if it falls short of abstinence. Abstinence remains the ultimate goal, but harm reduction programs recognize that many behavior change attempts and treatment episodes may take place before stable abstinence is achieved, if it occurs at all. In the interim, interventions can help substance abusers learn to drink or use drugs in less harmful ways, but they cannot benefit from them if total abstinence is required for participation, as is the case in most U.S. treatment programs. Relaxing the abstinence requirement for participation removes a known deterrent to treatment entry and is responsive to the often chronic, relapsing nature of substance abuse (Marlatt et al., 1997).

Harm reduction programs are controversial in the United States, even though scientific evidence indicates their positive effects in reducing drug-related harms. For example, providing clean needles for IV drug users reduces the spread of HIV without increasing drug use (NIH, 1997), but the use of federal monies to fund clean needle exchanges is prohibited. Perhaps our Puritan heritage with its admonitions to avoid temptation and forbidden fruit has drawn us to favor approaches that emphasize and value abstinence above all else and stigmatize those who fail. However, the economic, health, and social costs that have resulted from such a zero tolerance approach are now well documented and require us to entertain alternatives that may produce better outcomes at both the individual and societal levels.

## PURPOSE AND ORGANIZATION OF THE BOOK

Because the supply-side components of a comprehensive drug control strategy are well known and better developed than demand-side components, this volume was compiled in an effort to stimulate interest in an expansion of demand-side components, both with respect to availability and kind. In the United States, demand-side interventions have been equated with and limited to intensive treatments that are poorly suited for persons with mild to moderate problems and with school-based prevention programs such as DARE that are not highly effective (Ennet, Tobler, Ringwalt, & Flewelling, 1994). Although these interventions will continue to play a role, a major thesis of this book, which was originally articulated in a visionary statement by the Institute of Medicine (IOM; 1990), is that available interventions are not sufficiently diverse to address the heterogeneous needs of individuals with addictive behavior problems. The lack of diversity of interventions, coupled with their often punitive nature, deters help-seeking and, when it does occur, it often is late in problem development when substance abuse patterns are well established and harder to change (Marlatt et al., 1997).

In individuals with substance-related problems, considerable variability exists in drug use practices, in levels of physical dependence, and in the extent to which drug use impairs different domains of functioning (e.g., health, job, relationships). Each dimension lies along a continuum with respect to severity, the degree of severity usually is not uniform across dimensions, and positive change on one dimension can occur in the absence of changes on the others and contribute to improvements in overall functioning (Pattison, Sobell, & Sobell, 1977). This is true even among individuals who meet clinical criteria for a substance use disorder (Grant, Chou, Pickering, & Hasin, 1992). For example, one individual may experience negative legal consequences due to drinking (e.g., drunk driving arrests) without drinking excessively on a regular basis, another may drink heavily and develop tolerance and health problems without experiencing psychosocial problems due to drinking, and a third may drink heavily without incurring health problems but experience serious negative consequences at work and at home. Each presenting picture suggests different behavior change goals. The first person needs to stop drinking and driving but does not necessarily need otherwise to abstain. The second probably needs to abstain on a permanent basis, but will not require additional interventions to improve life–health functioning. The third requires assistance in improving areas of impaired functioning, but whether abstinence or moderation drinking is the goal will depend on the nature of the contingencies between drinking and resolving the life–health problems.

As articulated in the 1990 IOM report, *Broadening the Base of Treatment for Alcohol Problems,* traditional abstinence-oriented treatments do not easily accommodate the demonstrated variability in substance-related problems and tend to be most suitable for individuals with more severe problems in one or more dimensions (e.g., those with high physical dependence and health problems that are exacerbated by drinking, or those for whom any drinking would result in serious psychosocial or legal repercussions). Persons with severe problems are a highly visible segment of the population with substance-related problems, but they represent only a small minority of that population (< 10%). The majority have more circumscribed problems that are not well suited for traditional treatment, but they could benefit from interventions that are less intensive in scope, are problem specific, and may involve methods of service delivery that lie outside of clinical approaches to behavior change.

A major thesis of the book, which follows from the IOM report, is that *traditional clinical treatments should be complemented by less intensive interventions for persons with more circumscribed problems, thus forming an optimal continuum of care that combines clinical and public health approaches* (cf. Abrams, Emmons, Niaura, Goldstein, & Sherman, 1991). Traditional treatments and mutual help groups will continue to play a vital role in the continuum of care, but they should be supplemented by a range of interventions that (1) attract more substance abusers into helping environments, including the underserved majority with mild to moderate problems, as well as those with more severe problems who have little interest in giving up drug use but wish to reduce the harm associated with it (e.g., HIV infection); (2) are more accessible both within and outside of the formal health care system, thus reducing barriers to help-seeking and the stigmatizing effects of treatment participation; and (3) facilitate the natural forces that promote behavior change and make greater use of social and community resources.

The first half of this book, including the remainder of this chapter, elaborates the conceptual and empirical bases for these recommendations. They are predicated upon recent scientific advances in understanding the addictive behavior change process and the limited role of interventions in facilitating it, and they involve a reformulation of the change process that differs from dominant 12-step and disease model perspectives. Key components of the revised perspective include (1) recognizing that participation in treatment or mutual help groups is neither a necessary nor a sufficient condition for problem resolution, which can occur with or without interventions; (2) acknowledging the limitations of current interventions in promoting change and the often greater influence on long-term outcomes of motivational and environmental variables that surround efforts to change; and (3) viewing problem resolution as a dynamic behavioral process that is spread out in time, often over several years, and that may involve multiple attempts to change before new behavior patterns emerge and stabilize. Individual chapters in this volume address elements of the revised perspective, including influences on behavior change processes with and without interventions (Chapters 4–7), motivation for change

(Chapters 5 and 7), influences on help-seeking (Chapters 3–5), and the role of the environment in behavior change (Chapters 4 and 7; cf. Chapter 10). These topics are recent developments because addictive behavior change has long been viewed as dependent upon participation in intensive treatment or mutual help groups guided by the 12-step principles of AA.

Pursuing this expanded perspective on addictive behavior change requires knowledge of *public health approaches* that are not familiar to many treatment providers and clinical researchers, who have worked within the *clinical model* that is the hallmark of medical care and psychotherapy. Articulating the public health perspective and how interventions guided by it can be combined with clinical approaches to form an optimal continuum of care is the goal of the second half of the book. In brief, the clinical perspective targets individuals who have already developed a problem with interventions that are relatively intensive, expensive, and effective, and are delivered by professionals, typically in health care settings. The public health perspective targets populations or at-risk groups with interventions that typically are more preventive than palliative; are less intensive, costly, and effective; and can be delivered by nonprofessionals in a range of settings (e.g., primary care, work-site, or community settings) using dissemination methods that do not require extensive personal contact (e.g., using written materials, videotapes, television, or the Internet). Public health approaches also encompass regulatory and taxation measures aimed at protecting and improving health, although their consideration is beyond the scope of this book. Because public health interventions reach many more individuals than do clinical interventions, in the aggregate, they may be more effective overall, even though they are less effective on a case-by-case basis.

Medicine and public health have had a long-standing, complementary partnership to promote the health of the nation. A similar selective combination of the two approaches to address addictive behaviors seems long overdue, and it is an approach increasingly advocated by experts who originally worked within the clinical model (e.g., Abrams et al., 1991; Battle & Brownell, 1996; Heather, 1996; Marlatt, 1996; Sobell & Sobell, 1993; cf. Miller & Hester, 1989). The second half of the book discusses interventions needed in an expanded perspective on behavior change and begins to lay the groundwork for necessary evolutions in the roles of mental health professionals in today's health care environment. This section is aimed at empowering practitioners to expand their services beyond traditional psychotherapy and also to offer brief, problem-focused interventions and interventions that may be delivered in primary care, community, and other nontraditional settings.

Offering services that better span the continuum of care will require practitioners to blend clinical and public health approaches to behavior change. The public health approach and how it differs from the clinical approach is described in Chapter 8, this volume. Subsequent chapters present intervention approaches guided by a public health model for a range of addictive behaviors, often in concert with elements of a clinical approach, and suggest directions for expanding behavior change initiatives to form an optimal continuum of care. These include chapters on brief interventions (Chapter 9), the Community Reinforcement Approach and related contingency management procedures (Chapter 10), and stepped-care approaches to triaging and coordinating service delivery across the continuum of care (Chapters 11–12).

Because of the crucial importance of basing intervention development and dissemination on evaluation research, Chapter 13 presents an overview of program evaluation research in the era of managed care. In an expanded perspective on addictive behavior change, evaluation must occur on at least two levels. One level is familiar to researchers and practitioners who have worked within a clinical model and entails evaluating the efficacy of different therapies in promoting behavior change. The second level is less familiar and involves comparisons of the monetary costs and benefits of a range of demand reduction interventions. Such analyses can guide the selection of intervention components that collectively provide cost-effective coverage and rational resource allocation across the continuum of care required by addictive disorders. Cost-effectiveness, cost–benefit, and cost–utility analyses are becoming increasingly influential as health care in the United States moves to a managed care model (Yates, 1995).[2]

## A LOOK BACK: THE PSYCHOTHERAPY ERA AND RECIPROCAL INFLUENCES ON ADDICTIVE BEHAVIOR TREATMENT AND RESEARCH

To appreciate the innovative nature of these initiatives, it is useful to look back at what came before them. This is the focus of the remainder of the chapter, which selectively discusses clinical research and practice on addictive behaviors and the more general field of psychotherapy that guided them, and sets the stage for the topics covered later in the book.

### The Assumptions of Psychotherapy: A Clinical Model Exemplar

Huge literatures in psychology, psychiatry, and other mental health fields are devoted to describing and evaluating different forms of psychotherapy for an amazing array of disorders, including addictive behaviors. Despite loudly touted differences in the conceptual systems guiding the different therapies and in the technical aspects of their implementation, the various psychotherapies have been guided by a clinical model and thus share fundamental assumptions that are not widely recognized. Identifying them and understanding their influence on research and practice are important because they differ from the assumptions of the public health model. Effectively combining the two approaches requires that their similarities and differences be understood and respected. The major assumptions of psychotherapy and how they require revision in an expanded perspective on behavior change are summarized in Table 1.1 and are discussed, beginning with the assumptions of psychotherapy:

- *Assumption 1: The psychotherapy dyad or similar small-group interaction is the primary vehicle for behavior change.* The dyad originated in the doctor–patient relationship and was adopted and elaborated in psychoanalysis, the first formal psychotherapy. A fundamental assumption of psychoanalysis is

**TABLE 1.1. The Assumptions of Psychotherapy Contrasted with Reformulations in Service of an Expanded Perspective on Behavior Change**

| Original assumptions | Reformulated assumptions |
| --- | --- |
| 1. The psychotherapy dyad or similar small-group interaction is the primary vehicle for behavior change. | Behavior change methods and helping environments should be expanded beyond the psychotherapy vehicle to include initiatives guided by public health principles that can be applied outside of clinic and institutional settings. |
| 2. The therapeutic action of psychotherapy is akin to surgery or drug treatment, and the controlling variables of behavior change reside within the treatment experience. | The effects of psychotherapy are context dependent, and extratherapeutic variables play an important, but understudied role in the behavior change process. |
| 3. Psychotherapy outcomes should be related to in-session psychotherapeutic processes. | Process research should be expanded to investigate processes that operate outside of the therapy experience, interact with it, and are manifest over more extended time frames. |
| 4. Efficacy studies using randomized controlled clinical trials are the best research strategy for evaluating behavior change initiatives such as psychotherapy. | The research base on behavior change provided by treatment efficacy studies should be augmented by naturalistic studies of change among treated and untreated samples and by studies of treatment utilization and effectiveness in usual care settings. |

that all psychic conflicts and defense mechanisms will eventually be manifest within the therapeutic relationship and, hence, will be available therein for analysis and resolution. Although many later approaches to behavior change rejected other aspects of psychoanalysis, they almost universally adopted the dyad as the vehicle for change, even when their primary focus was on extratherapeutic behaviors and events, as in the case of behavior therapy. Part of the appeal of the dyad is the convenience it affords the practitioner and its easy accommodation of cultural and legal emphases on obtaining informed consent for treatment.

  • *Assumption 2: The therapeutic action of psychotherapy is akin to surgery or drug treatment, and the controlling variables of behavior change reside within the treatment experience.* This assumption also has its roots in psychoanalysis and contributed to the initial emphasis on technical differences between psychotherapies and to a continuing lack of interest in understanding how the broader context surrounding treatment delivery may influence treatment engagement and outcomes. The therapeutic action of psychotherapy is considered to resemble the action of intensive medical or drug treatments (Moos & Finney, 1983; Stiles & Shapiro, 1994), with the causes of change presumably emanating from technical features of the treatment procedures. If treatment is effective, then change should occur during or immediately after treatment, which is delivered intensively over a time-limited period. Long-term follow-ups thus are not conceptually meaningful from this perspective and were absent in the early evaluation literature, although they were phased in as the impermanence of behavior change became apparent. The failure of treatment effects to endure usually was attributed to extinction of the original treatment-produced changes (Shiffman, 1992), and little attention was paid to what was happening outside of treatment. Indeed, in psychoanalysis, patient focus on extratherapeutic events was considered to be a form of resistance.

  • *Assumption 3: Psychotherapy outcomes should be related to in-session psychotherapeutic processes.* This is a corollary of Assumptions 1 and 2. If the controlling variables of behavior change reside within the therapeutic interaction, then what happens during therapy sessions should be related to longer-term outcomes. Despite much research, only limited success has been achieved in relating in-session client and therapist behaviors to treatment outcomes (reviewed by Orlinsky & Howard, 1986).

  • *Assumption 4: Efficacy studies using randomized controlled clinical trials (RCTs) are the best research strategy for evaluating behavior change initiatives such as psychotherapy.* In a practice that follows from Assumption 2, RCTs have been adopted uncritically from medical and pharmacological evaluation research without questioning whether the design is well suited to studying the influences of psychotherapy on the behavior change process. Exclusive reliance on RCTs is defensible only to the extent that treatment effects are independent of the contexts surrounding help-seeking and treatment delivery.

## Reformulating the Assumptions in Service of an Expanded Perspective on Behavior Change

• *Assumption 1 reformulated: Behavior change methods and helping environments should be expanded beyond the psychotherapy vehicle to include initiatives guided by public health principles that can be applied outside of clinic and institutional settings.* Uncritical acceptance of the dyad as the proper vehicle for behavior change has discouraged mental health practitioners, especially psychologists and psychiatrists who follow a clinical model of practice, from offering services other than psychotherapy delivered in clinic, private practice, and other institutional settings. This has led to a passive, "high threshold" approach to service delivery. Providers wait for clients to present for services, often after passing through one or more system gatekeepers (e.g., primary care physicians, insurance authorization), and do not try to influence the help-seeking process or to bring services to those in need. As discussed in Chapter 8, this is quite different from the active, "low threshold" approach of the public health model, which attempts to lower barriers to services and to reach out to persons who are at risk or in need.

Also embedded in the clinical model are judgments about the strength of client motivation to change, depending on the circumstances that surround treatment entry (Miller, 1985; Pringle, 1982; see Chapter 5, this volume). Clients who have external pressures to seek help are viewed as being less (intrinsically) motivated to change compared to those who are self-referred. In the addiction treatment literature at least, this assumption has been largely unsupported. Coerced and self-referred clients have similar treatment outcomes, although it is true that coerced clients often have better attendance records and thus receive more care (De Leon, 1988; Stitzer & McCaul, 1987). The public health approach does not make such inferences about motivation from an absence of help-seeking and instead focuses on making services more accessible.

Even behavior therapists and applied behavior analysts who are directly concerned with modifying environment–behavior relationships have rarely worked outside of clinic or institutional environments, a fact that has influenced the course of development of behavior theory and applied research. For example, behavior therapists became cognitive-behavior therapists to accommodate the verbal behavior interface that the psychotherapy dyad imposed on their assessment and manipulation of environment–behavior relationships in outpatient settings (Kohlenberg, Tsai, & Dougher, 1993). Applied behavior analysts have favored institutional environments (e.g., mental retardation centers, schools, business organizations), where they can exercise control over activities and commodities that function as reinforcers. Thus, the two specialties in psychology that otherwise are best prepared to guide behavior change applications in the natural environment have avoided working in such settings extensively. Knowledge about environment–behavior relations outside of controlled environments has suffered accordingly but is fundamental to forming a continuum of care that spans institutional and community settings.

Much of what is known about behavior patterns in the natural environment comes from disciplines such as anthropology, sociology, social work, public health, behavioral medicine, and the community mental health movement of the 1960s. As mental health practitioners expand their approaches to care, it is critical that they use these sources of information about working in nontraditional environments and combine them with established principles of behavior change that range in application from individuals to communities to populations. One feature of behavior change programs that is the same across settings is the importance of developing trust and setting goals that are acceptable to all involved parties.

- *Assumption 2 reformulated: The effects of psychotherapeutic interventions are context dependent, and extratherapeutic variables play an important, but understudied role in the behavior change process.* The early psychotherapy era (1950s and 1960s) was a competitive, energetic time when therapy proponents of various persuasions were investigating the efficacy of their treatments, generally in the hope of demonstrating superior outcomes with their approach. The main players during the "psychotherapy wars" were proponents of psychodynamic, behavioral, and client-centered approaches. By the mid-1970s, sufficiently numerous and well-conducted comparative treatment outcomes studies forced the field to accept the "dodo bird" verdict ("Everyone has won and all must have prizes") regarding the equivalence of psychotherapy outcomes across the different approaches (Luborsky, Singer, & Luborsky, 1975).

The verdict was not conceptually satisfying, because it indicated that the technical attributes specific to different therapies were largely superfluous in determining outcomes. Outcomes were more reliably related to nonspecific factors that were common to all therapies, including the strength of the therapeutic alliance and certain client and therapist characteristics (reviewed by Beutler, Crago, & Arizmendi, 1986; Garfield, 1986). Originally, such nonspecific variables had been viewed as uninteresting nuisance variables, the effects of which needed to be separated from those of the specific, technical variables, a perspective that promoted the early widespread use of attention placebo control groups. The inadvertent discovery that nonspecific factors contributed to psychotherapy outcomes instead suggested that they should be objects of study in their own right.

Hence, they were renamed "common" factors, a development that stimulated attempts at rapprochement, integration, and eclecticism by proponents of the different therapy approaches (Garfield, 1994; Garfield & Bergin, 1986).

The verdict had methodological effects on psychotherapy research as well. Gordan Paul's (1967) famous litany—"What treatment, by whom, is most effective for this individual with that specific problem, under which set of circumstances?"—encouraged greater specificity in evaluation questions, and research quality improved as procedures aimed at reducing variance and increasing measurement sensitivity became standard practice. These included tactics to increase treatment integrity (e.g., treatment standardization and manualization), expansion and improvement of dependent measures beyond categorical outcome assessments, and adoption of the RCT as the sine qua non of outcome research (see Assumption 4). In a related development, statistical power problems were virtually eliminated by the introduction of meta-analysis (e.g., Smith, Glass, & Miller, 1980), a statistical technique for combining outcome data across studies to determine treatment effect sizes.

Despite the salutary effects of these innovations on research practice, they were introduced primarily in service of continuing to investigate the original question about the relative efficacy of different treatments, and the issue of whether this was a good question was not considered until later. The use of more sensitive and powerful designs and measures produced some minor qualifications of the dodo verdict (e.g., anxiety disorders are best treated with behavior therapy; Barlow, 1988; Smith et al., 1980), showed that treated participants fare better than untreated or minimally treated controls (e.g., Bowers & Clum, 1988) for some, but not all, disorders (addictive behaviors are such an exception; e.g., Sobell, Cunningham, & Sobell, 1996); and yielded improved methods for treatment dissemination and therapist training (e.g., through treatment manualization). These benefits notwithstanding, the variance explained by treatment effects in controlled outcome studies usually was modest and fairly constant across treatment modalities and psychological disorders. The equivalence of psychotherapy outcomes thus continues to stand as the preeminent generalization from this line of research.

Treatment outcome studies in the addictive behaviors field followed a similar, though not identical, course of development. First, methodologically adequate evaluations of addiction treatments have a truncated history relative to the psychotherapy field and were generally lacking until federal funding became available with the establishment of NIAAA and NIDA. Prior to the 1970s, addiction studies were an academic backwater, probably because addictive behaviors were heavily stigmatized and widely regarded as difficult to treat. The quality of addiction research improved quickly during the last quarter century (Morley, Finney, Monahan, & Floyd, 1996; Sobell & Sobell, 1989) by incorporating methodological improvements made in the general psychotherapy literature and, in some instances, by developing superior methodologies (e.g., for increasing the accuracy of verbal reports and for conducting lengthy follow-ups).

Second, as in the psychotherapy field, the initial questions addressed in addiction research were competitive outcome questions (see Emrick, 1975; Pattison et al., 1977), generally between behavior therapy and more traditional approaches, including psychotherapy and abstinence-oriented formal treatments guided by the principles of AA. AA, in its original form as a mutual help group, has not been widely investigated because of the impediments posed by its commitment to participant anonymity (McCrady & Miller, 1993). Initially promising results in favor of behavioral treatments were overshadowed, first, by the controlled drinking controversy and, second, by the high relapse rates found across a range of treatment approaches. The controlled drinking controversy centered on the issue of whether persons with drinking problems could resume moderation drinking without problems or whether they should maintain lifelong abstinence, as held by AA (for summaries, see Marlatt, 1983; Miller, 1983). Although predictors of moderation and abstinence outcomes remain elusive (Rosenberg, 1993), the evidence is clear that moderation is possible in a subset of cases (Armor & Meshkoff, 1983; Marlatt, Larimer, Baer, & Quigley, 1993; Sobell & Sobell, 1987). However, regardless of drinking goals and treatment orientation, treatment benefits tend to be short-lived for many clients with alcohol and other addictive behavior problems (reviewed by Miller & Hester, 1986; Tucker, Vuchinich, & Gladsjo, 1990/1991).

These issues have been difficult for the field, but they brought to the forefront conceptual issues and new research questions that moved the field beyond a singular focus on treatment-produced behavior change toward a broader conception of the change process that is not tied exclusively to participation in interventions. Treatment is now regarded as one of several variable classes that can influence the often lengthy change process, along with contextual and motivational variables that surround attempts to change. This broadened perspective, borne out of the humbling experiences of addiction treatment, is beginning to influence the general psychotherapy literature as well.

Five developments during the late 1970s and 1980s helped promote a broadened perspective. First, Marlatt's (e.g., 1978; Marlatt & Gordon, 1985) paradigm challenging work on relapse determinants and processes directed attention away from end-point treatment outcome evaluations toward the study of what was happening during the posttreatment interval when substance use episodes of varying severity took place. A large, process-oriented literature has since developed (reviewed by Tucker et al.,

1990/1991; see Chapters 4 and 7, this volume) and has shown how substance use varies with changing environmental circumstances. Relapses are associated with negative events and emotions, whereas maintenance of problem resolution is associated with positive events and greater personal and social resources (e.g., Sandahl, 1984; Shiffman, 1982; Vuchinich & Tucker, 1996a).

Second, treatment outcome studies with follow-ups of several years or more (e.g., Moos, Finney, & Cronkite, 1990; Polich, Armor, & Braiker, 1981; Simpson & Sells, 1982) have shown that outcomes are highly variable over time, ranging from abstinence, nonproblem substance use, to substance abuse, often by the same individuals at different points in time. Similar to the relapse literature, the variability in outcomes is related to individuals' life circumstances and psychosocial functioning during the posttreatment interval. Such contextual variables tend to account for more outcome variance than do many client or treatment characteristics (Brewer, Catalano, Haggerty, Gainey, & Fleming, 1998; Moos et al., 1990).

Third, Prochaska, DiClemente, and colleagues (e.g., Prochaska & DiClemente, 1983, 1986; Prochaska, DiClemente, & Norcross, 1992) developed the "transtheoretical" model of behavior change, with its central concept of the stages of change, to contend with issues raised by the dodo bird verdict. The model proposed that across disorders and treatments, the change process proceeds in identifiable stages that extend in time before and after active behavior change, which is traditionally, but not necessarily, associated with treatment participation. Addictive behaviors have been heavily represented in empirical applications of the model (e.g., Prochaska & DiClemente, 1983, 1986; see Chapter 6, this volume). Although the model has conceptual problems (Vuchinich & Tucker, 1996b), and inferences from it have outstripped the database (Davidson, 1992; see Chapter 6, this volume), the model has been very important in expanding the field's temporal view of behavior change beyond the psychotherapy experience and in relegating treatment to only one of several variable classes that may influence change.

Fourth, Miller's (1985) reconceptualization of motivation for treatment in situational, rather than trait, terms directed attention toward understanding and being responsive to the life circumstances and problems of clients as they present for treatment. Much like client-centered therapy, this approach meets clients "where they are" instead of requiring them to conform to a singular, treatment-dictated view of their problem, as is the case in 12-step programs (cf. Pringle, 1982). As discussed in Chapters 5 and 9 of this volume, Miller's reconceptualization of motivation has stimulated the development of interventions to enhance motivation for treatment and for behavior change (e.g., Miller & Rollnick, 1991).

Fifth, survey research has repeatedly shown that few substance abusers enter treatment (e.g., Hingson, Mangione, Meyers, & Scotch, 1982; Narrow et al., 1993; Regier et al., 1993) and that many resolve their problems without it (e.g., Stall & Bernacki, 1986; Sobell et al., 1996). In the case of alcohol problems, natural resolutions appear to be more common than treatment-assisted resolutions (Sobell et al., 1996) and are associated with environmental variables such as those found to influence positive treatment outcomes (e.g., Klingemann, 1991; Tucker, Vuchinich, & Pukish, 1995). These findings further question the usual emphasis on treatment-produced change and suggest the importance of separating influences on help-seeking patterns from influences on behavior change, which can occur with or without interventions (Tucker & Gladsjo, 1993).

These five developments have promoted revisions in earlier views that wedded addictive behavior change to treatment participation. As discussed further in the first half of this book, they have suggested new research questions about the role of extratreatment contextual and motivational variables in the change process and how influences on behavior change may differ from influences on help-seeking patterns. Another development that supports this trend away from focusing exclusively on treatment-produced change comes from the recent negative findings of Project MATCH (Project MATCH Research Group, 1997; see Chapter 2, this volume). In this multisite RCT, problem drinkers ($N = 1,726$) were randomly assigned to one of three individually delivered treatments (12-step facilitation, skills training, or motivational enhancement therapy) that were similar along nonspecific dimensions. The study sought to identify client variables assessed at treatment intake (e.g., readiness to change, psychiatric severity, gender) that enhanced outcomes in each treatment, with technical differences between treatments providing the basis for the matching hypotheses. One-year outcomes were similar across groups, and the matching hypotheses were largely unsupported. These negative findings cannot be attributed to low statistical power or to poorly conducted research or data analyses. This was excellent research conducted in the finest tradition of the clinical model and its assumptions about treatment-produced behavior change. However, like the general psychotherapy field before it, in Project MATCH, the substance abuse field now has a definitive dodo bird verdict (cf. McLellan et al., 1994), which makes consideration of alternative perspectives on behavior change all the more compelling.

• *Assumption 3 reformulated: Process research should be expanded to investigate processes that operate outside of the therapy experience, interact with it, and are manifest over more extended time frames.* The psychotherapy process literature has contributed elegant schemes for measuring, coding, and understanding interpersonal interactions, but the process variables identified within the confines of the psychotherapy dyad have proven notoriously difficult to relate to treatment outcomes. These difficulties have led to recent alternative approaches to addressing the process–outcome relationship that are either more molecular or molar in their unit of analysis. The "events paradigm" of Stiles, Shapiro, and Elliott (1986) exemplifies a more molecular approach. Within individual therapy sessions, the goal is to identify the immediate effects of discrete treatment procedures or therapist verbalizations. If such "micro" interventions are effective within sessions, they presumably will summate over sessions to produce enduring positive change. This approach takes the traditional view of treatment-produced change (per Assumptions 1 and 2) to its logical extreme by adopting the therapy session or single intervention tactic within a session as the unit of analysis. As Stiles and Shapiro later conceded (1994), the approach failed to resolve the process–outcome conundrum.

The five developments summarized earlier point in a different direction. They suggest that process-oriented studies of behavior change should become more molar in their temporal perspective and adopt a longer, rather than shorter, unit of analysis that extends in time well before and after any participation in time-limited treatments. The transtheoretical model and research on motivation and help-seeking highlight the role of processes and events that take place before active behavior change or treatment entry occurs. Marlatt's work on relapse, research on natural resolution, and treatment outcome studies with lengthy follow-ups point to the critical role of the environment, especially after the initiation of change, in determining outcomes. These developments suggest that meaningful regularities between addictive behavior patterns and environmental and motivational variables may not emerge when the unit of analysis is brief and focuses on temporally contiguous relationships between discrete events (e.g., treatment) that occur shortly before changes in drug use (Vuchinich & Tucker, 1996b).

For example, many substance abusers make repeated attempts to quit or control their use. Some attempts involve interventions, others do not, and behavior change can occur with or without them. Instead of focusing only on the effects on substance use of a single intervention experience, as is necessarily the case in treatment outcome studies, a more molar perspective seeks to identify covariation between substance use patterns, the surrounding environment, and help-seeking experiences over lengthier time frames. As another example, research on natural resolution has identified regularities between events and behavior patterns over a period of several years that surround the often circumscribed act of becoming abstinent or shifting from a problem to nonproblem pattern of substance use (Klingemann, 1991; Tucker, Vuchinich, & Gladsjo, 1994; Tucker et al., 1995; see Chapter 4, this volume). These environment–behavior relations are not always apparent if the assessment is limited to a briefer period immediately preceding the initiation of stable abstinence or moderation drinking (e.g., Sobell, Sobell, Toneatto, & Leo, 1993).

These research questions are very different from asking how in-session therapy processes relate to outcomes in a single treatment experience, but they are process-oriented questions nonetheless. Understanding the functional value of help-seeking within the context of individuals' life circumstances and how interventions may interact with those circumstances to facilitate change are process questions posed at a broader level of analysis. It is one that seems compatible with the temporally extended nature of addictive behavior patterns, which typically develop and change over many years. The contextual variables that influence those patterns also are spread out in time. However, as discussed next, addressing them requires the use of research methods that are out of step with the scientific preferences of psychology and other fields guided by a clinical model.

- *Assumption 4 reformulated: The research base on behavior change provided by treatment efficacy studies should be augmented by naturalistic studies of change among treated and untreated samples and by studies of treatment utilization and effectiveness in usual care settings.* RCTs are widely regarded as the gold standard for determining the "true" effects of an intervention (per Assumption 2) independent of patient and contextual variables that might contribute "error" variance. However, the design applies a medical treatment metaphor to the behavior change process, and it enhances internal validity through experimental control at the expense of reducing the generalizability of findings (Blacker & Mortimore, 1996; Johnson, 1996; Mechanic, 1978; Moos & Finney, 1983; Seligman, 1995).

RCTs strive to reduce error variance by studying homogeneous patient groups and by standardizing their research experiences except for variations in the interventions that are the focus of investigation. Several components of that "error" variance, however, are integral aspects of the behavior change process in real-world settings. For example, the randomization requirement of RCTs treats the processes and circumstances that lead people to seek care as a nuisance variable that requires statistical control (Mechanic, 1978; Moos & Finney, 1983). When a minimal treatment control group is included, the natural resolution process ("spontaneous remission") is treated as a nuisance variable, and when RCTs are conducted double-blind, patient and provider expectations about treatment outcomes are, too (Seligman, 1995). Participant noncompliance is another nuisance variable often handled in ways that promote sample bias; for example, samples are restricted to persons who are considered likely to comply with the protocol or who demonstrated compliance during a prerandomization "run in" period (Johnson, 1996). The standardization of treatment protocols also reduces fluctuations in treatment delivery, including those aimed at accommodating individual differences in patient preferences and responses to treatment (Seligman, 1995).

Exclusive reliance on RCTs is defensible only to the extent that Assumption 2 is correct and that the effects of treatment are independent of the contexts surrounding treatment seeking and treatment delivery. As discussed earlier, using a medical treatment metaphor to conceptualize the behavior change process and the role of psychotherapy in promoting it is highly questionable, because change is a process, not a discrete event, that typically unfolds over time and depends to a large degree on the surrounding context. This may be less of a concern with respect to some medical and drug treatments, but exclusive reliance on RCTs is being questioned in those literatures as well (e.g., Blacker & Mortimore, 1996; Johnson, 1996).

Other limitations of RCTs reflect feasibility issues and differences that may exist when a treatment is delivered in a research versus a clinical context (Blacker & Mortimore, 1996; Seligman, 1995). The use of standard treatment protocols in RCTs is methodologically appealing but precludes individualization of treatment based on patient responses or preferences, or as the contexts surrounding treatment participation change, as is usual in clinical practice. The sample bias common in RCTs in favor of compliant participants with well-defined problems leaves unknown the ease or difficulty which with a treatment can be delivered to the more heterogeneous clientele served in clinical practice ("A clinician's task would be easy indeed if all their patients were of the kind found in standard RCTs." Blacker & Mortimore, 1996, p. 354). Another concern is the extent to which efficacious but complex research treatment protocols can be disseminated to and implemented by practitioners who work in environments that are less well controlled or resourced. For these reasons, the overall utility of an intervention has come to be viewed as depending on both its *efficacy* as established in controlled research, and its *effectiveness*, as implemented in usual clinical practice (American Psychological Association, 1995).

As discussed throughout this book, the variables and processes that RCTs treat as nuisance factors (e.g., behavior change over time in the absence of interventions, compliance patterns, client expectations, and help-seeking processes) are key elements in behavior change and the delivery of care, and merit study in their own right. Indeed, the history of psychotherapy and addiction research is replete with instances where yesterday's nuisance variable became today's substantive research question. For example, investigating natural resolutions can reveal the processes and contingencies that support behavior change and thus can help improve treatments (Sobell et al., 1996). Studying compliance can suggest ways to reduce noncompliance with specific interventions and illuminate the complex relationships between compliance patterns and health status (Johnson, 1996). Studying help-seeking patterns and processes in the absence of random assignment may suggest ways to reduce barriers to service utilization and help identify naturally occurring matching variables that enhance treatment outcomes (De Leon, 1998; Mechanic, 1978; Moos & Finney, 1983).

It follows logically from these points that research on behavior change should be expanded beyond treatment efficacy studies to include naturalistic studies of behavior change among persons with a range of help-seeking experiences, including studies of treatment effectiveness when clients self-select their interventions (Mechanic, 1978; Seligman, 1995). This expanded research agenda requires that the different approaches be understood and respected, and be used to investigate the subset of empirical questions for which each is better suited. Attributes of the two approaches are summarized in Table 1.2.

Over the long run, confidence in generalizations about behavior change will increase if findings using each research approach converge on similar inferences. If the findings repeatedly diverge, however, then methodological features designed to handle variability due to "nuisance factors" may be influencing the outcome or may be a critical part of the phenomenon of interest. For example, suppose treatments $A$ and $B$ are compared extensively using designs that do and do not involve the random assignment of participants to treatments. In one scenario, assume that treatment $A$ consistently outperforms treatment $B$, regardless of the design used. In another scenario, suppose that treatment $A$ outperforms $B$ when participants are not randomized, but that the two treatments produce similar outcomes when they are (i.e., a dodo bird verdict). The first scenario suggests that $A$ is the better treatment regardless of whether clients self-select their treatment. The second scenario suggests that allowing clients to self-select their treatment improves outcomes from treatment $A$ and that a natural "treatment matching" process may be an important part of the difference.

Rather than trivializing the latter finding as evidence of selection bias that is undermining a comparative test of the "true effects" of the treatments (the efficacy viewpoint), a broadened perspective suggests the utility of investigating this naturally occurring self-selection process to understand the appeal of treatment $A$ for some clients and to identify variables that contribute to their improved outcomes. Variables so identified then could be verified as treatment matching variables in studies that involve random assignment, but it must be appreciated that such designs remove the element of consumer choice and thus do not fully model the natural treatment-seeking and engagement process. Randomly assigning

**TABLE 1.2. Selected Attributes of Randomized Controlled Clinical Trials (RCTs) That Assess Treatment Efficacy Compared with Naturalistic Studies of Treatment Effectiveness and Health Services Utilization**

| Efficacy studies using RCTs | Effectiveness and health services utilization studies |
|---|---|
| Goal is to detect the "true" effects of treatment by minimizing all other sources of variation. | Goal is to assess the feasibility and effectiveness of interventions delivered in usual care settings and the variables that influence utilization patterns, outcomes, and costs. |
| Participants are randomly assigned to treatment conditions; their only choice is whether or not to participate in the RCT and to accept random assignment. | Providers and health care consumers choose clinical procedures based on recipient needs and preferences within the constraints of their mutual health care resources. |
| Care is standardized within treatment conditions and is not adjusted based on recipient responses, except when life-threatening developments occur. | Care is adjusted as consumer needs, preferences, and resources change over the course of treatment. |
| Study groups are selected to represent homogeneous, "pure" forms of disorders that are uncommon in practice. | Samples better represent the heterogeneity of client populations and medical and psychological disorders, including comorbidities. |
| Measurement focuses on hypothesized treatment-produced changes assessed at predetermined intervals; protocols are not modified until the end of the study, except in extreme cases when the treatment is either very good or very bad. | Measurement sensitivity and integrity are vital, but the timing of assessments and the use of data may be more closely tied to the service delivery process and used to improve it, including as regards client satisfaction. |
| To establish the true effects of treatment, data from compliant participants who complete treatment and thus are fully "dosed" are considered most informative. | Why participants do not comply fully with treatment or seek alternative sources of help are central research questions, rather than nuisance variables in need of statistical control as in RCTs. |
| Efficacy studies have high internal validity, but selection bias is a serious potential problem, and the generalizability of findings collected under highly controlled conditions is problematic. | Effectiveness studies have lower internal validity but a higher potential for generalization if threats to internal validity are not excessive. |
| This research strategy embodies a paternalistic approach to the delivery of care and to the dissemination of research findings to practitioners in a "top down" fashion. | This research strategy tends to operate within the worldview of practitioners and health care consumers and to yield more easily applied findings. |

*Note.* These points were variously derived from the papers cited in the section on Assumption 4.

clients to choice and no-choice conditions does not solve the problem, because the resulting sample is necessarily limited to treatment seekers who are willing to be research participants under these restricted choice conditions.

This recommendation to broaden the base of behavior change research is straightforward but will be resisted in some disciplines for at least two reasons. First, naturalistic studies typically are descriptive and correlational in nature, and a bias favors experimental research in psychology, medicine, and related fields that are guided by a clinical model. Mackenzie (1977) has argued convincingly, however, that the uncritical use of experimental methods and their often associated reliance on hypothetico-deductive approaches to theory construction are premature without a solid descriptive database. This certainly characterizes the state of knowledge about the human behavior change process, especially in environments that are not highly controlled. Adherence to an experimental approach may provide a (false) sense of scientific viability, but it is at odds with the development of knowledge in other life sciences such as biology, where conceptual advances often followed, rather than preceded, extensive observational studies. Naturalistic research methods offer several advantages, including being directly applicable to the species of interest (humans) and allowing efficient investigation of rare and common events, including those that occurred in the distant past (Cole, 1980). The ability to study behavior patterns over lengthy time frames is central to broadening the base of behavior change research.

Second, methodologies for naturalistic observation are unfamiliar and underutilized in many disciplines dominated by a clinical model. Fields such as anthropology and public health that routinely use these methods can provide guidance in their conduct, including in research on drug abuse (e.g., Lambert, Ashery, & Needle, 1995). The behavior therapy and behavioral medicine literatures also offer naturalistic observation methods (e.g., self-monitoring), including methods for assessing addictive behaviors (e.g., Donovan & Marlatt, 1988). However, skepticism continues about the accuracy of such methods and about the value of naturalistic research in general, and it is a bias the field must set aside in an expanded perspective on addictive behavior change.

## A LOOK AHEAD: EXPANDING ROLES FOR MENTAL HEALTH AND ADDICTION PROFESSIONALS IN THE 21ST CENTURY

These themes suggest that dominant clinical approaches to changing addictive behavior and many other psychological disorders probably have reached an asymptote with respect to effectiveness when delivered in the usual psychotherapeutic context. Innovations and improvements in substance abuse services will likely come from an expansion of demand-side interventions beyond those predicated on the psychotherapeutic vehicle and will also include approaches that are guided by a public health model and that take service utilization issues into account. Continued efforts to develop and improve clinical therapies without a concomitant concern with understanding the broader contexts in which they are delivered, and in which behavior change and help-seeking processes take place, are not likely to produce anything more than small incremental gains in effectiveness and will continue to fail to reach the majority of persons who do not seek help.

Improving access to addiction services in the health care system and expanding the range of services available therein will be an important part of this expanded initiative. These changes alone, however, will not solve the help-seeking problem, because interventions tied to the heath care system will continue to be stigmatizing as long as the United States pursues the War on Drugs. As recommended by the IOM (1990) and by harm-reduction proponents (e.g., Marlatt, 1998; Marlatt et al., 1997), a key piece in developing a more optimal continuum of care is bringing low-threshold interventions to substance abusers and expanding community involvement in addressing drug-related problems. As discussed next, each of these recommended avenues of change in the delivery of services for addictive behaviors offers opportunities for mental health professionals.

## Opportunities within the Health Care System

After decades of being poorly integrated into mainstream health care, mental health and substance abuse (MH/SA) services are now being integrated somewhat, and their future will be increasingly tied to forces that influence the health care system. Contributing to this change is the growing evidence that MH/SA problems adversely affect health status and health care costs and that treating them can produce positive economic returns (Fiedler & Wight, 1989; Fuller, 1995; Mechanic, 1994; Putnam, 1982). The process of integration is far from complete, however, and most health care plans contract or "carve" out MH/SA services to behavioral health programs or providers who are not well integrated into usual medical care (Frank, McQuire, & Newhouse, 1995). Much remains to be worked out in developing organizational patterns that promote coordinated care and accessible MH/SA services (Mechanic, Schlesinger, & McAlpine, 1995).

Doctoral-level mental health and addiction professionals have much to contribute to this organizational process, but continuing to function as a generic service provider—that is, as a therapist—is not likely to be a growth area in the future. Functioning autonomously as a therapist was the goal of a generation of psychologists, who fought to gain professional and financial independence from psychiatry, and was a driving force behind the competitive era of psychotherapy outcome research. However, the same arguments and evidence produced and used by psychologists in their initiative vis-à-vis psychiatry are now being used effectively against them (see Dawes, 1994) by subdoctoral therapists, who want similar professional privileges, and by managed care companies, who want to drive down costs by reimbursing all therapists at rates tied to the lowest rung of the provider ladder. Subdoctoral therapists far outnumber doctoral providers, especially in the addictions area, and this fact will continue to drive reimbursement for therapy down to rates acceptable to the lowest competent provider.

Several alternative roles make better use of the training and skills of doctoral level professionals. In health care organizations and plans that cover medical, mental health, and addiction services, doctoral professionals with comprehensive mental health training and expertise in sorting out mental health and medical problems (e.g., psychiatrists, psychologists) can function effectively as triage agents and as coordinators of care, working as needed in collaboration with primary care physicians (e.g., Blount, 1998). Related roles will involve participation in interdisciplinary health care teams and supervision of subdoctoral therapists, who will be doing more of the direct service delivery. Proficiency in assessing and coordinating the care of common mental health disorders (i.e., anxiety, depressive, and substance use disorders) will be essential, because many medical visits involve psychological distress, not a physical problem (Mechanic, 1994). In addition to promoting better care, utilization rates and health costs could be reduced if medical and mental health problems are properly diagnosed and treated earlier in the help-seeking cycle.

In the addiction field, for example, doctoral professionals can coordinate the assessment and referral of individuals to levels of care that are commensurate with the nature and severity of their problems, including those with dual diagnoses, and can monitor their progress and adjust the level of care depending upon their treatment response. The chapters in this volume on stepped-care approaches (11 and 12) discuss this process. The coordination of care can both involve substance-focused services and facilitate receipt of needed medical care and human services.

Another area in which mental health professions have much to contribute is in prevention and health promotion (IOM, 1994; Winett, King, & Altman, 1989). These initiatives have enjoyed some much-deserved attention, especially in health maintenance organizations, but it remains true that American health care continues to emphasize curing disease over preventing it (Mechanic, 1994). This is unlikely to change much until the managed care industry, which is rapidly changing, stabilizes. Currently, most individuals remain in a particular plan for only a brief time, which eliminates economic incentives for prevention in favor of attracting plan members who are relatively healthy (i.e., promoting favorable selection). Once the market stabilizes, individuals covered in a given plan will likely stabilize as well, and economic incentives should then exist to keep plan members healthy and shift services somewhat in the direction of preventive care. Under these circumstances, consumer preferences should begin to exert more influence on health plan configurations. An incipient interest in consumer choice and satisfaction is apparent in the health insurance literature (e.g., Ullman, Hill, Scheye, & Spoeri, 1997; see the Winter 1996 issue of *Health Affairs*) and contrasts with the restrictions on consumer choice that are the hallmark of managed care.

If these predicted developments take place, mental health and addiction professionals will have opportunities to redefine and expand their roles. The organizational changes created in the health care system by managed care will close some doors, while opening others. To navigate the opportunities that arise, nonphysician professionals must operate in an entrepreneurial fashion and position themselves so that their marketable services complement those of other health care providers, especially primary care physicians. They must be responsive to market forces operating on health care consumers, provider organizations, and third-party payers, and become comfortable with the organizational culture of contemporary health care (see Belar & Deardoff, 1995). These themes are discussed further in the second half of this book.

## Opportunities in Community and Other Nonmedical Settings

Expanding the base of interventions for addictive behaviors also requires developing interventions that are not tied to the health care system, because interventions delivered in that system will remain somewhat stigmatizing and high threshold (IOM, 1990; Marlatt, 1998; Marlatt et al., 1997). Lower threshold alternatives can serve multiple functions that operate at different points along the continuum of care, including the following:

- Prevention and early case finding, including greater use of naturally occurring contact points for problem identification and referral (e.g., through the informal social network or accessible professionals like pharmacists).
- Self-initiated assessment and brief interventions for individuals

with mild to moderate problems (e.g., through written or video-taped literature or Internet access, sometimes with limited professional or paraprofessional oversight).

- Motivational enhancement for behavior change and help-seeking among persons with a range of problem severity, with opportunities for onward referrals to different kinds and levels of care depending on interest and need.
- Harm reduction programs for persons with no immediate interest in giving up substance use, but who are receptive to reducing the harm, or risk of harm, associated with it (e.g., driving under the influence, HIV transmission).
- Case management of treatment and human services for persons with serious substance abuse and pervasive problems of living (e.g., the homeless).
- Community enrichment interventions that increase the availability of attractive, nondrug alternative activities that compete with drug use.
- Provision of a range of interventions for addictive disorders in health care, work-site, and other community settings, with mechanisms for "treatment sampling" by consumers.
- Media campaigns to heighten awareness of the prevalence and heterogeneity of addictive disorders and (with time) the accessibility and diversity of interventions for them.

These initiatives address different points along a continuum of care but share several common characteristics and goals, including (1) expanding intervention options beyond those now provided as part of the dominant clinical approach to treatment; (2) providing services that are responsive to the needs and preferences of individuals with a range of problems, rather than continuing the "one size fits all" approach of most treatments; (3) working within the natural environments in which addictive behavior patterns occur to reduce drug use and drug-related problems, and to increase the accessibility of services; and (4) encouraging a less coercive approach to helping persons with problems and working to reduce the associated stigma, thereby reducing barriers to help-seeking.

The harm reduction programs enacted during the past 10–15 years in several Western European countries (most notably the Netherlands and Great Britain), Canada, and Australia illustrate these goals in action and how they differ from the abstinence-oriented treatments that dominate the United States. These interventions variously include free needle exchanges to reduce the spread of HIV among IV drug users and to promote onward referrals for drug and medical treatment (e.g., Brettle, 1991; Carvell & Hart, 1990), providing methadone "by bus" to addicts in the street instead of requiring attendance at a clinic (Buning, Van Brussel, & Van Santen, 1990), and providing vouchers for free and immediate treatment (Levine, 1991). At the policy and organizational levels, changes have been made to decriminalize individual drug use and to make treatment available upon demand. These initiatives have helped reduce rates of HIV transmission, have reached heretofore inaccessible segments of the drug abusing community, have come to function as low-threshold gateways to receipt of needed drug and medical treatment, and have reduced criminal activity associated with drug abuse (Marlatt, 1998; NIH, 1997). An important feature is that they involve collaborations between the addict community, treatment providers, policymakers, and the government.

Contrary to the fears of some, these initiatives have not increased drug use or abuse or needle sharing (e.g., Guydish, Bucardo, Young, Woods, Grinstead, & Clark, 1993; NIH, 1997). Nevertheless, harm reduction measures remain controversial in the U.S., even in light of the growing database that supports their utility (NIH, 1997). Although it is doubtful that all elements of harm reduction programs in other countries will work equally well in the United States, the general approach deserves more consideration as part of an overall drug control strategy.

As another example of resistance in the United States to interventions that are not punitive and abstinence-oriented in a direct sense, consider the fate during the first Clinton administration of the midnight basketball program that was to have been introduced into urban ghetto areas with high drug use and crime rates. The proposal was ridiculed and quickly abandoned, even though evidence suggests that introducing this kind of competing nondrug activity into a drug-rich environment is precisely the kind of environmental enrichment required to reduce drug taking (see Chapter 7, this volume). It was good science but bad politics, and illustrates the schism in the United States between scientific knowledge on the one hand and drug control policy and lay views of addiction on the other. The gap is less acute in many other countries, including those with harm reduction programs.

## CONCLUDING COMMENTS: THE FUNDAMENTAL ISSUE OF STIGMA IN U.S. APPROACHES TO ADDICTIVE BEHAVIOR CHANGE

The limited role of science in U.S. drug policy and interventions will not be solved easily, but it is important to recognize that the limitation exists and continues to impede the development and implementation of many of the demand reduction strategies discussed in this book and elsewhere (Levine & Reinarman, 1994; NIH, 1997). The limited impact of science on policy and popular thinking is partly due to the recency of development of a relevant scientific knowledge base, but powerful, cultural notions about the nature of addiction and how to deal with the drug problem have almost certainly been more influential. Almost without exception, attempted solutions to date, whether emanating from the policy, legal, health care, or mutual help arenas, have been based on stigmatizing drug use and the drug user (Des Jarlais, 1995). The demand-side interventions discussed in this book generally reject this social control tactic and seek to reduce the stigma of drug use and abuse and its treatment. It thus is important to consider how the two approaches differ.

As discussed by Jones and colleagues (1983), the use of stigma as a behavior control tactic serves several social functions. First, by defining individuals with the stigmatized characteristic (the "marks") as members of a social out-group who are denied advantages of the dominant in-group, stigmatization seeks to maintain the dominant social order and to promote greater cohesiveness among the in-group. Second, it promotes identification of the marks, thus allowing them to be segregated in stigma-defined groups that are sufficiently visible, so that they can be monitored and controlled by the dominant group.[3] Third, unlike permanent exclusions such as exile or execution, opportunities are afforded the marks to regain at least some of the advantages of the dominant group if they repent and adhere to rules of conduct dictated by the in-group (Gusfield, 1967). Otherwise, the marks remain an enemy of the dominant social order (e.g., the "outlaw addict").

This process helps maintain dominant social norms while providing a mechanism for some stigmatized individuals to reenter mainstream social groups, thereby assuring that not all stigmatized persons are lost permanently to the dominant group. The need for a reentry mechanism varies directly with the size of the stigmatized group, which is large in the case of persons with addictive behaviors, thus giving them a measure of power in the process. The need for and success of stigmatization also depend on characteristics of the physical attribute or behavior that is the basis for the stigma. As discussed by Jones et al. (1983), stigmatization will vary with (1) the ease or difficulty of concealing the stigmatized attribute or behavior, (2) its course over time, (3) how disruptive it is, (4) its aesthetic qualities, (5) its origins, and (6) the extent to which it imperils the larger group. It is easier to stigmatize individuals with attributes that are hard to conceal; that are enduring, disruptive, and aesthetically unappealing; that can be blamed on the stigmatized person; and that imperil the larger group.

Success in initiating and maintaining a stigma also depends on the social distance between the mark and the marker (Jones et al., 1983). Initially, the tendency to stigmatize will be greater when social group boundaries are not well defined and the mark attribute threatens the cohesiveness of the dominant group. Once the stigma is established, however, it is easier to maintain the greater the social distance between the mark and the marker. Stigma is reduced when the mark becomes familiar and humanized.

Although a power differential exists in the relationship between marks and markers in favor of the dominant group, stigma can serve social functions for the marks. Depending on views about the changeability and origins of the stigmatized attribute, stigma can reduce personal blame and responsibility for some problems (Brickman et al., 1982), while augmenting positive attributions for favorable outcomes (Jones et al., 1983). Stigma-defined groups also promote social comparison processes within the group, rather than with the dominant group, thus supporting value shifts that emphasize positive attributes of the stigmatized group, while devaluing dimensions on which they fare poorly (Crocker & Major, 1989).

It is useful to consider the U.S. approach to the drug problem from this perspective. Conventional views incorporated into the War on Drugs and 12-step principles of recovery assume that addicts will conceal and deny their drug abuse (Dimension 1), but will be unable to do so indefinitely because the course of addiction is progressive (2), increasingly disruptive (3), and socially and morally offensive (4). Although the addict cannot be blamed for the disease of drug addiction (5), he or she endangers society through addictive behavior patterns and by exposing others, especially youths, to the seductive appeal of drugs (6). The attraction and function of the repentant pathway of 12-step programs need little explication in this context (see Trice & Roman, 1970), and seeking help is a "stigmatizing confession of a state of . . . illness sufficiently extreme to be beyond self-help" (Jones et al., 1983, p. 304).

In contrast to an approach based on stigmatization, an expanded perspective on addictive behavior change seeks to maintain many affected individuals as contributing members of mainstream, rather than drug-defined, social communities, while they attempt to resolve their problem (Des Jarlais, 1995). This obviously is not possible or desirable in all cases, particularly when the problem is severe and chronic or imperils others (e.g., as in the case of chronic drunk drivers). Nevertheless, it is a realistic alternative for the majority with less severe problems, many of whom will "mature out" of their drug career in their 40s and 50s, often without formal interventions. Thus, unlike traditional views that stigmatize addiction, an expanded perspective strives to reduce incentives for concealment (Dimension 1) that emanate from stigmatization and to promote help-seeking and behavior change early during problem development; assumes that the course of addiction is variable and changeable (2) and does not inevitably result in pervasive problems that are disruptive (3) and repugnant (4); assumes that addictive behaviors are multidetermined by complex social, environmental, and biological factors, and are not reducible to a single physical cause or character flaw (5); and evaluates the harm of component behaviors from the perspective of both the individual and group without assuming a priori that either party is inevitably imperiled (6).

By reducing stigmatization, the need for a systematic pathway for repentance and redemption also is reduced, and intervention avenues can be pursued that entail fewer coercive social controls and more of a partnership between helpers and help recipients. This analysis suggests that the terms of the relationship between marks and markers are subject to negotiation and change, and that the marks have some power in the process, depending on the nature of the stigmatized attribute and the size of the stigmatized group. For example, regarding the emergence of AA in the aftermath of Prohibition, one could speculate that AA's embracement of the stigma of alcoholism and its commitment to abstinence were traded for (1) greater public acceptance of alcohol problems as a disease deserving of treatment, rather than as a moral or criminal problem deserving of punitive action; and (2) an opportunity to recover anonymously in a supportive fellowship that placed no demands on the larger community, thus discouraging any incursions from it (i.e., "taking care of one's own").

The current debate about the War on Drugs and harm reduction alternatives appears to involve similar social negotiations about how drug abusers will be treated by the dominant group, which is once again heavily criminalizing drug-taking and stigmatizing the drug abuser. This time, the marks have relatively more power in the negotiation. First and probably most important, the risk that AIDS poses to the entire population means that the dominant power group cannot afford to remain indifferent to the needs and preferences of drug abusers. Effective HIV risk reduction requires cooperation between the two communities, and continuing a punitive, stigmatizing, and coercive approach to dealing with drug abusers will not enlist their essential cooperation. It probably is this peril to the dominant group that will force concessions from them to provide less stigmatizing and more accessible interventions that allow for harm reduction without insisting upon universal abstinence.

Second, compared to when Prohibition was enacted, considerably more knowledge exists about the failure of supply-reduction strategies to curb the drug problem, while producing a range of untoward effects, and about the heterogeneous nature of addictive disorders and the need to intervene accordingly. Supply-side approaches have been tried in the United States twice this century and have failed both times, but demand reduction approaches continue to receive only marginal funding. Evidence of more positive effects is accruing in other countries that have placed greater emphasis on demand reduction strategies (Marlatt, 1998).

Third, the current debate is taking place at a time when a generation of Americans who were heavily exposed to recreational drugs during their youth are coming into positions of power and influence. The social distance between the drug abusing community and the dominant group is thus somewhat reduced. On the one hand, the literature on stigma suggests that this may intensify efforts to stigmatize drug use if the reduced social distance threatens the cohesiveness of the dominant group, which may be a factor motivating the War on Drugs. On the other hand, a large segment of the baby-boom generation has firsthand knowledge, based on their experiences and those of their friends, of the continuum along which drug use and drug problems vary, at least with respect to commonly used drugs such as alcohol, marijuana, and cigarettes. Their collective familiarity with drugs may help reduce the stigma associated with drug use and drug treatment, and may promote a more nuanced and sophisticated view of the drug problem and solutions to it. For example, it seems likely that attempts to demonize soft drugs such as marijuana will continue to fail, whereas legitimate popular consensus is growing about the health hazards of smoking, the risks to mother and fetus of drug use during pregnancy, and the need to sharply reduce drunk driving.

A more pessimistic view is that the stigma of drug abuse has taken such firm root that individuals will be ridiculed as being "soft on drugs" when they attempt to make rational distinctions about the dangerousness of different drugs and drug-related problems—and base drug laws and policies accordingly—and attempt a more balanced allocation of resources between demand- and supply-side approaches. To be sure, many Americans do not find individuals with drug and other addictive behaviors to be deserving of help, or they naively assume that punitive, zero tolerance approaches are effective. Although not widely discussed or analyzed, there also are stakeholders with strong financial and political interests in continuing the War on Drugs. Law enforcement and many government agencies benefit from the money flowing from the War on Drugs (Dreyfuss, 1997). Politicians get considerable mileage out of taking tough, antidrug positions, and corporations pay large sums of money to drug-testing companies. Such forces will impede shifting resources toward demand reduction strategies, but the dollars needed to expand them pale by comparison to those spent on the War on Drugs.

By articulating a range of demand reduction approaches to addictive behavior change, this book illustrates what the mental health professions and related social and behavioral sciences can contribute to an expanded approach to the drug problem. It is more than therapy and more than research on therapy process and outcome. It is time to give up our characteristically American war metaphor for solving the drug problem and to approach it as the complex social and public health problem that it is, bringing the best resources to bear on it from the social and behavioral sciences and medicine, in collaboration with persons who suffer from addictive behavior problems. Supply-side interventions will be a part of the approach, but their exclusive pursuit can no longer be justified. Finding a more effective combination of supply- and demand reduction strategies is the challenge before us.

## ACKNOWLEDGMENTS

Preparation of this chapter was supported by Grant Nos. R01 AA08972 and K02 AA00209 from the National Institute on Alcohol Abuse and Alcoholism. I thank Joe Buckhalt, Dennis Donovan, Alan Marlatt, and Rudy Vuchinich for their comments on an earlier draft.

## NOTES

1. Racial issues also were intertwined with Prohibition, which some view as a white Protestant effort to control the drinking of Irish and German immigrants in the Northeast and Midwest, and blacks in the South. Industrialists such as Henry Ford wanted a sober workforce, and their support was important for the passage of the 18th Amendment (Wiebe, 1967). In a related vein, the lengthy campaign for Prohibition by the Women's Christian Temperance Union probably delayed the passage of the 19th Amendment that gave women the right to vote because of fears among "wets" that franchising them would speed the adoption of Prohibition.

2. A third level of analysis that is beyond the scope of the book involves cost-related analyses of different supply- and demand-side interventions that can inform policy decisions and resource allocation across the two general drug control strategies. The Rand Corporation research brief (1995) described earlier exemplifies this level of analysis.

3. The segregation of mental deviants has a long-standing history in Western cultures. The asylum movement of the Victorian era, for example, continued to influence interventions for mental and behavioral disorders well into the 20th century (Grob, 1991). The community mental health movement of the 1960s and the deinstitutionalization of the mentally ill after the development of major tranquilizers have not erased earlier, entrenched tendencies to segregate the mentally ill. Some of the ways in which they are segregated have changed, sometimes to their greater detriment (e.g., the homeless who have mental health or substance abuse problems), but the social dynamics remain largely unchanged in the United States.

## REFERENCES

Abrams, D. B., Emmons, K. M., Niaura, R., Goldstein, M. G., & Sherman, C. B. (1991). Tobacco dependence: An integration of individual and public health perspectives. In P. E. Nathan, J. W. Langenbucher, B. S. McCrady, & W. Frankenstein (Eds.), *Annual review of addictions research and treatment* (pp. 391–436). New York: Pergamon.

Alcoholics Anonymous World Services. (1985). *Alcoholics Anonymous comes of age.* New York: Author.

American Psychological Association. (1995). *Template for developing guidelines: Interventions for mental disorders and psychosocial aspects of disease.* Washington, DC: APA Task Force on Psychological Interventions.

Armor, D. J., & Meshkoff, J. E. (1983). Remission among treated and untreated alcoholics. In N. K. Mello (Ed.), *Advances in substance abuse: Behavioral and biological research* (Vol. 3, pp. 239–269). Greenwich, CT: JAI Press.

Barlow, D. H. (1988). *Anxiety and its disorders: The nature and treatment of anxiety and panic.* New York: Guilford Press.

Battle, E. K., & Brownell, K. (1996). Confronting a rising tide of eating disorders and obesity: Treatment vs. prevention vs. policy. *Addictive Behavior, 21,* 755–765.

Belar, C. D., & Deardorff, W. W. (1995). *Clinical health psychology in medical settings: A practitioner's guidebook.* Washington, D.C.: American Psychological Association.

Bennett, L. A. (1988). Alcohol in context: Anthropological perspectives. *Drugs and Society, 2,* 89–131.

Beutler, L. E., Cargo, M., & Arizmendi, T. G. (1986). Research on therapist variables in psychotherapy. In S. L. Garfield & A. E. Bergin (Eds.), *Handbook of psychotherapy and behavior change* (pp. 257–310). New York: Wiley.

Blacker, C. V. R., & Mortimore, C. (1996). Randomized controlled trials and naturalistic data: Time for a change? *Human Psychopharmacology, 11,* 353–363.

Blount, A. (Ed.). (1998). *Integrated primary care: The future of medical and mental health collaboration.* New York: Norton.

Boardman, B. (1989). *Flappers, bootleggers, "Typhoid Mary" and the bomb: An anecdotal history of the United States from 1923–1945.* New York: Harper & Row.

Bowers, T. G., & Clum, G. A. (1988). Relative contribution of specific and nonspecific treatment effects: Meta-analysis of placebo-controlled behavior therapy research. *Psychological Bulletin, 103,* 315–323.

Brettle, R. P. (1991). HIV and harm reduction for injection drug users. *AIDS, 5,* 125–136.

Brewer, D. D., Catalano, R. F., Haggerty, K., Gainey, R. R., & Fleming, C. B. (1998). A meta-analysis of predictors of continued drug use during and after treatment for opiate addiction. *Addiction, 93,* 73–92.

Brickman, P., Rabinowitz, V. C., Karuza, J., Coates, D., Cohn, E., & Kidder, L. (1982). Models of helping and coping. *American Psychologist, 37,* 368–384.

Britt, C. L., Gottfredson, M. R., & Goldkamp, J. S. (1992). Drug testing and pretrial misconduct: An experiment on the specific deterrent effects of drug monitoring defendants on pretrial release. *Journal of Research in Crime and Delinquency, 29,* 62–78.

Buning, E. C., Van Brussel, G. H. A., & Van Santen, G. (1990). The "methadone by bus" project in Amsterdam. *British Journal of Addiction, 85,* 1247–1250.

Carvell, A. M., & Hart, G. J. (1990). Help-seeking and referrals in a needle exchange: A comprehensive service to injecting drug users. *British Journal of Addiction, 85,* 235–240.

Cole, P. (1980). The analysis of case-control studies (Introduction). In N. E. Breslow & N. E. Day (Eds.), *Statistical methods in cancer research* (Vol. 1, pp. 14–40). Lyon, France: World Health Organization.

Coombs, R. H., & Ryan, F. J. (1990). Drug testing effectiveness in identifying and preventing drug use. *American Journal of Drug and Alcohol Abuse, 16,* 173–184.

Courtland, D. T. (1996/1997). The Drug War's hidden toll. *Issues in Science and Technology, 13,* 71–77.

Crocker, J., & Major, B. (1989). Social stigma and self-esteem: The self-protective properties of stigma. *Psychological Review, 96,* 608–630.

Davidson, R. (1992). Prochaska and DiClemente's model of change: A case study? *British Journal of Addiction, 87,* 821–822.

Dawes, R. M. (1994). *House of cards: Psychology and psychotherapy built on myth.* New York: Free Press.

De Leon, G. (1988). Legal pressure in therapeutic communities. *Journal of Drug Issues, 18,* 625–640.

De Leon, G. (1998). Commentary: Reconsidering the self-selection factor in addiction treatment research. *Psychology of Addictive Behaviors, 12,* 61–77.

DeRios, M. D., & Smith, D. E. (1977). The function of drug rituals in human society: Continuities and changes. *Journal of Psychedelic Drugs, 9,* 269–275.

Des Jarlais, D. C. (1995). Harm reduction: A framework for incorporating science into drug policy (editorial). *American Journal of Public Health, 85,* 10–12.

Donovan, D. M., & Marlatt, G. A. (Eds.). (1988). *Assessment of addictive behaviors: Behavioral, cognitive, and physiological procedures.* New York: Guilford Press.

Dreyfuss, R. (1997). The Drug War: Where the money goes. *Rolling Stone, 775,* 37–44, 87–88.

Emrick, C. D. (1975). A review of psychologically oriented treatment of alcoholism: II. The relative effectiveness of different treatment approaches and the effectiveness of treatment versus no treatment. *Quarterly Journal of Studies on Alcohol, 36,* 88–108.

Ennett, S. T., Tobler, N. S., Ringwalt, C. L., & Flewelling, R. L. (1994). How effective is drug resistance education? A meta-analysis of Project DARE outcome evaluations. *American Journal of Public Health, 84,* 1394–1401.

Fiedler, J. L., & Wight, J. B. (1989). *The medical offset effect and public health policy: Mental health industry in transition.* New York: Praeger.

Fink, P. J., & Tasman, A. (Eds.). (1992). *Stigma and mental illness.* Washington, DC: American Psychiatric Association Press.

Frank, R. G., McQuire, T. G., & Newhouse, J. P. (1995). Risk contracts in managed mental health care. *Health Affairs, 14,* 50–64.

Fuller, M. G. (1995). More is less: Increasing access as a strategy for managing health care costs. *Psychiatric Services, 46,* 1015–1017.

Garfield, S. L. (1986). Research on client variables in psychotherapy. In S. L. Garfield & A. E. Bergin (Eds.), *Handbook of psychotherapy and behavior change* (pp. 213–256). New York: Wiley.

Garfield, S. L. (1994). Eclecticism and integration in psychotherapy: Developments and issues. *Clinical Psychology: Science and Practice, 1,* 123–137.

Garfield, S. L., & Bergin, A. E. (1986). Introduction and historical overview. In S. L. Garfield & A. E. Bergin (Eds.), *Handbook of psychotherapy and behavior change* (pp. 3–22). New York: Wiley.

Gavin, D. V., Harland, R. D., Michaelis, R. C., & Holloway, F. A. (1989). Caffeine–phenylethylamine combinations mimic the cocaine discriminative cue. *Life Sciences, 44,* 67–73.

Gavin, D. V., Moore, K. R., Youngblood, B. D., & Holloway, F. A. (1993). The discriminative stimulus properties of legal over-the-counter stimulants administered singly and in binary and tertiary combinations. *Psychopharmacology, 110,* 309–319.

Glasner, P. D., & Kaslow, R. A. (1990). The epidemiology of human immunodeficiency virus infection. *Journal of Consulting and Clinical Psychology, 58,* 13–21.

Grant, B. F., Chou, S. P., Pickering, R. P., & Hasin, D. S. (1992). Empirical subtypes of DSM-III-R alcohol dependence: United States, 1988. *Drug and Alcohol Dependence, 30,* 755–784.

Grob, G. N. (1991). *From asylum to community: Mental health policy in modern America.* Princeton, NJ: Princeton University Press.

Gusfield, J. R. (1967). Moral passage: The symbolic process in public designations of deviance. *Social Problems, 15,* 175–188.

Guydish, J., Bucardo, J., Young, M., Woods, W., Grinstead, O., & Clark, W. (1993). Evaluating needle exchange: Are there negative effects? *AIDS, 7,* 871–876.

Harding, W. M., Zinberg, N. E., Stelmark, S. M., & Berry, M. (1980). Formerly-addicted-now-controlled opiate users. *International Journal of the Addictions, 15,* 47–60.

Heath, D. B. (1987). Anthropology and alcohol studies: Current issues. *Annual Review of Anthropology, 16,* 99–120.

Heather, N. (1996). The public health and brief interventions for excessive alcohol consumption: The British experience. *Addictive Behaviors, 21,* 857–868.

Heather, N., Wodak, A., Nadelmann, E. A., & O'Hare, P. (Eds.). (1993). *Psychoactive drugs and harm reduction: From faith to science.* London: Whurr.

Hingson, R., Mangione, T., Meyers, A., & Scotch, N. (1982). Seeking help for drinking problems: A study in the Boston metropolitan area. *Journal of Studies on Alcohol, 43,* 273–288.

Hoffman, N. R., & Miller, N. S. (1992). Treatment outcomes for abstinence-based programs. *Psychiatric Annals, 22,* 402–408.

Holder, H. D., & Blose, J. O. (1992). The reduction of health care costs associated with alcoholism treatment: A 14 year longitudinal study. *Journal of Studies on Alcohol, 53,* 293–302.

Institute of Medicine. (1990). *Broadening the base of treatment for alcohol problems.* Washington, DC: National Academy Press.

Institute of Medicine (1994). *Reducing risks for mental disorders: Frontiers for preventive intervention research.* Washington, D.C.: National Academy Press.

Jellinek, E. M. (1960). *The disease concept of alcoholism.* Highland Park, NJ: Hillhouse Press.

Johnson, S. B. (1996, May). *Compliance behavior: Implications for biomedical research.* Paper presented at the NIH Seminar Series on Health and Behavior, National Institutes of Health, Bethesda, MD.

Jones, E. E., Farina, A., Hastorf, A. H., Markus, H., Miller, D. T., & Scott, R. A. (1983). *Social stigma: The psychology of marked relationships.* New York: Freeman.

Jordan, C. M., & Oei, T. P. (1989). Help-seeking behaviour in problem drinkers: A review. *British Journal of Addiction, 84,* 979–988.

Klingemann, H. K.-H. (1991). The motivation for change from problem alcohol and heroin use. *British Journal of Addiction, 86,* 727–744.

Kohlenberg, R. J., Tsai, M., & Dougher, M. J. (1993). The dimensions of clinical behavior analysis. *Behavior Analyst, 16*, 271–282.
Lambert, E. Y., Ashery, R. S., & Needle, R. H. (Eds.). (1995). *Qualitative methods in drug
abuse and HIV research* (NIDA Research Monograph No. 157). Rockville, MD: National Institute on Drug Abuse, U.S. Department of Health and Human Services,
Public Health Service, National Institutes of Health.
Leigh, B. C., & Stall, R. (1993). Substance use and risky sexual behavior for exposure
to HIV: Issues in methodology, interpretation, and prevention. *American Psychologist, 48*, 1035–1045.
Levine, C. (1991). AIDS prevention and education: Reframing the question. *AIDS Education and Prevention, 3*, 147–163.
Levine, H. G., & Reinarman, C. (1994). When science and medicine are ignored: The
case of U.S. drug policy. *Addiction, 89*, 535–536.
Luborsky, L., Singer, B., & Luborsky, L. (1975). Comparative studies of psychothera-
pies: Is it true that "everyone has won and all must have prizes"? *Archives of Gener-
al Psychiatry, 32*, 995–1008.
MacAndrew, C., & Edgerton, R. B. (1969). *Drunken comportment.* Chicago: Aldine.
Mackenzie, B. D. (1977). *Behaviourism and the limits of scientific method.* Atlantic Highlands,
NJ: Humanities Press.
Makela, K., Arminen, I., Bloomfield, K., Eisenbach-Stangl, I., Bergmark, K. H., Ku-
rube, N., Mariolini, N., Ólafsdóttir, H., Peterson, J. H., Phillips, M., Rehm, J.,
Room, R., Rosenqvist, P., Rosovsky, H., Stenius, K., Swiatkiewicz, G., Woronow-
icz, B., & Zieliński, A. (1996). *Alcoholics Anonymous as a mutual-help movement: A study
in eight societies.* Madison: University of Wisconsin Press.
Maloff, D., Becker, H. S., Fonaroff, A., & Rodin, J. (1979). Informal social controls and
their influence on substance use, *Journal of Drug Issues, 9*, 161–184.
Marlatt, G. A. (1978). Craving for alcohol, loss of control, and relapse: A cognitive-
behavioral analysis. In P. E. Nathan, G. A. Marlatt, & T. Loberg (Eds.), *Alcoholism:
New directions in behavioral research and treatment* (pp. 271–314). New York: Plenum.
Marlatt, G. A. (1983). The controlled drinking controversy: A commentary. *American
Psychologist, 38*, 1097–1110.
Marlatt, G. A. (1996). Harm reduction: Come as you are. *Addictive Behaviors, 21*,
779–788.
Marlatt, G. A. (Ed.). (1998). *Harm reduction: Pragmatic strategies for managing high-risk behav-
iors.* New York: Guilford Press.
Marlatt, G. A., & Gordon, J. R. (Eds.). (1985). *Relapse prevention: Maintenance strategies in
the treatment of addictive behaviors.* New York: Guilford Press.
Marlatt, G. A., Larimer, M. E., Baer, J. S., & Quigley, L. A. (1993). Harm reduction for
alcohol problems: Moving beyond the controlled drinking controversy. *Behavior
Therapy, 24*, 461–504.
Marlatt, G. A., Tucker, J. A., Donovan, D. M., & Vuchinich, R. E. (1997). Help-seeking
by substance abusers: The role of harm reduction and behavioral–economic approaches to facilitate treatment entry and retention. In L. S. Onken, J. D. Blaine,
& J. J. Boren (Eds.), *Beyond the therapeutic alliance: Keeping the drug dependent individual in
treatment* (NIDA Research Monograph, No. 165, pp. 44–84). Rockville, MD: U.S.
Department of Health and Human Services, Public Health Service, National Institutes of Health.

McCrady, B. S., & Miller, W. R. (Eds.). (1993). *Research on Alcoholics Anonymous: Opportunities and alternatives.* New Brunswick, NJ: Rutgers Center of Alcohol Studies.

McLellan, A. T., Alterman, A. I., Metzger, D. S., Grissom, G. R., Woody, G. E., Luborsky, L., & O'Brien, C. P. (1994). Similarity of outcome predictors across opiate, cocaine, and alcohol treatments: Role of treatment services. *Journal of Consulting and Clinical Psychology, 62,* 1141–1158.

Mechanic, D. (1978). Sociocultural and social-psychological factors affecting personal responses to psychological disorder. *Journal of Health and Social Behavior, 6,* 393–404.

Mechanic, D. (1994). *Inescapable decisions: The imperatives of health reform.* New Brunswick, NJ: Transaction Press.

Mechanic, D., Schlesinger, M., & McAlpine, D. D. (1995). Management of mental health and substance abuse services: State of the art and early results. *Milbank Quarterly, 73,* 19–55.

Miller, W. R. (1983). Controlled drinking: A history and critical review. *Journal of Studies on Alcohol, 44,* 68–83.

Miller, W. R. (1985). Motivation for treatment: A review with special emphasis on alcoholism. *Psychological Bulletin, 98,* 84–107.

Miller, W. R., & Hester, R. K. (1986). The effectiveness of alcoholism treatment: What research reveals. In W. R. Miller & N. Heather (Eds.), *Treating addictive behaviors: Processes of change* (pp. 121–174). New York: Plenum.

Miller, W. R., & Hester, R. K. (1989). Treating alcohol problems: Toward an informed electicism. In R. K. Hester & W. R. Miller (Eds.), *Handbook of alcoholism treatment approaches: Effective alternatives* (pp. 3–13). New York: Pergamon Press.

Miller, W. R., & Rollnick, S. (Eds.). (1991). *Motivational interviewing: Preparing people to change addictive behavior.* New York: Guilford Press.

Moos, R. H., & Finney, J. W. (1983). Expanding the scope of alcoholism treatment evaluation. *American Psychologist, 38,* 1036–1044.

Moos, R. H., Finney, J. W., & Cronkite, R. C. (1990). *Alcoholism treatment: Context, process, and outcome.* New York: Oxford University Press.

Morley, J. A., Finney, J. W., Monahan, S. C., & Floyd, A. S. (1996). Alcoholism treatment outcome studies, 1980–1992: Methodological characteristics and quality. *Addictive Behaviors, 21,* 429–443.

Nadelmann, E. A. (1998). Commonsense drug policy. *Foreign Affairs, 77,* 111–126.

Narrow, W. E., Regier, D. A., Rae, D. S., Manderscheid, R. W., & Locke, B. A. (1993). Use of services by persons with mental and addictive disorders. *Archives of General Psychiatry, 50,* 95–107.

National Institutes of Health. (1997). *Interventions to prevent HIV risk behaviors* (NIH Consensus Statement No. 15(2), pp. 1–41). Bethesda, MD: Author.

Orlinsky, D. E., & Howard, K. I. (1986). Process and outcome in psychotherapy. In S. L. Garfield, & A. E. Bergin (Eds.), *Handbook of psychotherapy and behavior change* (3rd ed., pp. 311–381). New York: Wiley.

Pattison, E. M., Sobell, M. B., & Sobell, L. C. (Eds.). (1977). *Emerging concepts of alcohol dependence.* New York: Springer.

Paul, G. (1967). Outcome research in psychotherapy. *Journal of Consulting Psychology, 31,* 109–118.

Peele, S. (1991). *Diseasing of America: Addiction treatment out of control.* Boston: Houghton Mifflin.

Polich, J. M., Armor, D. J., & Braiker, H. B. (1981). *The course of alcoholism: Four years after treatment.* Santa Monica, CA: Rand Corporation.

Pringle, G. H. (1982). Impact of the criminal justice system on the substance abusers seeking professional help. *Journal of Drug Issues, 12,* 275–283.

Prochaska, J. O., & DiClemente, C. C. (1983). Stages and processes of self-change of smoking: Toward an integrative model of change. *Journal of Consulting and Clinical Psychology, 51,* 390–395.

Prochaska, J. O., & DiClemente, C. C. (1986). Towards a comprehensive model of change. In W. R. Miller & N. Heather (Eds.), *Treating addictive behaviors: Processes of change* (pp. 3–28). New York: Plenum.

Prochaska, J. O., DiClemente, C. C., & Norcross, J. C. (1992). In search of how people change: Applications to addictive behaviors. *American Psychologist, 47,* 1102–1114.

Project MATCH Research Group. (1997). Matching alcoholism treatment to client heterogeneity: Project MATCH posttreatment drinking outcomes. *Journal of Studies on Alcohol, 58,* 7–29.

Putnam, S. (1982). Alcoholism, morbidity and care seeking: The inpatient and ambulatory service utilization and associated illness experience of alcoholics and matched controls in a health maintenance organization. *Medical Care, 20,* 97–121.

RAND Corporation. (1995). *Projecting future cocaine use and evaluating control strategies* (Research Brief No. 6002). Santa Monica, CA: Rand Drug Policy Research Center.

Regier, D. A., Narrow, W. E., Rae, D. S., Manderscheid, R. W., Locke, B. Z., & Goodwin, F. K. (1993). The de facto U.S. mental and addictive disorders service system. *Archives of General Psychiatry, 50,* 85–94.

Reuter, P., & Caulkins, J. P. (1995). Redefining the goals of national drug policy: Recommendations from a working group. *American Journal of Public Health, 85,* 1059–1063.

Robert Wood Johnson Foundation. (1993). *Substance abuse: The nation's number one health problem: Key indicators for policy.* Princeton, NJ: Author.

Rosenberg, H. (1993). Prediction of controlled drinking by alcoholics and problem drinkers. *Psychological Bulletin, 113,* 129–139.

Sandahl, C. (1984). Determinants of relapse among alcoholics: A cross-cultural replication study. *International Journal of the Addictions, 19,* 833–848.

Sax, L., Dougherty, D., Esty, K., & Fine, M. (1983). *The effectiveness and cost of alcoholism treatment* (Health Technology Case Study No. 22). Washington, DC: Office of Technology Assessment.

Seligman, M. E. P. (1995). The effectiveness of psychotherapy: The Consumer Reports study. *American Psychologist, 50,* 965–974.

Shiffman, S. (1982). Relapse following smoking cessation: A situational analysis. *Journal of Consulting and Clinical Psychology, 50,* 71–86.

Shiffman, S. (1992). Relapse process and relapse prevention in addictive behaviors. *Behavior Therapist, 15,* 9–11.

Simpson, D. D., & Sells, S. B. (1982). Effectiveness of treatment for drug abuse: An overview of the DARP research program. *Advances in Alcohol and Drug Abuse, 2,* 7–29.

Smith, M. L., Glass, G. V., & Miller, T. I. (1980). *The benefits of psychotherapy.* Baltimore, MD: Johns Hopkins University Press.

Sobell, L. C., Cunningham, J. A., & Sobell, M. B. (1996). Recovery from alcohol problems with and without treatment: Prevalence in two population studies. *American Journal of Public Health, 86,* 966–972.

Sobell, L. C., & Sobell, M. B. (1989). Treatment outcome evaluation methodology with alcohol abusers: Strengths and key issues. *Advances in Behavioral Research and Therapy, 11,* 151–160.

Sobell, L. C., Sobell, M. B., Toneatto, T., & Leo, G. I. (1993). What triggers the resolution of alcohol problems without treatment? *Alcoholism: Clinical and Experimental Research, 17,* 217–224.

Sobell, M. B., & Sobell, L. C. (Eds.). (1987). *Moderation as a goal or outcome of treatment for alcohol problems: A dialogue.* New York: Haworth Press.

Sobell, M. B., & Sobell, L. C. (1993). Treatment for problem drinking: A public health priority. In J. S. Baer, G. A. Marlatt, & R. J. McMahon (Eds.), *Addictive behaviors across the lifespan: Prevention, treatment, and policy issues* (pp. 138–157). Beverly Hills, CA: Sage.

Stall, R., & Bernacki, P. (1986). Spontaneous remission from the problematic use of substances: An inductive model derived from a comparative analysis of the alcohol, opiate, tobacco, and food/obesity literatures. *International Journal of the Addictions, 21,* 1–23.

Stiles, W. B., & Shapiro, D. A. (1994). Disabuse of the drug metaphor: Psychotherapy process–outcome correlations. *Journal of Consulting and Clinical Psychology, 62,* 942–948.

Stiles, W. B., Shapiro, D. A., & Elliott, R. (1986). Are all psychotherapies equivalent? *American Psychologist, 41,* 165–180.

Stitzer, M. L., & McCaul, M. E. (1987). Criminal justice interventions with drug and alcohol abusers. In E. K. Morris & C. J. Braukmann (Eds.), *Behavioral approaches to crime and delinquency: A handbook of application, research and concepts* (pp. 331–361). New York: Plenum.

Szasz, T. S. (1992). *Our right to drugs: The case for a free market.* Westport, CT: Praeger.

Trice, H. M., & Roman, P. M. (1970). Delabeling, relabeling, and Alcoholics Anonymous. *Social Problems, 17,* 538–546.

Tucker, J. A., & Gladsjo, J. A. (1993). Help-seeking and recovery by problem drinkers: Characteristics of drinkers who attended Alcoholics Anonymous or formal treatment or who recovered without assistance. *Addictive Behaviors, 18,* 549–542.

Tucker, J. A., Vuchinich, R. E., & Gladsjo, J. A. (1990/1991). Environmental influences on relapse in substance use disorders. *International Journal of the Addictions, 25,* 1017–1050.

Tucker, J. A., Vuchinich, R. E., & Gladsjo, J. A. (1994). Environmental events surrounding natural recovery from alcohol-related problems. *Journal of Studies on Alcohol, 55,* 401–411.

Tucker, J. A., Vuchinich, R. E., & Pukish, M. M. (1995). Molar environmental contexts surrounding recovery from alcohol problems by treated and untreated problem drinkers. *Experimental and Clinical Psychopharmacology, 3,* 195–204.

Ullman, R., Hill, J. W., Scheye, E. C., & Spoeri, R. K. (1997). Satisfaction and choice: A view from the plans. *Health Affairs, 16,* 209–217.

Vuchinich, R. E., & Tucker, J. A. (1996a). Alcoholic relapse, life events, and behavioral theories of choice: A prospective analysis. *Experimental and Clinical Psychopharmacology, 4,* 19–28.

Vuchinich, R. E., & Tucker, J. A. (1996b). The molar context of alcohol abuse. In L. Green & J. H. Kagel (Eds.), *Advances in behavioral-economics: Vol. 3. Substance use and abuse* (pp. 133–162). Norwood, NJ: Ablex.

Weibe, R. H. (1967). *The search for order (1877–1920)*. New York: Hall & Wang.

Winett, R. A., King, A. C., & Altman, D. G. (1989). *Health psychology and public health: An integrative approach*. New York: Pergamon Press.

Yates, B. T. (1995). Cost-effectiveness analysis, cost–benefit analysis, and beyond: Evolving models for the scientist-manager-practitioner. *Clinical Psychology: Science and Practice, 2,* 385–398.

Zinberg, N. E., & Harding, W. M. (1979). Control and intoxicant use: A theoretical and practical overview. *Journal of Drug Issues, 9,* 121–143.

Zinberg, N. E., Harding, W. M., & Winkeller, M. (1977). A study of social regulatory mechanisms in controlled illicit drug users. *Journal of Drug Issues, 7,* 117–133.

# 2

## From Hindsight to Foresight: A Commentary on Project MATCH

### G. ALAN MARLATT

The purpose of this chapter is to provide a commentary and critique of Project MATCH, the largest and most expensive treatment research study ever conducted in the alcoholism field. The long-awaited results of this study, first initiated and funded by the National Institute on Alcohol Abuse and Alcoholism (NIAAA) in 1989, were finally published early in 1997. Project MATCH has been fraught with controversy over the past decade, a debate that reached its peak after the preliminary results were announced. The chapter begins with an overview of the design and findings of Project MATCH. The second section reviews a number of critical misinterpretations about the study and the ultimate meaning of its findings. Much of this controversy centers around potential limitations of the research design employed by MATCH investigators (discussed in the third section). The final section is devoted to a discussion of alternatives to treatment matching, with an emphasis on client choice or self-selection factors. In terms of addictive behaviors such as alcohol dependence, it may be more productive to view individuals who seek or are referred for treatment as "consumers" who are capable of selecting among viable treatment options, rather than as "patients" who are assigned to a particular treatment by a professional utilizing treatment-matching criteria.

### PROJECT MATCH: METHODS AND RESULTS

For those who still might be unfamiliar with Project MATCH, which stands for "Matching Alcoholism Treatments to Client Heterogeneity," here is a summary of the procedures and results. In the largest and most expensive clinical trial of any psychotherapies undertaken to date, a total of 1,726 patients were recruited at nine treatment facilities throughout the United States to take part in Project MATCH (Project MATCH Research Group, 1993). The purpose of this large study, funded by the NIAAA, was to learn whether certain types of patients respond best to specific forms of psychological treatment for alcoholism. If so, future patients could be "matched" to a particular type of treatment in order to maximize positive treatment outcomes. Most of the patients were white males (25% were women, and 15% were from minority populations). Patients were drawn from two parallel arms: an outpatient arm (with patients selected directly from the community) and an aftercare arm (consisting of patients who had recently completed inpatient or intensive day hospital treatment). Patients in both arms of the study were extensively assessed, using interviews and tests, to gather data on demographic characteristics, drinking behavior, personality, predisposing factors for alcohol problems, and personal and medical effects of drinking.

Ten patient matching characteristics were assessed, based on promising findings already reported in the existing literature (consisting of over 30 prior studies) on treatment matching: severity of alcohol involvement, cognitive impairment, conceptual level, gender, meaning seeking, motivation, psychiatric severity, social support for drinking versus abstinence, sociopathy, and alcoholic typology. As might be expected, assessment of all these variables at baseline, prior to treatment, took considerable time: "On average the entire assessment battery, including self-report questionnaires, took about 8 hours to complete" (Project MATCH Research Group, 1997a, p. 11). During the five follow-up sessions conducted every 90 days following treatment completion, a core set of procedures and instruments were readministered by the same individual who conducted the baseline assessment. More than 90% of patients completed all five of the follow-up data sessions during the year following treatment.

The three treatment conditions evaluated in the randomized clinical trial were chosen because they all showed potential for matching and had promising outcomes in prior treatment outcome studies. Treatment conditions included the following:

1. *Twelve-step facilitation* (TSF): This treatment consisted of 12 weekly sessions in which the therapist introduced patients to the first 5 of the 12 steps of Alcoholics Anonymous, and encouraged them to become involved in AA. As stated in the NIAAA description in *Alcohol Alert* (April 1997, p. 2), "Although grounded in the 12-Step principles, it was a professionally delivered, individual therapy different from the usual peer-organized AA meetings and was not intended to duplicate or substitute for traditional AA."

2. *Cognitive-behavioral therapy* (CBT): In this condition, therapists taught coping skills to enable patients to cope with high-risk situations and emotional states known to precipitate relapse (i.e., relapse prevention). Patients practiced drink-refusal skills, learned to manage negative moods, and were taught to cope with urges to drink, in 12 individual treatment sessions.

3. *Motivational enhancement therapy* (MET): Patients assigned to this condition received four individual sessions in which therapists used principles of motivational psychology; rather than teaching them coping skills, therapists encouraged patients to consider their situation and how alcohol affected their lives, and to develop and implement a plan to stop drinking. In all three conditions, the procedures for administering treatment were provided in detailed treatment manuals, and the treatment sessions were delivered by carefully trained and supervised professionals in individual therapy sessions.

As documented here, the results of Project MATCH stimulated considerable controversy in the field of alcoholism treatment and research. Much was expected from the results of this large, expensive study that cost $27 million to conduct over an 8-year period (divided by the $N$ of 1,726 patients, this cost represents an investment of $15,643 per patient). The research group, headed by Thomas Babor, of the University of Connecticut Department of Psychiatry, consisted of two NIAAA coordinators (NIAAA initiated and funded the study as a cooperative contract), 15 Clinical Research Unit staff, 8 collaborating investigators, and a 5-person Monitoring Board. As stated by the Project MATCH Research Group (1997a), "Project MATCH is the largest, statistically most powerful, psychotherapy trial ever conducted" (p. 25).

The long-awaited results of Project MATCH were published in the January 1997 issue of the *Journal of Studies on Alcohol* (Project MATCH Research Group, 1997a). In summarizing these results and subsequent interpretations of the findings by other commentators, extensive quotations are cited from original sources. This is a deliberate editorial strategy, designed to minimize the potential bias associated with presenting summaries that may not capture the original intent of the authors.

The overall results as presented in the Abstract show that all three treatment conditions were equally effective in terms of reducing drinking rates and that little evidence for a treatment matching effect was found:

> Significant and sustained improvements in drinking outcomes were achieved from baseline to 1-year posttreatment by the clients assigned to each of these well-defined and individually delivered psychosocial treatments. There was little difference in outcomes by type of treat-

ment. Only one attribute, psychiatric severity, demonstrated a significant attribute by treatment interaction: In the outpatient study, clients
low in psychiatric severity had more abstinence days after 12-step facilitation treatment than after cognitive-behavioral therapy. Neither treatment was clearly superior for clients with higher levels of psychiatric
severity. . . . The lack of other robust treatment effects suggests that,
aside from psychiatric severity, providers need not take these client
characteristics into account when triaging clients to one or the other of
these three individually delivered treatment approaches, despite their
different treatment philosophies. (Project MATCH Research Group,
1997a, p. 7)

Later in the paper, the results for drinking from baseline to follow-up are
given in more detail:

Prior to entry into their inpatient or day hospital treatment, aftercare
subjects were abstinent around 20% of the days per month. In the
month immediately following Project MATCH treatments they were
abstinent more than 90% of the time and at Month 15 [one year after
treatment completion] there was only a slight decrement in abstinence.
Outpatient subjects averaged slightly more abstinent days per month at
baseline, but were abstinent more than 80% of the days at posttreatment, with only a slight decrement at the 15-month follow-up. . . . In
the aftercare arm, approximately 35% of subjects reported continued
complete abstinence throughout the 12 follow-up months; 65% slipped
or relapsed during that period. . . . For the outpatient subjects, 19%
maintained complete abstinence throughout the follow-up and approximately 46% had a heavy-drinking period of three consecutive days by
the end of the follow-up period. (Project MATCH Research Group,
1997a, p. 14)

Despite noting the absence of a no-treatment control group as a
caveat in interpreting the results, the authors come to the firm conclusion
that all three treatment conditions are equally effective and therefore in-
terchangeable in terms of assigning patients to treatment type:

Although the efficacy of the three treatments cannot be demonstrated
directly since the trial did not include a no-treatment control group,
the striking differences in drinking by clients from pretreatment levels
to all follow-up points suggest that participation in any of these treatments will be associated with substantial and sustained changes in
drinking. . . . One important conclusion of this trial is that individually delivered psychosocial treatments embodying very different treatment philosophies appear to produce comparably good outcomes. (p.
23)

Another caveat presented by the MATCH authors concerned the possible impact of the high compliance rate shown by patients in the study on both overall treatment efficacy and any potential matching effects:

> In fact, the sustained, positive improvement for clients in all three treatment conditions may have left little room for matching effects to emerge. . . . The treatment compliance of the individuals in this trial was high. Subjects received substantial amounts of the specified treatments. Compliance enhancement procedures (i.e., calling clients between sessions, sending reminder notes and contacting collateral sources) and the greater attention of individual treatment may have produced a level of overall compliance that made it difficult for differences between treatments to emerge. It is possible that previous matching studies may have reflected variations in treatment compliance. (p. 23)

As the MATCH authors acknowledge, the results of the study are difficult to interpret (or easy to misinterpret) because of the lack of a control group and because of the high compliance rate shown by clients. Despite such caveats, the "bottom line" of the paper clearly discourages matching clients to different treatment approaches in order to enhance outcome: "The limited matching findings may disappoint many who have believed in the efficacy of matching treatments to subject characteristics and they certainly challenge the existing view that treatment matching is a key to improved treatment effectiveness" (p. 25).

## INTERPRETATIONS AND CRITIQUES OF MATCH RESULTS

Project MATCH results were officially released to the public at a press conference held in Washington, DC, on December 17, 1996, timed with the release of the January 1997 issue of *Journal of Studies on Alcohol*. An article published in the December 18 issue of *The New York Times*, entitled, "Responses of Alcoholics to Therapies Seem Similar," presented the results as perceived by the public media:

> Trying to match types of alcoholics with specific therapies has little effect on the results, according to a major Government study released today [December 17]. Researchers said the eight-year study of the concept of treatment matching, which is done, for example, on the basis of severity of drinking or personality traits, shows that patients seeking help through different psychological therapies get good results, in most cases, from each approach. . . . Based on the results of 30 smaller studies, *the researchers matched patients who displayed certain characteristics with the*

*approach that seemed best for them, said the study to be published* in the January issue of *The Journal of Studies on Alcohol.* (Leary, 1996, p. A4; emphasis added)

Based on the previous statement that "researchers matched patients who displayed certain characteristics with the approach that seemed best for them," most readers unfamiliar with the study probably assumed patients were intentionally matched to one or another of the three treatment conditions based on the results of "30 smaller studies." No where in the article is it mentioned that the patients were randomly assigned and not deliberately matched to treatment conditions.

Other published accounts of the Project MATCH results announced at the December 17 news conference appeared to view the study as a comparative treatment efficacy or outcome study, and not as an investigation of various matching hypotheses. For example, *The Seattle Times* carried the following headline in its December 18 article entitled, "Study: Three Alcohol Treatments Found Equally Effective":

> A ground-breaking study of alcoholism treatment has reached the surprising conclusion that all three leading behavioral approaches work equally well for a wide variety of patients. . . . The findings undermine long-held beliefs about alcoholism. Treatment professionals have long thought that each of the three therapies was most effective on patients who showed certain traits. . . . But the ambitious eight-year study sponsored by the National Institute on Alcohol Abuse and Alcoholism (NIAAA) showed that those considered best served by 12-step programs—and others—appeared to do equally well using any of the three therapeutic approaches. (*The Seattle Times,* December 18, 1996, p. B1)

Neither in *The New York Times* nor in *The Seattle Times* was the experimental design (random assignment to treatment conditions and testing of a priori matching hypotheses) clearly described or explained. Depending on the story one reads, the purpose of the study appears to be either (1) an investigation of treatment matching in which "researchers matched patients . . . with the approach that seemed best for them" (*The New York Times*), or (2) a study of comparative treatment efficacy that "reached the surprising conclusion that all three leading behavioral approaches work equally well" (*The Seattle Times*). In an attempt to clarify this discrepancy, I wrote a Letter to the Editor of *The New York Times* on December 18, 1996. Although it was not published, the letter reads as follows:

> To the Editor,
>     The Dec. 18 article reporting equal effectiveness of three types of therapy for alcohol dependence ("Responses of Alcoholics to Thera-

pies Seem Similar") draws an unfair conclusion about treatment matching. Although the report states that researchers matched patients who displayed certain characteristics with the approach that seemed best for them, the design of the study actually called for random assignment of patients to one of the three treatment conditions (12-step facilitation, cognitive-behavioral treatment, or motivational enhancement therapy). Given that assignment to treatment was based on a randomized selection procedure (based on a computerized "urn-balancing program") and not by professionals who matched patients to the most promising type of treatment, it is misleading to conclude that treatment matching does not work—i.e., that "one size fits all" when it comes to selecting a treatment program.

A better test of the treatment matching hypothesis would be first to match patients to the best possible treatment program (based on matching characteristics such as gender, age, motivation for change, and presence of associated psychological or health problems), and compare their outcomes to those who were not matched (all of whom receive the same treatment). As a way of assigning patients to treatment, nothing could be more opposite than random assignment (assigning patients on a random basis similar to a coin toss) and treatment matching (assigning patients based on a professional therapist's knowledge and skills).

Another problem in interpreting the results is that the design for this randomized clinical trial failed to include a control-group, such as a group of patients that received only the extensive personal assessment and follow-up interviews that patients in all three treatment conditions received. The similarity of treatment outcome results reported may simply reflect the impact upon the patients' commitment to change due to their being enrolled in an important and expensive ($27 million) national research study and their willingness to be randomly assigned to treatment and to complete multiple diagnostic assessment and follow-up interviews during the year following treatment.

Given the plethora of competing treatment approaches for alcohol and drug dependence, ranging from aversion therapy to spiritual conversion, to conclude from the results of this study that treatment matching does not work and that "a patient can do equally well with any treatment method" is both misleading and scientifically unsound.

The long-awaited results were actually first presented on June 25, 1996 (6 months before the published report appeared in the January issue of the *Journal of Studies on Alcohol*, 1997), at the Scientific Meeting of the Research Society on Alcoholism (RSA) held in Washington, DC. Dr. Jeffrey Schaler, an adjunct professor of justice, law, and society at American University, was asked to provide a report on the June meeting by Dr. Tom Horvath, President of SMART Recovery, an alcohol and addiction treatment and self-help group. In Dr. Schaler's report on June 25, 1996, the day of the RSA conference in Washington, he came to this visceral conclusion:

> The bottom, bottom line: There's no difference in effectiveness among AA, Cognitive-Behavior Therapy and Motivational Enhancement Training for creating abstinence and reducing drinking. Or, the most comprehensive, contemporary cognitive-based, scientifically proven effective approaches to therapy are no more effective than old time religion. Major implication: Since there's no different between AA and the other two, why should anyone pay for Cognitive Behavior Therapy or Motivational Enhancement Training? That's a MAJOR implication, as far as I'm concerned. It could drive all substance-abuse treatment out of business. (personal communication, June 1996)

Schaler later elaborated his comments in an opinion column published in the August/September 1996 issue of *Psychnews International* entitled, "Selling Water by the River: The Project MATCH Cover Up" (Schaler, 1996). Dr. Schaler was interviewed about his views by Bruce Bower for an article on Project MATCH published in the January 25, 1997, issue of *Science News*: "'The Project MATCH findings support the idea that selling treatment for heavy drinking alongside free self-help programs such as AA is like selling water by the river, to coin a Zen saying,' contends psychologist Jeffrey A. Schaler of American University in Washington, D.C. 'Why buy when the river gives it for free'" (Bower, 1997). From the perspective of Dr. Schaler and others in the alcoholism treatment arena, Project MATCH was designed primarily as a treatment efficacy study in which all three conditions were found to be equivalent. In a commentary on this misinterpretation, NIAAA Director Enoch Gordis stated:

> The major finding from Project MATCH—that matching patients to treatments added little benefit to treatment results—was a surprise to clinical investigators and to service providers alike. . . . After the findings from Project MATCH were publicized, it appeared clear from comments received by NIAAA that these findings, in some instances, had been misinterpreted. Therefore, I believe it is useful to clarify again what Project MATCH was and what it was not. Project MATCH was a study of patient–treatment matching; it was not a study of treatment efficacy. While it is heartening to learn that patients who participated in all three treatment arms of Project MATCH did well, this study was not designed to test whether treatment (versus no treatment) works but whether patients, based on their characteristics, responded better to one therapy versus another. Although the one match found . . . is of interest, on the whole, it is likely that patients in

competently run alcoholism treatment programs will do as well with one of three treatments studied as with the others. (National Institute of Alcohol Abuse and Alcoholism, 1997, pp. 3–4)

Subsequent commentaries on the results of Project MATCH also noted problems in the study design and interpretation of results. In the January 25, 1997, issue of *Science News*, a two-page summary of the study was presented under the headline, "Alcoholics Synonymous" (Bower, 1997):

> The coordinators of Project MATCH have finally served up their findings, but with a shot of disappointment and a twist of irony. At a press conference held last December in Washington, D.C., they announced that alcoholics reduce their drinking sharply and to roughly the same degree after completing any of three randomly assigned treatments. . . . Opinions diverge sharply regarding the study's implications and the adequacy of its design. . . . The absence of a control group of alcoholics who received no specific intervention raises the likelihood that volunteers improve because of intensive personal attention and encouragement rather than any specific treatment techniques. . . . The data suggest that AA and other free self-help groups prove effective enough to replace professionally administered alcoholism treatments that command big insurance bucks. A third perspective holds that flaws in the design of Project MATCH leave open the possibility that many alcoholics benefit from treatment matching or could abandon their addiction on their own, outside the world of clinical interventions and AA. (p. 62)

One of the most vocal critics of Project MATCH has been psychologist Stanton Peele. In an essay entitled, "All Wet," published in *The Sciences* (Peele, 1998), a publication of the New York Academy of Sciences, Peele first criticizes the extensive exclusionary criteria used to select the subjects who participated in the research:

> Going deeper into the MATCH methodology shows why its results could differ so dramatically from those of other research. Virtually all the subjects were alcohol dependent. But people simultaneously diagnosed with a drug problem were excluded from the study. . . . Initially, 4,481 potential subjects were identified; fewer than 1,800 of them were actually included. The MATCH participants were volunteers. Yet in real life, patients are increasingly being referred for treatment by the courts, by their employers or by social agencies. They are threatened with prison, loss of a job or loss of benefits if they do not get help. Furthermore, Project MATCH dropped potential subjects for reasons such as lack of permanent home address and for legal or probation problems. Others declined to participate because of the "inconvenience" of treatment. Compared with the volunteers excluded from the study,

those who participated in MATCH were motivated, stable and free of criminal or severe drug problems—all of which predict a greater likelihood of success. (p. 20)

Peele concludes his essay with a commentary on the need for alternatives to abstinence as the sole criterion for evaluating treatment effectiveness:

But perhaps the biggest heresy that MATCH supports—inadvertently so—is the value of reduced drinking as a goal in alcoholism treatment. The MATCH organizers chose to present their success in terms of the number of drinking days and the amount imbibed on those days. They did not trumpet the news of their subjects' abstinence rates. . . . The data from Project MATCH and other mainstream research conflict in many ways, but they make this much clear: Since the majority of alcoholics do not stop drinking, whether treated or untreated, whether measured in the general population or following a gold-standard set of treatments, the ironclad insistence on abstinence as the only goal of therapy is perverse indeed. (p. 21)

## LIMITATIONS OF THE PROJECT MATCH DESIGN

What was the rationale behind the design and implementation of Project MATCH? As stated in the NIAAA published newsletter, *Alcohol Alert*:

To build on studies of patient–treatment matching that had already been conducted and to make recommendations about appropriate patient–treatment matches, the NIAAA initiated Project MATCH (Matching Alcoholism Treatment to Client Heterogeneity) in late 1989. By the time Project MATCH began, the Institute of Medicine (IOM) had urged systematic and definitive studies of the patient–treatment matching hypothesis to improve treatment out-comes and better utilize scarce resources. (National Institute on Alcohol Abuse and Alcoholism, 1997, pp. 1–2)

In this Institute of Medicine report, *Broadening the Base of Treatment of Alcohol Problems* (Institute of Medicine, 1990), the committee voiced concern about selection of the randomized controlled trial (RCT) as the sole criterion for conducting treatment matching studies:

Although the randomized controlled trail (RCT) has many advantages and should be more broadly used to answer questions of clinical relevance, it has disadvantages that tend to limit its widespread application in clinical treatment settings. Alternative methodologies, if less powerful in terms of the demonstration of treatment efficacy, may nevertheless be more widely applicable and can provide information to complement that derived form RCTs. (p. 149)

In Chapter 11 of the Institute of Medicine report, an alternative approach to the RCT design is recommended:

> Simple outcome monitoring often demonstrates a close association between some particular variable and successful outcome. Of course, this method does not definitely prove that a matching effect has occurred, but it is certainly suggestive. As a next step, the variable (or variables) identified from outcome monitoring as associated with positive outcome can be used as a guide to the matching of a subsequent group of individuals to treatment. The outcomes from the subsequent group can then be compared with those of the previous group. A higher proportion of positive outcomes suggests that (other factors being equal between the two trials) an effective match has been identified. This "bootstrapping" strategy has been used effectively in the treatment of persons with alcohol and drug problems. . . . It does not involve the random assignment of individuals to treatment . . . but instead is a methodology that is more readily implemented in clinical treatment settings. (Institute of Medicine, 1990, p. 281)

Despite these concerns about the randomized controlled trail as a means of testing treatment matching hypotheses, the Project MATCH research group nevertheless selected this experimental design for their study (Project MATCH Research Group, 1993). In a description of the rationale for selecting a randomized trail design over a design in which patients would be intentionally matched to specific treatment modalities, two Project MATCH researchers stated their case for utilization of what they call a "hindsight" matching study:

> Although a standard randomized clinical trail of treatments is prospective with respect to time, from the viewpoint of matching under discussion here it is a retrospective design because no decision rules are employed to assign cases to treatment prospectively. The matches and mismatches in a clinical trial are seen only in looking back after randomization and treatment. For purposes of the present discussion, this type of design will be termed a "hindsight" matching study. (Miller & Cooney, 1994, p. 38)

Whether Project MATCH is viewed as a prospective treatment efficacy study or as a retrospective investigation of patient–treatment matching variables, the experimental design leaves many questions unanswered. For those who interpret it as a treatment efficacy study, the results are difficult to interpret because of the lack of a no-treatment, assessment-only control condition. One cannot conclude that "treatment works" on the basis of the study findings, because it may have been the case that many patients would have done well on the basis of their prior treatment experience (aftercare arm patients) or in response to the very intensive individual assessment sessions that all patients received prior to and following participation in the relatively brief therapy component (outpatient and aftercare arm patients). The Project MATCH Research Group acknowledged this possibility in their published report:

> Finally, research follow-up compliance was remarkable, reflecting an intensive effort on the part of the research staff and payment of clients as an incentive to return for follow-up. The overall effect of being a part of Project MATCH, with its extensive assessment, attractive treatments and aggressive follow-up, may have minimized naturally occurring variability among treatment modalities, and may, in part, account for the favorable treatment outcomes. (Project MATCH Research Group, 1997a, p. 24)

Apart from the lack of an assessment-only control group, the design of Project MATCH does indeed meet many of the criteria of a treatment efficacy study. Seligman (1995) distinguished between two types of methods for determining whether treatment works. In a *treatment efficacy* study, patients are randomly assigned to different treatment conditions, and considerable control is often exerted over the nature and duration of the treatment interventions (in order to enhance internal validity and establish causative relationships between type of treatment and assessed outcomes). In a *treatment effectiveness* study, patients are free to pursue whatever treatment they prefer, and the nature of the treatment is left uncontrolled.

Other researchers have also argued that efficacy studies are often so constrained that they provide little practical or useful information as to what actually happens in clinical practice (Blacker & Mortimore, 1996; Moos, Finney, & Cronkite, 1990). Goldfried and Wolfe (1996) criticized the generalizability of results obtained from treatment efficacy studies based on the clinical trial paradigm:

> In the typical clinical trails paradigm, one "pure form" theoretical approach is compared with another. . . . Unlike clinical practice, in which we as therapists often find it more effective to use interventions associated with different therapeutic orientations, our current research methodology allows little room for taking into account the relevant patient determinants/dynamics that may influence what we should do clinically. Instead, different therapy interventions are administered, which typically focus on the preferred variables associated with a given theoretical orientation (e.g., cognition, behavior, affect, and interper-

sonal systems). These different therapy approaches are compared, often resulting in findings that fail to result in differential effectiveness between orientations. Moreover, our outcome research is characterized by a basic dilemma with respect to the type of patients that eventually participate in treatment efficacy studies. This quandary might be called the interpretability/generalizability dilemma. In order to improve the interpretability of findings, rigorous inclusion and exclusion criteria are used for the selection of research patients. As the number and rigor of these criteria increase, the generalizability of the findings from treatment efficacy research decreases. (pp. 1010–1011)

Project MATCH met many, although not all of the criteria for a treatment efficacy study. Among them, it carefully addressed a number of critical methodological and design issues that often threaten the internal and external validity of clinical trials, including "clearly articulated a priori hypotheses, successful random assignment, use of manuals for all conditions, monitoring treatment delivery, assessment of treatment fidelity, delivery of an adequate amount of treatment, limiting attrition, and reliable outcome assessment" (Project MATCH Research Group, 1997a, p. 25).

Generalization of the results of Project MATCH to treatment as conducted in the "real world" is limited for the reasons outlined above by Goldfried and Wolfe (1996). In order to enhance the internal validity of Project MATCH, the external validity of the study is seriously compromised. The extent of the screening and recruitment process, along with the intensive and extensive number of individual assessment and personalized follow-up sessions received by patients in Project MATCH is most unlikely to occur in the naturalistic treatment environment. Many otherwise "typical" patients in alcoholism or substance abuse treatment were excluded from the study:

> Exclusion criteria were: a DSM-IV diagnosis of current dependence on sedative/hypnotic drugs, stimulants, cocaine or opiates; any intravenous drug use in the prior 6 months; currently a danger to self or others; probation/parole requirement that might interfere with protocol participation; lack of clear prospects for residential stability; inability to identify at least one "locator" person to assist in tracking for follow-up assessments; acute psychosis; severe organic impairment; or involvement (current or planned) in alternative treatment for alcohol-related problems other than that provided by Project MATCH. . . . Other general admission requirements for all subjects were: willingness to accept randomization to any of the treatment conditions; residence within reasonable commuting distance, with available transportation to sessions; and completion of prior detoxification when medically indicated. (Project MATCH Research Group, 1997a, pp. 9–10)

The strictness of these criteria for inclusion or exclusion from the study raises questions about the generalizability of the findings to other patient populations. The highly homogeneous sample of patients who met these criteria may be quite different from the known heterogeneity of the alcohol-dependent population. Even if the results had revealed evidence of treatment matching effects, the generalization of these findings to other populations would be dubious at best.

As several commentators have also noted, alcoholism and other addiction treatment programs typically employ group therapy and self-help groups, rather than conducting individual therapy sessions with patients. In this sense, the TSF condition differs in drastic ways from the spiritual fellowship of AA. There is no therapist in AA, a mutual self-help group whose members share a commitment to sobriety. As noted by NIAAA Director Enoch Gordis:

> Project MATCH also was not a study of the efficacy of simply attending Alcoholics Anonymous (AA) meetings. Although based on the principles of the AA, the Project MATCH Twelve-Step Facilitation (TSF) treatment used intensive one-one-one sessions between patients and professional therapists, rather than the AA peer-led group experience, to introduce the initial steps of and encouragement involvement in AA. (Gordis, 1997, p. 3)

In Project MATCH, AA attendance was allowed to vary, leading to the possibility of overlap with other conditions. In a recent analysis of the internal validity of the Project MATCH treatments, Carroll et al. (1998) noted the extent of overlapping AA attendance across the three treatment conditions, particularly in the aftercare arm:

> For the outpatient study, participants assigned to TSF reported attending AA meeting an average of 21% of treatment days versus 4% for CBT and 7% for MET. . . . For the aftercare arm of the study, percentage of days of AA attendance was 41% for TSF versus 28.2% for CBT and 29% for MET. The higher overall rate of AA attendance for aftercare participants very likely reflects substantial encouragement to attend AA meetings as part of the inpatient or day hospital treatment which preceded their involvement with Project MATCH treatments. (p. 296)

## ALTERNATIVE RESEARCH DESIGNS
## FOR TREATMENT MATCHING STUDIES

Given these concerns, what alternative designs are recommended to assess treatment matching effects? One possible design would randomly assign

patients to either (1) a matched treatment conditions, in which each patient would be assigned to a particular treatment condition based on the
best available evidence (based on prior matching studies), or (2) a non-
matched condition, in which all patients would receive a standardized,
"one-size-fits-all" treatment program. This design has been successfully
employed by McClelland and his colleagues (1997) in their research on
drug treatment effectiveness. McClelland et al. found that when treatment
was individually matched to patient needs (as assessed by the Addiction
Severity Index, a diagnostic interview that elaborates several area of potential patient problems in addition to level of substance abuse, including
health, family, economic problems, etc.), patients had better overall outcomes compared to when patients were assigned to a standard "treatment
as usual" condition. This type of design was described as a "foresight
matching design" by Miller and Cooney (1994), who rejected it in favor of
the "hindsight" design utilized in Project MATCH:

> In "foresight" matching designs, in contrast, the compared groups are
> defined by treatment-assigned procedures. Within one experimental
> group, at least, individuals are assigned to treatments not at random,
> but according to a priori matching criteria, and its is precisely this as-
> signment procedure (not the treatments themselves) that is the subject
> of experimental evaluation. On closer examination, however, a hind-
> sight matching design is logically equivalent (under many conditions)
> to a foresight matching study with subjects assigned to be matched or
> mismatched to treatments. . . . The point is that from a methodological
> standpoint, it is irrelevant whether subjects were matched (or mis-
> matched) by chance or by intent. Within both designs one can analyze
> for main effects of treatments, of subject characteristics or of matched
> versus mismatched status. (Miller & Cooney, 1994, p. 39)

This comment, that the "foresight" design permits the investigator to
evaluate the matching or assignment procedures (vs. the treatments themselves), is at the heart of the controversy over Project MATCH. When
therapists consider matching someone to treatment, other matching criteria are also involved over and above the nature of the treatment type itself.
Such factors as credibility of the therapist ("I think you would work particularly well with this therapist") and the potential for therapeutic alliance
are critical. Other factors include perceived need for group support (self-
help groups may be recommended for this reason), the existence of other
life problems besides alcohol or drug abuse, and coexisting mental health
problems. In addition, there are such practical factors as access to treatment, cost and reimbursement, legal constraints, as well as a host of other
individual client factors (age, gender, ethnic identity, motivation to change,
etc.).

An important point to consider is the issue of *consumer choice* or self-selection as an alternative to treatment matching. In the treatment-matching paradigm, patients are "assigned" to a particular treatment based on the perspective of the professional treatment provider. In the consumer choice paradigm, prospective consumers of treatment services are allowed to "shop around" and select a treatment or self-help group of their own choosing (Seligman, 1995). When first told about the design for Project MATCH, Klaus Maukela of the Center for Alcohol Studies in Finland remarked, "I'm not sure about this treatment matching stuff. If I want to buy a new car, the last thing I need is for some 'expert' to tell me which car would be best for me for whatever reason. I like to be the one who decides which car is for me. The same is true for selecting a treatment for alcoholism" (personal communication, August, 1996).

How could a study be designed to evaluate the difference between consumer choice in the selection of treatment options and random assignment of patients to treatment conditions in a clinical trial? In a comment on this possibility in conducting psychotherapy efficacy trials, Hollon (1996) noted:

> Seligman (1995) argued that randomization itself may be "worse than useless for the investigation of the actual treatment of mental illness in the field" (p. 974). With this I do not agree, although I think that there is an interesting point embedded in his argument, one that could be addressed by randomly assigning one group of patients to a condition in which they are allowed to choose among the various treatment options to which other groups of patients are randomly assigned. (p. 1027)

In the same special issue of the *American Psychologist,* dedicated to outcome assessment of psychotherapy (October 1996), Jacobson and Christensen suggested a research design to evaluate consumer treatment selection:

> However, the utility of shopping for therapists can be easily studied within a clinical trial, simply by varying the degree of active shopping the clients are allowed and doing so in a systematic way. To take an extreme example, in one condition, clients would have no opportunity to shop, both the treatment and the therapist would be assigned to them, as in most efficacy studies; in the other condition, clients would receive a great deal of information about therapists and treatments and choose the one that felt most comfortable. (p. 1037)

Still, use of a randomized control procedure to investigate consumer "shopping" for treatment as compared to professional treatment matching may not provide the best answer to this question. It could be the case that the process of how clients come to seek help is a central feature of the behavior change process itself (Marlatt, Tucker, Donovan, & Vuchinich, 1997). As Seligman noted (1995), clients who actively seek a particular treatment approach or therapist are different from clients who enter treatment studies by the "passive process of random assignment to treatment and acquiescence with who and what happens to be offered in the study" (p. 967).

Many factors enter into the equation when it comes to understanding consumer selection among treatment options, including such factors as the client's perceived suitability for treatment, availability of relevant services, effort required for participation in treatment, as well as externally mediated incentives such as court-mandated treatment or availability of housing or vouchers (De Leon, 1998). In a recent review of the "self-selection factor" in addiction treatment, De Leon concludes:

> On the basis of clinical experience, developing theory, and research on motivation and recovery stages, a new perspective can be outlined that redefines the importance of self-selection in interpreting the effectiveness of treatment. In this perspective, the impact of intervention (treatment) depends on client selection factors (such as motivation or readiness for treatment), and these factors are necessary contributors to outcomes. Rather than a problem, self-selection represents a prerequisite for treatment effectiveness. (p. 72)

## HARM REDUCTION AS A MEANS OF PROMOTING TREATMENT CHOICE

Recent developments in the addictions research field have illustrated the importance of harm reduction as a consumer-based approach to treatment (Erickson, Riley, Cheung, & O'Hare, 1997; Marlatt, 1998). Based on a public-health approach and founded by "grassroots" advocacy groups (including active drug users), harm reduction offers a pragmatic yet compassionate set of principles and procedures designed to reduce the harmful consequences of addictive behavior (Marlatt, 1996).

Five basic principles of harm reduction have been identified (Marlatt, 1996, 1998). The first principle is that harm reduction, with its philosophical roots in pragmatism and its compatibility with a public health approach, offers a practical alternative to either the moral or disease models of addiction. Unlike traditional approaches, harm reduction shifts the focus of treatment from alcohol or drug use itself to the consequences or effects of these behaviors. Such effects are evaluated primarily in terms of whether they are harmful or helpful to the drug consumer and to the larger society, and not on the basis of whether the behavior itself is considered morally right or wrong.

A second principle of harm reduction is that this approach accepts alternatives to abstinence in the client's selection of treatment goals. Examples include needle-exchange programs for intravenous (IV) drug users (to reduce the risk of HIV infection from sharing drug injection equipment), methadone maintenance for opiate addiction, controlled or moderate drinking for those dependent on alcohol, and nicotine replacement therapies for addicted smokers (Marlatt & Tapert, 1993). These harm reduction procedures stand in sharp contrast to the goals of most traditional alcohol and drug treatment programs. In these programs, abstinence is almost always required as a precondition for treatment. For a potential consumer of treatment services, there is an essential "catch-22" involved here: One must first abstain in order to receive treatment designed to maintain abstinence!

A third principle is that harm reduction has emerged as a "bottom-up" approach based on consumer input and demand, in contrast with the authoritarian or "top-down" policy assumed by most traditional treatment programs. For example, needle-exchange programs for IV drug users began in the Netherlands in response to input from addicts who belonged to a "Junkiebond" union and advocated for policy changes that would permit the legal exchange of needles to reduce the risk of HIV infection. Harm reduction programs are very consumer-oriented and often establish a partnership or collaborative arrangement with the client group involved. By seeking input from members of the group in need of services, clients are more likely to feel like "stakeholders" who are committed to a shared treatment plan.

The fourth principle that characterizes the harm reduction model is the support for "low-threshold" access to treatment. Rather than setting abstinence as a high-threshold requirement of receiving treatment services, advocates of harm reduction are willing to reduce such barriers by meeting clients "where they are" in the process of change. Such "user-friendly" approaches make it easy for people with problems to "get on board," get involved, and get started. Low-threshold programs do this by reaching out and achieving partnership and cooperation with the population in need, by reducing stigma associated with getting help, and by providing an integrative, normalized approach to high-risk drug and alcohol use (Marlatt, 1996).

The fifth and final principle is that harm reduction is based on the tenets of compassionate pragmatism, and not on the requirements of moral idealism. Rather than labeling the person who uses drugs as morally weak or bad, harm reduction asks the question: To what extent are the consequences of this individual's behavior harmful or helpful? The next question is: What can be done to reduce these harmful consequences? Harm reduction is a compassionate approach because it does not denigrate people who engage in high-risk behaviors. Instead of pejorative terms used to label people as "substance abusers" or "chemically dependent," harm reduction shifts the focus to the individual's behavior and its consequences. Here the shift is from labeling someone as a "drug abuser" to a "consumer" who experiences harmful or helpful consequences. The word "consumer" seems particularly apt, because people consume both substances and services.

In a recent review of determinants of help-seeking by individuals with substance abuse problems, it was found that the primary factor that motivates people to seek treatment is their experience of the negative consequences of harmful effects of using drugs (e.g., health problems, interpersonal difficulties, financial problems), rather than by identifying "substance abuse" itself as the central problem (Marlatt et al., 1997). By switching the focus to reducing the harm associated with alcohol or drug use, prospective help seekers are more likely to come "out of the closet" and seek assistance. The link between consumer choice and the harm reduction model may be mediated by the psychology of "behavioral economics" as elucidated by Vuchinich (see Chapter 7, this volume). The field of behavioral economics has provided an elegant analysis of determinants of consumer choice.

## WHITHER TREATMENT MATCHING?

In addition to the primary results of Project MATCH as presented in the 1997 paper in the *Journal of Studies on Alcohol* (Project MATCH Research Group, 1997a), several additional publications have appeared based on this research study including a report of 3-year drinking outcomes (Project MATCH Research Group, 1998) and another paper that provides an analysis of the secondary a priori hypotheses generated by the Project MATCH group (Project MATCH Research Group, 1997b). In brief, these results show that (1) outpatients high in anger and treated with MET had better posttreatment drinking outcomes than those in CBT, and (2) aftercare clients high in alcohol dependence had better outcomes in TSF, whereas those with low alcohol dependence did better in CBT. The authors concluded:

> Considered together with the results of the primary hypotheses, matching effects contrasting these psychotherapies are not robust. Possible explanations include: (a) among the client variables and treatments tested,

matching may not be an important factor in determining client outcomes; (b) design issues limited the robustness of effects; and (c) a more
fully specified theory of matching is necessary to account for the complexity of results. (Project MATCH Research Group, 1997b, p. 1671)

Another recent paper published by the Project MATCH group supports the idea that therapeutic alliance is a critical factor in predicting
treatment outcome, over and above the specific type of treatment condition involved:

> The main finding regarding the therapeutic alliance in [Project
> MATCH] was its consistent prediction among outpatient alcoholics
> clients of treatment participation and positive drinking-related out-
> comes, whether the alliance was rated from the client or therapist per-
> spective. We found this effect even after controlling for a number of co-
> variates, including the client's pretreatment drinking history. Consis-
> tent with our hypotheses, the effect was generally consistent with a
> larger body of literature indicating the contribution of the therapeutic
> alliance to psychotherapy treatment outcome. (Connors, Carroll, Di-
> Clemente, Longabaugh, & Donovan, 1997, pp. 594–595)

These findings fit nicely with the preceding discussion of consumer
choice in selecting treatment or self-help options. When consumers look
for a therapist, they are more likely to stay in treatment if a therapeutic alliance is established, regardless of the therapist's school of training or theoretical orientation. This brings us back to basics. The best way to establish a good therapeutic alliance is for consumers to shop around to find a
good match, whether this is a friend or a therapist, group or counselor, an
inspiring book on how to change, or through the help of medication or
meditation.

Despite the many caveats about Project MATCH as a reliable and
valid test of treatment matching, the NIAAA is sponsoring a sequel study,
entitled "Project COMBINE." The new matching study will randomly assign alcohol-dependent clients to one or both of two pharmacotherapies
(naltrexone or acomprasate, both considered to be anticraving agents) or
placebo medications combined with either a behavioral intervention (to be
selected from among the three treatment in the original Project MATCH
study) or a program designed to enhance medication compliance. Since
this new study is currently still in the early stages, the results will not be
known for some time to come. For those of us who are uncertain about
the future of treatment matching, there may be a glimmering light at the
end of the tunnel. In the meantime, for those who are still in the dark
about all this, the best question for now may be: Anyone got a match?

# REFERENCES

Blacker, C. V. R., & Mortimore, C. (1996). Randomized controlled trials and naturalistic data: Time for a change? *Human Psychopharmacology, 11*, 353–363.

Bower, B. (1997). Alcoholics Synonymous: Heavy drinkers of all stripes may get comparable help form a variety of therapies. *Science News, 151*(4), 52–63.

Carroll, K. M., Connors, G. J., Cooney, N., DiClemete, C. C., Donovan, D. M., Kadden, R. R., Longabaugh, R. L., Roundsaville, B. J., Wirtz, P. W., & Zweben, A. (1998). Internal validity of Project MATCH treatments: Discriminability and integrity. *Journal of Consulting and Clinical Psychology, 66*, 290–303.

Connors, G. J., Carroll, K. M., DiClemente, C. C., Longabaugh, R., & Donovan, D. M. (1997). The therapeutic alliance and its relationship to alcoholism treatment participation and outcomes. *Journal of Consulting and Clinical Psychology, 65*(4), 588–598.

De Leon, G. (1998). Commentary: Reconsidering the self-selection factor in addiction treatment research. *Psychology of Addictive Behaviors, 12*(1), 761–777.

Erickson, P. G., Riley, D. M., Cheung, Y. W., & O'Hare, P. A. (Eds.). (1997). *Harm reduction: A new program for drug policies and programs.* Toronto: University of Toronto Press.

Goldfried, M. R., & Wolfe, B. E. (1996). Psychotherapy practice and research: Repairing a strained alliance. *American Psychologist, 51*, 1007–1016.

Gordis, E. (1997, April). Patient–treatment matching—a commentary. *Alcohol Alert, 26*, pp. 1–3.

Hollon, S. (1996). The efficacy and effectiveness of psychotherapy relative to medications. *American Psychologist, 51*(10), 1025–1030.

Institute of Medicine. (1990). *Broadening the base of treatment for alcohol problems.* Washington, DC: National Academy Press.

Jacobson, N. S., & Christensen, A. (1996). Studying the effectiveness of psychotherapy: How well can clinical trials do the job? *American Psychologist, 51*(10), 1031–1039.

Leary, W. E. (1996, December 18). Responses of alcoholics to therapies seem similar. *The New York Times,* p. A4.

Marlatt, G. A. (Ed.). (1996). Harm reduction: Come as you are. *Addictive Behaviors, 21*(6), 779–788.

Marlatt, G. A. (1998). *Harm reduction: Pragmatic strategies for managing high-risk behaviors.* New York: Guilford Press.

Marlatt, G. A., & Tapert, S. F. (1993). Harm reduction: Reducing the risks of addictive behaviors. In J. S. Baer, G. A. Marlatt, & R. McMahon (Eds.), *Addictive behaviors across the lifespan* (pp. 243–273). Newbury Park, CA: Sage.

Marlatt, G. A., Tucker, J. A., Donovan, D. M., & Vuchinich, R. E. (1997). Help-seeking by substance abusers: The role of harm reduction and behavioral–economic approaches to facilitate treatment entry and retention. In L. S. Onken, J. D. Blaine, & J. J. Boren (Eds.), *Beyond the therapeutic alliance: Keeping the drug-dependent individual in treatment* (NIDA Research Monograph No. 165, pp. 44–84). Rockville, MD: U. S. Department of Health and Human Services, Public Health Service, National Institutes of Health.

Mattson, M. E., Allen, J. P., Longabaugh, R., Nickless, C. J., Connors, G. J., & Kadden, R. M. (1994). A chronological review of empirical studies matching alcoholic clients to treatment. *Journal of Studies on Alcohol,* (Suppl. 12), pp. 16–29.

McLelland, A. T., Grissom, G. R., Zanis, D., Randall, M., Brill, P., & O'Brien, C. P. (1997). Improved outcomes from problem service "matching." *Archives of General Psychiatry, 54*(8), 730–735.

Miller, W. R., & Cooney, N. D. (1994). Designing studies to investigate client–treatment matching. *Journal of Studies on Alcohol,* (Suppl. 12), 38–45.

Moos, R. H., Finney, J. W., & Cronkite, R. C. (1990). *Alcoholism treatment: Context, process, and outcome.* New York: Oxford University Press.

National Institute on Alcohol Abuse and Alcoholism. (1997). Patient–treatment matching. *Alcohol Alert, 36,* 1–4.

Onken, L. S., Blaine, J. D., & Boren, J. J. (Eds.). (1997). *Beyond the therapeutic alliance: Keeping the drug-dependent individual in treatment* (NIDA Research Monograph No. 165). Rockville, MD: U. S. Department of Health and Human Services, Public Health Service, National Institutes of Health.

Peele, S. (1998). All wet. *The Sciences, 38*(2), 17–21.

Project MATCH Research Group. (1993). Project MATCH: Rationale and methods for a multisite clinical trial-matching patients to alcoholism treatment. *Alcoholism: Clinical and Experimental Research, 17*(6), 1130–1145.

Project MATCH Research Group. (1997a). Matching alcoholism treatment to client heterogeneity: Project MATCH posttreatment drinking outcomes. *Journal of Studies on Alcohol, 58,* 7–29.

Project MATCH Research Group. (1997b). Project MATCH secondary a priori hypothesis. *Addiction, 92*(12), 1671–1698.

Project MATCH Research Group. (1998). Matching alcoholism treatments to client heterogeneity: Project MATCH three-year drinking outcomes. *Alcoholism: Clinical and Experimental Research, 22*(6), 1300–1311.

Schaler, J. A. (1996). Selling water by the river: The Project Match cover up. *Psychnews International, 1*(5). (Electronic publication; mailbox: *pni@badlands.nodak.edu*)

Seligman, M. E. P. (1995). The effectiveness of psychotherapy: The Consumers Report Study. *American Psychologist, 50,* 965–974.

# 3

# Public Health Perspectives on Access and Need for Substance Abuse Treatment

LAURA A. SCHMIDT
CONSTANCE M. WEISNER

The main objective of this chapter is to identify key issues and open questions in our current understanding of how people gain access to alcohol and drug treatment services when they are needed. We begin with a general discussion on the measurement of the need for services, on the interplay between need and demand, and on how these factors relate to service access and utilization. Taking a public health perspective, need and access are viewed in the context of interacting community service systems. We take a broad view of the service system that includes not only specialty programs such as methadone maintenance programs and recovery homes, but also generalist health and social service agencies such as primary health clinics, prisons, and welfare programs. Our view of the potential treatment populations for substance abuse services is equally broad. Depending on the target goals of interventions, populations in need can be defined in a variety of different ways and measured by drawing upon a variety of different sources of data.

Following an overview of these key issues, we critically evaluate the current state of research, suggesting that it is useful to organize explanatory variables according to a scheme that includes individual level, organizational level, and sociocultural factors affecting service access and utilization. If one views all three levels of explanation as equally relevant, then it quickly becomes apparent that we have a much better understanding of the individual-level factors than of determinants of utilization operating at the organizational and sociocultural levels. Help-seeking has been traditionally viewed as a voluntary process where individuals and families recognize a drinking or drug problem and eventually seek help from professionals or mutual aid organizations to solve it. However, the rise of managed health care and growing emphasis on criminal justice and workplace referrals to substance abuse treatment have profoundly altered pathways to care by placing professionals and organizations in critical gatekeeping roles. These recent developments in the organization and financing of addiction treatment call for a view of access and utilization that reaches well beyond the dynamics of individual help-seeking.

## OVERVIEW OF THE ISSUES: MEASURING NEED

Selecting the most relevant and accurate measures for estimating the need for alcohol and drug services in defined communities is important for planning health services and for establishing equity, or for making services equally accessible to all consumer groups. An additional reason for studying need is to make projections of potential utilization levels if barriers to service use were eliminated. Such projections for the U.S. population would be very helpful in evaluating the adequacy of existing treatment capacity and provider manpower. Finally, patterns of access can influence the clinical outcomes of alcohol and drug treatment programs. Certain types of clients—women or individuals with severe addictions—may do better if they have access to appropriate types of treatment programs or services of a particular intensity (Gottheil, McLellan, et al., 1992; Institute of Medicine, 1990; Mattson, Allen, et al. 1994; McLellan, Alterman, et al., 1994).

A broad range of measures have been used in epidemiological research to evaluate the size of populations potentially in need of services. The most common measures, including alcohol and drug dependence, abuse, and individual social indicators of problem drinking or drug abuse, represent a range of degrees of severity, operationalization, and time frame. More fundamentally, measurement approaches differ in terms of how they conceptualize alcohol and drug problems, or represent different vantage points on what constitutes need (for a discussion on the ambiguities in defining need, see Room, 1980, pp. 214–215). Dependence implies that the individual would experience great difficulty in stopping drug use either due to the physiological (e.g., tolerance, withdrawal) or psychological (e.g., craving) consequences. Abuse implies a different level of treatment readiness—that while social functioning is impaired, physiological and psychological compulsions are not yet a major aspect of the problem. Problem drinking measures, which are increasingly being used in alcohol research, typically consist of a combination of heavy drinking, dependence symptoms, and alcohol-related social consequences, and imply that yet a lower severity threshold may be appropriate for intervention (Institute of Medicine, 1990). A final approach to measuring need focuses on the "disaggregation" of alcohol or drug problems into specific health, psychological and social consequences such as liver cirrhosis, drunken driving, and alcohol- or drug-related crimes. Unlike psychological and psychiatric measures, the disaggregated approach implies no assumptions about an underlying condition or disease entity such as "alcoholism" or "addiction," but rather simply takes the various manifestations and problems associated with regular alcohol or drug use at face value (for discussions, see Cahalan, Cisin, et al., 1969; Room, 1977).

Measures of need also differ with regard to the severity of the condition, how explicitly and consistently measures are operationalized in research, and in terms of the time frames during which symptoms must have been present in order to be deemed significant. Measures of problem drinking have been less consistently operationalized across studies than psychiatric diagnoses of abuse and dependence (see, e.g., minor differences in measures used by Weisner & Schmidt, 1992; Wilsnack, Klassen, et al., 1991). But it is also true that the components of alcohol dependence and abuse diagnoses have changed across periodic revisions of the American Psychiatric Association's *Diagnostic and Statistical Manual of Mental Disorders* (DSM) and the World Health Organization's *International Classification of Diseases* (ICD), the official sources on psychiatric nomenclature on addictive disorders. In practice, even slight differences in levels of severity, operationalization, and time frame can give rise to considerable differences in results on the magnitude of need. This suggests that the details of different measurement approaches should be taken quite seriously in evaluating need and, especially, in comparing results across different empirical studies. For example, according to the U.S. National Alcohol Survey, 12-month estimates of alcohol dependence, as defined by the fourth edition of the American Psychiatric Association's DSM (DSM-IV), suggest that about 3.9% of the U.S. adult general population in 1990 was clinically in need of alcohol treatment (Caetano & Room, 1994). In contrast, projections of need for the United States using the DSM-IV alcohol dependence measure in the combined Epidemiologic Catchment Area (ECA) Studies—which used a 6-month time frame—were 2.8% (Regier, Narrow, et al., 1993). Estimates of need using measures of problem drinking on a 12-month basis yield significantly higher rates, or suggest much greater levels of need. For instance, the Community Epidemiology Laboratory (CEL) studies suggest that 11.3% of the population of a Northern California county meet problem drinking criteria (Weisner & Schmidt, 1993).

In order to illustrate how different measures can produce sizable differences in estimates of need, Table 3.1 compares a variety of different indicators of the need for alcohol services in a general population survey, ranging from disaggregated, alcohol-related problems to more formal measures of problem drinking and alcohol dependence based on DSM-IV. Alcohol dependence, a condition that implies a high level of severity, suggests a fairly low level of need, as do some individual indicators of dependence, such as alcohol-related hallucinations and delirium tremens. In contrast, heavy- and problem-drinking measures suggest much higher levels of need, as do some health indicators, such as alcohol-related heart disease. An additional point illustrated by these data is that measures involving outside responses to drinking behaviors can sometimes yield lower rates of alcohol problems than self-reports of the same behaviors. For example, when individuals were asked whether they ever committed certain alcohol-related criminal behaviors—whether or not they had been caught by authorities—lifetime rates of criminal behavior were much higher than they would have been if one were only to consider lifetime rates of arrest (34.3% vs. 11.6%). However, in this survey, only about half as many individuals who were diagnosable as problem drinkers appeared willing to label themselves as such (11.3% vs. 5.4%). Although not shown here, the prevalences yielded by these different measures also varied substantially when groups within the population were compared across categories of

**TABLE 3.1. General Population Prevalence (%) of Alcohol-Related Medical and Social Problems**

|  | % |
| --- | --- |
| Alcohol-dependent | 2.3 |
| Heavy drinker | 13.8 |
| Problem drinker | 11.3 |
| Self-labeled alcoholic or problem drinker | 5.4 |
| Heart disease | 8.1 |
| Alcohol-related liver problems | 0.4 |
| Delirium tremens | 0.4 |
| Hallucinations | 0.2 |
| Criminal behaviors | |
| 12 months | 8.9 |
| Lifetime | 34.3 |
| Lifetime arrests | 11.6 |
| DUI arrests | 1.3 |
| Public drunkenness arrests | 0.5 |
| Alcohol-related traffic accidents | 0.4 |

*Note.* Data from the Community Epidemiology Laboratory 1989 General Population Survey, unweighted $N = 3,069$ (for details on survey methodology, see Weisner & Schmidt, 1995).

gender and ethnicity (see Weisner & Schmidt, 1993). This sort of sub-group variation clearly adds further complexity to the comparative analysis of different measures of need.

Measures of need can also vary due to differences in the coverage of sampling frames of surveys. Improving the coverage of population-based samples, in fact, would constitute a significant step forward in the improved accuracy of needs assessment. General population research in the substance abuse field—one of the preferred needs assessment approaches—has increasingly come under attack on the grounds that sampling frames usually lack coverage of some of the most crucial population groups residing within the areas studied (General Accounting Office, 1993). Populations living in residential treatment facilities, jails, board and care facilities, university and military housing, homes for the elderly, welfare hotels, as well as homeless populations, represent an increasing proportion of the U.S. population. Alcohol and drug abuse are often overrepresented within these groups. Studies such as the National Household Drug Survey's DC*MADS project (U.S. National Institute on Drug Abuse, 1990) have attempted to provide coverage of some of these groups, as have the institutional samples covered in the ECA project sponsored by National Institute of Mental Health (NIMH) and the CEL studies sponsored by National Institute on Alcohol Abuse and Alcoholism (NIAAA). To evaluate the magnitude of bias introduced into estimates of need based on incomplete sampling frames, we measured problem drinking in a California county's general population, as well as in most of its health and welfare system populations (see Weisner, Schmidt, et al., 1995). We found that a substantial number of individuals entering alcohol, drug, mental health, welfare, and criminal justice agencies (17%) did not live in settings typically covered in general population sampling frames. The prevalence of problem drinking among this group was 43.8%, as compared with 11.3% in the general population, suggesting that excluding nonhousehold populations from general population studies is likely to produce downwardly biased estimates of need. Statistics on the county's population size further suggested that the combined size of these excluded nonhousehold populations was large enough to introduce meaningful bias into general population survey estimates of the need for alcohol services.

The choice to use one conceptualization of alcohol and drug problems over another should be mainly determined by the context in which assessments of need are to be used. While measures of dependence are usually seen as the most appropriate for evaluating the need for intensive treatment services, disaggregated indicators of alcohol and drug problems seem particularly conducive to harm reduction approaches that allow for different target goals within a range of intervention options. Problem drinking and alcohol abuse imply lower thresholds of clinical severity and therefore have often been used to evaluate the need for screening, referral and early intervention programs within health services. Indeed, the National Drug and Alcohol Treatment Utilization Survey (NDATUS) suggests that many programs promoting early intervention are already targeting problem drinkers who come through their doors on workplace and criminal justice referrals (Institute of Medicine, 1990; Weisner & Schmidt, 1993). Of course, practical constraints—most notably, the availability of data—often place serious limitations on measurement choices. In planning situations at the county and state level, where resources to conduct broadscale research are typically quite limited, institution-based social indicators such as alcohol- and drug-related mortality and hospital discharge statistics, may be the only data available that are available for measuring need. Once the context and practical circumstances have determined what measures are relevant and logistically possible, then one is often left in the position of mainly taking other measurement issues, such as bias due to sample coverage and time frame, into account at the point of interpreting results.

## Distinguishing Need from Demand

It is difficult to make accurate estimates of the need for substance abuse services without taking important confounding factors into account, particularly those involving the interplay between the demand and need for services. Clearly, not all individuals who might be considered in need of alcohol or drug services by clinical or survey measures actually obtain help, and there are likely to be at least some people engaged in treatment whose symptoms are below clinical thresholds. Understanding demand can thus be useful in explaining the dynamics of unmet need.

The interconnections and complexity of the relationship between need and demand are issues that have only begun to be touched upon by researchers. It seems particularly important to consider the role of coercion preceding entry into alcohol and drug treatment. As observers increasingly point out, entry into substance abuse treatment usually involves some degree of external coercion, perhaps through encounters with the criminal justice system, employer requirements, government regulations that require addicted welfare recipients to cooperate with treatment in order to maintain entitlements, or social pressure from family and community (Gerstein & Harwood, 1990; Schmidt, Weisner, et al., 1998; Stitzer & McCaul, 1987; Weisner, 1990). Additional factors that may influence the interplay of need and demand are as wide-ranging as shifting norms about the seriousness of alcohol problems (Room, Greenfield, et al., 1991), general attributions of problems to alcohol (Institute of Medicine, 1990), treatment capacity and the marketing and advertising of alcoholism services (Schmidt & Weisner, 1993a), geographic and economic access to treatment services (Institute of Medicine, 1990), and effects of the growing availability of population- or problem-specific programs, such as those focused on women or ethnic minorities (Schmidt & Weisner, 1995).

There are very few empirical studies that explicitly examine the relationship between need and demand, with the notable exception of econometric analyses comparing need and demand curves in the U.S. population (Harwood, in press). A significant impediment to the development of improved estimates of need and demand is the limited availability of epidemiological data on the alcohol treatment population at the level of the client. Such data would make it possible to adjust national projections of need by the size of the population in services, thus producing better accuracy. The only widely available national data consist of agency-level data, the NDATUS, but this data set lacks information on individual clients beyond aggregate census counts (U.S. National Institute on Drug Abuse, 1990). Recent national agency studies, primarily using case records, have predominately focused on the drug treatment system, with alcohol-only units not included.

## Evaluating the Fit between Need and Access

A public health approach to evaluating the fit between need and access takes a broad view of the resources in communities available for responding to alcohol and drug problems, and it also emphasizes diversity in the population in need of services. In the past, research on substance abuse primarily focused on specialty treatment programs, such as alcohol and drug detoxification centers, methadone maintenance programs, outpatient counseling agencies, recovery homes, and therapeutic communities (Alterman, Droba, et al., 1992; Batten, 1993; Hayashida, Alterman, et al., 1989; Price & D'Aunno, 1992; Weisner, 1985; Wheeler, Fadel, et al., 1992). We, however, suggest viewing these specialty services as situated within broader networks of health and human services that interact and establish interorganizational dependencies, comprising a rather more complex, sprawling, "de facto" system of substance abuse treatment (Regier, Narrow, et al., 1993; Weisner & Schmidt, 1995).

Analyses of the CEL studies point to the important role of agencies outside the specialty treatment sector in responding to alcohol and drug problems in the community. The prevalence of problem drinking and illicit drug use is not insignificant in the caseloads of many community agencies and varies quite significantly across service populations. For example, based on representative samples of the caseloads in community service systems as measured at admission, rates of problem drinking varied from a low 15% in primary health clinics to a high of 40% in the drug treatment system. Standardized rates in other service systems fell somewhere in between these two extremes: emergency rooms, 19%; the welfare system, 24%; the mental health system, 26%; criminal justice system, 54% (Weisner & Schmidt, 1993). Within each of these institutional settings, a range of severity was found across measures of problem drinking, alcohol dependence, and illicit drug use. Not only professionals in generalist health and social services play significant roles in handling substance abuse problems, but also mutual aid organizations, including Alcoholics and Narcotics Anonymous, as well as other voluntary groups, such as Women for Sobriety and Rational Recovery. Indeed, these segments of substance abuse treatment systems are so significant that respondents in the National Alcohol Survey who had sought help for a drinking problem reported having gone to Alcoholics Anonymous and nonspecialty providers more often than to specialized treatment agencies, such as detoxes and recovery centers (Weisner, Greenfield, et al., 1995).

So far, we have descriptive studies that point to the important roles of mutual aid and generalist health and social service organizations in responding to substance abuse. However, many questions remain about how the dynamics of treatment entry are played out in this context of multiple treatment options. It remains an open question whether individuals seek help from generalist health and social service providers out of preference or due to a perceived lack of access to specialty treatment agencies. Another open question is whether or not AA and other mutual aid groups play a role of reducing demand for professional treatment services. Nor is it clear that those who receive care from specialty treatment organizations are best served by those settings. There is, for example, some evidence that problems of excessive hospitalization and the misutilization of services are more acute in substance abuse facilities than in other health services (Strumwasser, Patanjpe, et al., 1991). Substance abuse problems may play a role in determining pathways to services outside specialty alcohol and drug treatment services as well. For example, one study (Schmidt, 1995) found that alcohol involvement in admissions to mental health services was a strong predictor of a case being routed to a locked hospital ward as opposed to a psychiatric outpatient program. While heavy drinking and symptoms of alcohol dependence among psychiatrically disturbed individuals did not predict psychiatric admissions, serious social consequences related to drinking—such as criminal justice involvement and family or workplace confrontations about drinking—increased a person's chances of being admitted to a locked hospital ward by sixfold. This suggests that one important function of the mental health system vis-à-vis alcohol problems is to contain social disruptions due to problem drinking in the community.

Broadening the frame of research to include services outside the specialty treatment sector is important for three main reasons. First, in evaluating the fit between need and access to services, it is important to take into account the appropriateness of the services made available. Community agencies outside the specialty treatment sector clearly serve important functions in screening and referral for alcohol and drug problems, as well as, in some cases, providing on-site services for substance abuse. Such services may be particularly appropriate for problem drinkers and moderate drug users experiencing a lower severity of symptoms. Recent interest in matching populations characterized by particular sociodemographic or symptom characteristics to particular types of services underscores the value of considering the appropriateness of services when evaluating the fit between need and access (see Institute of Medicine, 1990). Second, it would be extremely useful for the purposes of planning alcohol and drug services to be able to project potential levels of utilization given that all barriers to access were removed. However, it is likely that some individuals in generalist health and social service agencies might be referred to, or might prefer, specialized services if they were more available. To estimate the outer limits of utilization rates, researchers should consider not only untreated substance abusers in the general population, but also substance abusers being served by a range of health and human service agencies.

Finally, considering the fit between service need and access means taking account of variation in need among different population groups, particularly different ethnic and gender groups. Utilization varies by gender and ethnic groups according to the NDATUS and national survey data, but we do not know if this is due to discrimination at the agency door, a lack of interest and denial of the problem among potential clients, or the fact that the kinds of services that would attract such groups are not available. The issue of fitting services to needs is particularly relevant to access by ethnic minorities and women. For example, there is some evidence that women resist entering alcohol services and instead seek care from private counselors and mental health programs, perhaps because the latter seem more suitable and less stigmatizing (Schmidt & Weisner, 1995; Thom, 1986; Weisner & Schmidt, 1992; Wilsnack & Beckman, 1984).

## A MULTILEVEL APPROACH FOR RESEARCH ON ACCESS AND NEED

Variables related to need, demand, and access can be usefully classified into a scheme comprised of micro-level and organization-level factors, and factors operating at the level of the sociocultural environment. One of the main goals of research on access and need should be to take into account *factors operating across multiple levels of explanation.* While there is an extensive body of research on individual help-seeking, there are far fewer studies of organizational and societal-level factors affecting access and need. It is quite plausible that there are important interactions among variables that crosscut different levels of analysis. For example, there are likely to be interactions between patterns in health insurance policy and variables such as age, socioeconomic status, and social network responses to substance abuse that have important bearing on access to services.

At the micro level, models of medical utilization and help- seeking have drawn attention to sociodemographic characteristics, as well as "illness behaviors" and "health beliefs" that positively or negatively predispose individuals to seek services. In substance abuse research, examples of the latter include the individual's perceptions of the severity of symptoms and beliefs about the appropriateness and efficacy treatment. The literature on medical care seeking has also isolated chief demographic or "predisposing" factors at the individual level that contribute to the demand for services and willingness to seek help, independent of the severity and nature of symptoms (Aday, 1972; Aday & Anderson, 1974); for substance abuse applications, see also Bannenberg, Raat, et al. (1992). Many studies have also incorporated attributes of the informal social networks surrounding individuals in need of services, and some have specifically tested competing hypotheses about the roles of family members, friends, and members of the immediate community in facilitating, as opposed to hindering, help-seeking by individuals in their social networks (Horwitz, 1977). Studies of the help-seeking process often tacitly assume a voluntaristic model of treatment utilization—an assumption that is not in line with the realities of how people usually get to substance abuse treatment. Entry into substance abuse treatment services usually involves some degree of coercion, including sanctions from the criminal justice system, the workplace, the welfare office, or pressure from family and community (Weisner, 1990; Schmidt & Weisner, 1993a).

Relevant research at the level of treatment organizations has examined the effects of professional gatekeeping, including organizational barriers to admission, the effects of particular screening and diagnostic routines, provider attitudes toward clients, and consumer satisfaction as it relates to caseload retention. Of special interest in our current health care system are the ways that particular funding approaches and reimbursement schemes used in public- and private-sector organizations influence who obtains services and the particular kinds of services they receive (Browne, Browne, et al., 1987; Feldstein, Wickizer, et al., 1988; Levin, Glasser, et al., 1984; Ridgely, Goldman, et al., 1990). Organizational research has, however, only begun to examine how different aspects of managed care impact access to substance abuse services (see, e.g., Altman &

Goldstein, 1988; England & Vaccaro, 1991; Levin, Glasser, et al., 1984; Mechanic, 1979; Rogowski, 1992; Schlesinger, Bentkover, et al., 1987). Such studies are of immediate importance, since managerial strategies oriented around cost containment can easily compete with the goals of improving the accessibility and quality of health services. With a few exceptions (e.g., Keeler, Manning, et al., 1988) studies of managed care typically have not included randomized assignment, a research strategy that would help to shed light on how differences in reimbursement systems affect access.

Sociocultural factors, including public norms and cultural change, influence the organization of substance abuse treatment systems and the attitudes and behavior of the individuals seeking help within them. Cultural change potentially influences individual readiness to seek help for alcohol and drug problems, perhaps by altering awareness of alcohol problems in social networks (Room, Greenfield, et al., 1991). Also, secular change in the governing images of these problems during periods of heightened public concern and temperance sentiment, such as the War on Drugs, can influence the social costs and stigmatization associated with admitting to a drinking or drug problem, as well as the extent to which coercion characterizes pathways to professional help (Bardsley & Beckman, 1988; Hingson, Mangione, et al., 1982; Mechanic, 1976). Finally, cycles of change in public opinion about alcohol and drug problems may also influence the supply of services indirectly by affecting political commitments to providing accessible services (e.g., see Room, Graves, et al., 1995; Schmidt & Weisner, 1995). The organization of treatment systems is also influenced by institutional pressures arising from their organizational environments, especially the state, professions, and market. Public regulatory and economic policies influence incentives for treatment organizations in both the public and private sectors to open their doors to particular pools of clients. Factors that are under less direct government control, such as treatment provider supply, prevailing clinical paradigms of intervention, levels of health insurance coverage in the public at large, and the accessibility of services in the voluntary and for-profit sectors, are critical factors in shaping the market for services and the resources available to organizations.

Some of the most important effects in the organization of alcohol and drug treatment systems also may interact with individual-level dynamics of help-seeking and coercion. For example, it appears that coercion in the workplace is more common in treatment entry to private sector agencies, whereas coercion through the police and courts predominates in public sector or government-sponsored treatment agencies (Roman, 1988; Yahr, 1988; Institute of Medicine, 1990; Schmidt & Weisner, 1993a). Yet so far, no studies have systematically examined the direct influences of such selection processes on the marked differences in demographic and clinical characteristics of populations in public- and private-sector treatment programs. Studies of the role of coercion in treatment entry have often focused almost exclusively on commitments and court mandates to treatment, to the exclusion of studying "softer" forms of coercion such as social pressuring by family and employers (Weisner, 1990). Employee assistance and other workplace referral policies greatly impact referral pathways and the sorting of clients across different types of services (Ames, 1993; Janes & Ames, 1993; Walsh, Hingson, et al., 1991). Such analyses may confront the fact that distinctions between the extent of coercion and self-referral and motivation are difficult to determine (Institute of Medicine, 1990; Roman, 1988). But there is a clear need here to integrate knowledge about social policy and organizational- and individual-level factors more deeply into research on health care utilization, and to design studies that can test interrelationships among these variables, as well as among competing hypotheses, about their effects.

While there are very few empirical studies that exemplify this kind of crosscutting research, some researchers have illustrated how such multi-level studies could be theorized and analyzed. Anderson and Newman (Newman, 1973) examined societal, health system, and individual-level determinants of treatment entry (described as predisposing, enabling, and illness factors). And Aday and Anderson's (1974) work on access to health care (e.g., health policy, characteristics of health delivery systems, characteristics of population at risk, and consumer satisfaction) involved some of the first health service studies to address divisions in research between individual-level and structural factors. Although limited, adaptations of the model of medical care seeking to the substance abuse field have been attempted (see Padgett, Struening, et al., 1990; Weisner & Schmidt, forthcoming). Mechanic (Mechanic, 1979) has discussed some of the methodological issues involved in drawing conclusions about interaction effects in multivariate modeling. More recently, Aday (Aday, Begley, et al., 1993) has examined conceptual issues regarding equity of access, such as the assumptions underlying policies on access, the issue of access to appropriate services, and actual versus potential need.

## A CRITICAL REVIEW OF EXISTING RESEARCH

In this section, we review findings on micro-level determinants of help-seeking, organizational-level influences, and environmental factors in more detail to sort out important themes and to open questions for future work on substance abuse treatment access. Although, for discussion purposes, we have grouped variables into three separate levels of explanation, we wish to emphasize that some of the most interesting and relevant hypotheses for empirical studies are likely to crosscut levels of analysis.

## Individual- or Micro-Level Determinants of Treatment Entry

The best-developed aspect of the literature on access to substance abuse services focuses on individual-level factors influencing treatment entry. Since individual-level determinants of utilization are the focus of Chapter 3, we confine our discussion here to briefly reviewing the coverage of a few key issues. This body of work builds on broader theories of help-seeking in medical, psychological and psychiatric research (Aday, 1972; Aday & Anderson, 1974; Greenley & Mechanic, 1976; McKinlay, 1972; Mechanic, 1975, 1976). Micro-level models of help-seeking often group determinants of help-seeking measured at the individual level by their roles as predisposing (sociodemographic) characteristics, perceptions and beliefs, personal enabling traits (e.g., drinking and treatment history), social enabling characteristics (support networks, health insurance, access, and availability), and need (severity) factors. Most theories of help-seeking integrate elements of the "health belief model," which focuses on social-psychological factors that trigger help-seeking, such as individuals' perceptions of symptom severity and social cues to taking action on health problems (Bardsley & Beckman, 1988).

Help-seeking studies have identified some of the key demographic predictors of substance abuse treatment entry, independent of patterns of alcohol or drug consumption (Bannenberg, Raat, et al., 1992). One of the better-studied of these dimensions is gender. There is considerable evidence of differences between women and men with regards to factors influencing entry (Ames, 1982; Beckman, 1975; Farid & Clarke, 1992; Hingson, Scotch, et al., 1980; Jackson, 1954; Jackson & Kogan, 1963; Jordan & Oei, 1989; Lindbeck, 1972; Roman, 1988; Thom, 1986; Vannicelli, 1984; Wilsnack, Klassen, et al., 1991; Wiseman, 1980), but those differences have not been widely examined using comparable populations and measures (Jordan & Oei, 1989). While there has been extensive work on gender differences in help-seeking, there are very few studies that inform differences in service use by ethnicity. Distributions of utilization across treatment agencies do vary significantly by ethnicity. For example, national data suggest that African Americans are overrepresented in public sector alcohol treatment programs, as compared to their proportions in the general population; in contrast, Hispanics are not overrepresented, except in drinking-driver programs (U.S. National Institute on Drug Abuse, 1990;

Weisner & Schmidt, 1993). There are also indications that some ethnic minority groups differ from whites in the "health beliefs" that trigger treatment seeking (Bardsley & Beckman, 1988), perhaps reflecting broader subcultural differences among ethnic groups. The public health research infrastructure poses some barriers to completing more in-depth studies of ethnicity and access to treatment. Survey sample sizes are usually too small to study minority groups separately, and data on race are often not available in insurance claims data sets, since some states have barred their collection.

While measures of substance abuse and psychiatric comorbidity have not been extensively integrated into the literature on access, there are indications that combined problems may affect treatment entry and may be associated with distinctive patterns of utilization. A variety of epidemiological studies have demonstrated high rates of comorbidity among drug, alcohol, and mental health diagnoses (Clayton, 1986; Helzer, Burnam, et al., 1991; Helzer & Pryzbeck, 1988; Lesswing & Dougherty, 1993; Magruder-Habib, Hubbard, et al., 1992; McLellan, Luborsky, et al., 1983a; Norton & Noble, 1987; Regier, Farmer, et al., 1990; Ross, 1989; Weisner & Midanik, 1993). Woody and associates (Woody, McLellan, et al., 1984, 1991) and McLellan and associates (McLellan, Alterman, et al., 1993; McLellan, Luborsky, et al., 1983a) found that higher rates of multiple problems are found in alcohol treatment populations over time. And Regier, Farmer, et al. (1990) demonstrated that individuals with multiple disorders have greater incentives to seek treatment and seek higher-intensity services (Wolfe & Sorenson, 1989).

Finally, the role of informal social networks in triggering treatment entry—including networks of friends, family, and colleagues—has been a major area of investigation in micro-level studies. Evidence on the effects of social networks on treatment entry is complex. Some investigators (Bailey & Leach, 1965; Finlay, 1975; Hingson, Mangione, et al., 1982) report that the pressure to get help following detection of a problem by family and friends is one of the major factors leading individuals to seek help. However, there is evidence that social networks can also hinder help-seeking for substance abuse treatment to the extent that they may deny or cover up the problem (Beckman & Amaro, 1986).

Micro-level variables—including health beliefs and attitudes, severity of problems, sociodemographic characteristics, and social network characteristics—are often partitioned in analytic models by the functions they purportedly play in the help-seeking process (Aday & Anderson, 1974). Sociodemographic characteristics, in particular, age, marital status, and employment status, are usually grouped under the rubric of demand characteristics and are viewed as independent of the individual's pattern of illness symptoms (e.g., Bannenberg, Raat, et al., 1992). There are, however, likely to be important interactions between sociodemographic characteristics and "enabling" factors in the process of treatment entry for alcohol and drug problems. Ethnicity and socioeconomic status may absorb the variance of larger organizational and social structural effects in multivariate models, such as the effects of uneven insurance coverage and coerced treatment entry. Specific population groups, or "target populations," distinguished by their age, gender, and ethnic statuses, are likely to be singled out for criminal justice interventions or coerced treatment because they are viewed as "at-risk"; meanwhile, service use by other groups may tend to be more discretionary. It is therefore plausible that sociodemographic characteristics interact with environmental tendencies toward coercive interventions or other organizational and environmental factors, thus moderating the role that sociodemographic variables play in predisposing individuals to seek help.

## Organizational-Level Factors Influencing Access

Potentially important organizational-level factors in access to alcohol and drug treatment include government and private-sector initiatives to contain the costs of treatment, trends in interorganizational linkages, program gatekeeping, and the privatization of health services. Over the past two or three decades, service systems responding to alcohol and drug problems have undergone profound change, both in their character and in their proportions. Changes in the financing of treatment have included a growing emphasis on delivering services through private, for-profit health systems, and bifurcation of public- and private-sector services into a "two-tiered" system of services for those with and without insurance coverage (D'Aunno, Sutton, et al., 1991; Morgan & Weisner, 1991; Price & D'Aunno, 1992; Wheeler, Fadel, et al., 1992; Yahr, 1988). The growing emphasis on cost containment throughout the health sector has justified the spread of managed care organizations and a trend toward providing substance abuse services in nonmedical and outpatient settings, which are generally less costly alternatives to traditional fixed-length-of-stay, hospital-based, inpatient programs. Other influential factors at the organizational level originate in the relationship of the substance abuse treatment system with other health and human service systems. Alcohol and drug treatment services tend to be outside the mainstream health system, and referral between different systems of services is infrequent (Weisner & Schmidt, 1995). Because substance abuse is associated with a range of other health and social problems, problem drinkers and drug users often come in contact with a variety of institutions in the community (Tam, Schmidt, et al., 1996). Important trends in relations among service systems include the recent merger of alcohol and drug treatment services

(Weisner, 1992), the growing role of employee assistance programs (Blum, Roman, et al., 1993; Roman, 1988) and the increasing role of criminal justice services as primary agencies of referral to alcohol services (Institute of Medicine, 1990).

These significant changes in the organization and financing of alcohol and drug services are likely to have important effects on access, particularly when these major trends in treatment systems impinge on patterns of professional gatekeeping within organizations. Gatekeeping procedures include formal organizational routines for screening, identifying, and referring-out prospective clients, but can also be influenced by the attitudes and biases of providers toward particular kinds of clients (Morgenstern & McCrady, 1992). The concept of professional gatekeeping comes out of societal reaction research in sociology, a body of theory and empirical research that included studies on the various roles that professionals (such as police officers, social workers, and the courts) play in client selection (Kitsuse, 1962; Lemert, 1972; Scheff, 1964). Patterns in the social handling of troubled persons have obvious consequences for service access, especially for behavioral problems such as mental illness and substance abuse, which elicit strong public reactions (Kitsuse, 1962; Scheff, 1964). Empirical studies have shown that the process of treatment entry is powerfully conditioned by factors such as the social visibility of illness symptoms, by the attitudes and "typifications" that providers hold about their clients, and the degree of surveillance of deviance in communities (Chambliss, 1973; Mendel & Rapport, 1969; Room, 1980; Rushing, 1972; Wilde, 1968). More visible, stigmatized, and easily labeled forms of deviance are expected to result in more intensive formal intervention. Recent studies (Lipsky, 1980; Schmidt & Weisner, 1993b) have argued that organizational characteristics, such as bureaucratic structure, may help to shape patterns of provider discretion in admissions. By and large, studies of gatekeeping that draw on the societal reaction perspective have not done much to integrate individual-level variables associated with help-seeking into research at a broader, organizational level. Rather, these studies have tended to view the individual receiving services as rather passive in the hands of gatekeepers; in other words, they have tended to hold individual-level factors constant (Lemert, 1972).

An important new development in research on professional gatekeeping within mainly private sector treatment programs is the appearance of case management and managed care systems (Clark & Fox, 1993; Lehman, 1987). Managed care approaches include strategies such as utilization review, selective contracting, and financial mechanisms such as prospective payment, all of which are used to achieve improved economic efficiency and, ideally, more comprehensive services (Intagliata, 1982; Keeler, Manning, et al., 1988; Levin, Glasser, et al., 1984; Tischler, 1990;

Wells, Hosek, et al., 1992). While the research on managed care in alcohol and drug services is very limited, the prevailing view is that many of the new gatekeepers under managed care do not routinely evaluate and refer potential cases to specialty alcohol and drug treatment programs (Schmidt & Weisner, 1993a). Moreover, there are presently few formal controls and regulations governing managed care organizations that would provide assurances that efforts to contain costs do not adversely affect the accessibility and quality of services (Borenstein, 1990; England & Vaccaro, 1991).

Managed care's effects on alcohol and drug treatment systems are understudied (Mechanic, Schlesinger, et al., 1995), although there are a number of studies of managed mental health care (Freund, Rossiter, et al., 1989). However, it can be dangerous simply to generalize what is known from the more extensive research on managed health and mental health care to substance abuse treatment. For example, managed care may have more consequences for access to substance abuse services than mental health services because problems of excessive hospitalization and other inappropriate treatment are much more prevalent in the treatment of substance abuse (Strumwasser, Patanjpe, et al., 1991). Moreover, establishing standardized treatment criteria for limiting payments for substance abuse are more difficult as compared with mental health treatments (Mechanic, Schlesinger, et al., 1995). Finally, the cyclical, relapsing nature of chronic alcohol and drug problems means that ongoing monitoring of clients is often necessary and a broader range of social, legal, and general health services may be needed in substance abuse treatment systems.

Given the rapid diffusion of managed care, it will be particularly important to conduct research that teases out the impact on access of different managed care strategies, such as utilization review, selective contracting, and financing incentives. There are at least four ways that managed care systems could *theoretically* influence the accessibility of alcohol and drug services. However, we wish to emphasize that none of these areas has been thoroughly researched in its implications. First, through selective reimbursement, managed care could influence the balance of different types of services made available. There is some early indication, for example, that prospective payment systems often provide financial incentives weighted in favor of a general hospital model emphasizing brief-stay detoxification and outpatient treatment (Mezochow, Miller, et al., 1987). Second, increased incentives for "patient dumping"—where less profitable, more severe cases are excluded from services—potentially place some substance abuse treatment clients at risk for receiving inadequate services due to shortened lengths of stay or transfers to inappropriate facilities. Third, because schedules of prospective payment are not always adjusted to provide adequate coverage of individuals with psychiatric and medical comorbidities, clients with multiple problems may receive less than adequate treatment for all of their needs, or may be vulnerable to exclusion from services. Fourth, because the "health maintenance" aspect of managed care tends to emphasize the prevention of chronic, severe conditions (that prove more costly to third-party payers in the long run), there is the positive potential for managed care to reduce the progression of problem drinking and drug addiction in covered populations through improved access to early case-finding and intervention programs.

In addition to these quite tangible influences of professional gatekeeping related to the formal organization and financing of services, there are some more intangible aspects of alcohol and drug service organizations, such as clinical philosophy and organizational culture, that are potentially influential in access to services. While it is logical that there may be discernible effects in these areas, they are relatively unresearched. For example, much has been written on the dominant model or "governing image" of abstinence as a treatment model and goal in the alcoholism field (Hubbard, 1990; Institute of Medicine, 1990; Room, 1978). While recent research has provided encouragement for the development of alternative strategies, such as brief intervention and moderation drinking approaches, we know very little about the degree to which alternatives to the abstinence approach have been integrated into alcohol and drug treatment, or about their impact on attracting new groups of clients to treatment.

Other organizational-level influences include the funding status and reimbursement mechanisms of alcohol treatment agencies, which may have an impact on the availability of treatment slots, the types of services (prevention, inpatient, outpatient, detoxification) available, and whether ancillary services that support treatment are offered, such as child care and vocational services. For example, the growing trends toward privatization in substance abuse treatment—that is, the growing emphasis on delivering services through private nonprofit and for-profit programs rather than governmental ones—may have different effects on the accessibility of services for individuals with and without private insurance coverage. Given the fixed amount of public dollars allocated for substance abuse, there are clear limits on the numbers of services that can be provided at low or no cost by government-sponsored agencies. Services therefore must be rationed whether or not explicit policies for rationing are put in place by government. In the absence of explicit policies, such rationing usually takes place by default in the public sector through waiting lists (Rogowski, 1992). These are hardly rational instruments for sorting out those clients most in need, or for assuring that clients will be matched to programs that best suit their needs.

A few empirical studies have examined the contracting-out of government services to private agencies and, more generally, how the privatization of alcohol treatment programs during the past 15 years has influenced who receives treatment and who does not (Morgan & Weisner, 1991; Price & D'Aunno, 1992; Schmidt & Weisner, 1993a; Weisner & Room, 1984; Yahr, 1988). A recent study of contracting-out mental health services found important differences in practices between public and private agencies but did not find evidence that these differences were associated with reduced access for low-income clients (Clark, Dorwart, et al., 1994). The study indicated that intervening factors, especially competition between contract agencies, affected the kinds of services those agencies provided. Research on public–private differences is limited by the lack of data sets that capture both types of organizations within the same sampling frame. It is possible, however, to make comparisons of private-sector substance abuse programs (Hoffman & Harrison, 1986) with data on public programs drawn from separate sampling frames (Polich & Orvis, 1979; Schmidt & Weisner, 1993b), although the shortcomings of this approach are obvious. Such comparisons suggest some important differences between the populations of clients who make it into treatment in the public and private sectors. For example, clients in private, for-profit programs appear to be younger and to have fewer psychological problems (Chopra, Preston, et al., 1979; Jacob, 1985).

## Sociocultural Influences on Access

The broader sociocultural environment creates a context in which individuals reflect on their own drinking and drug use and potentially seek help for what they believe is a problem. Broad trends in the culture and in public opinion can potentially influence social demands for action on alcohol and drug problems as well as affect social policies that define how services are financed and legally restricted. In this area, the research is quite limited; to our knowledge, there exist no studies that directly relate broad changes in public opinion to help-seeking on the individual level. However, there is some indirect evidence that, independent of other factors, cultural change can directly influence both the need for and supply of substance abuse services. For example, growing antidrug sentiment during the 1980s appears to have led to aggregate decreases in middle-class alcohol and drug consumption (Harrison, 1992; Midanik & Clark, 1994; Caetano & Kaskutas, 1995). Heightened awareness of alcohol and drug problems also coincided with aggregate increases in treatment utilization (Weisner, Greenfield, et al., 1995). During this period, there was also a dramatic expansion of publicly funded treatment programs as government responded to growing public demand for action on substance abuse problems (Schmidt & Weisner, 1993a).

Contemporary organizational theory also points to the potential importance of institutional pressures in the sociocultural environments of organizations, and particularly to the roles that the state, professions, and other organizational systems play in shaping them (for introduction, see Scott, 1987). Governmental policies oriented around containing costs and reforming the health system have altered access to services for groups funded through both public- and private-sector insurance (Freeman & Trabin, 1994; Lo & Woodward, 1993; McGuire, Dickey, et al., 1987; Mitchell, Dickey, et al., 1987). For example, the "diagnostic-related groups" approach to regulating Medicare reimbursements appears to have reduced general mental health expenditures, though this is generally achieved by reducing lengths of stay and inpatient bed days. Other studies have found that decreasing inpatient days increased the number of detoxification days, but not outpatient visits in managed care organizations (Mechanic, Schlesinger, et al., 1995). It is unclear, however, whether reductions in length of stay reflect increased efficiency or rather, undertreatment and reduced access. Though inconclusive, some recent studies have suggested that beneficial alcohol treatment outcomes are sometimes related to longer lengths of stay (Gottheil, McLellan, et al., 1981).

Treatment demand and access may also be influenced by the growing degree of government involvement in mandating treatment for particular populations and by government-sanctioned strategies for involuntary commitment. Researchers have examined the effects of mandated treatment on client compliance and treatment effectiveness, yielding findings that generally support mandated treatment as appropriate and effective within some client groups (Gerstein & Harwood, 1990; Hubbard, Marsden, et al., 1989; Leukefeld & Tims, 1993; Stitzer & McCaul, 1987). However, what has not been examined is the overall impact of the trend toward mandated treatment in terms of its impact on increased stigmatization of clients and on how communities and social networks respond to alcohol and drug problems. Furthermore, the number of referrals entering treatment from criminal justice settings has increased significantly, without a parallel increase in public-sector treatment capacity. But only a few studies have examined the impact on access for traditional clients of the system, such as individuals being brought in on charges of public drunkenness (Institute of Medicine, 1990).

Social policies and more diffuse policy environments can also be influential in determining the availability of alcohol and drug treatment resources nationally. For example, federal policies introduced during the 1980s appear to have initiated important developments in utilization patterns. The implementation of major federal budget legislation in 1982 effectively decentralized and deregulated service delivery for alcohol and drug problems. This was achieved through the introduction of relatively unrestricted block grants to states that encouraged local autonomy and responsibility in treatment systems. One result of this decentralization in decision-making powers was growing fragmentation in the organization of treatment services and, ultimately, in an uneven distribution of resources across geographic regions and social classes. For example, the distribution of substance abuse resources across states in the United States bears no apparent relation to indicators of the need for services (Institute of Medicine, 1990).

Alcohol and drug programs are also influenced by the policies and practices of other types of organizations operating in their environments, and changes in the relations between substance abuse treatment systems and other systems of services have had important implications for who has access to treatment. Tightening legal sanctions for alcohol and drug-related offenses during the 1980s led to a disproportionate increase in substance abusers in some criminal justice settings (Mauer, 1992; U.S. Bureau of Justice Statistics, 1991). Indirectly, this has resulted in a growing role for criminal justice as the predominant system delivering referrals to therapeutic agencies in alcohol and drug treatment systems (Gerstein & Harwood, 1990; Stitzer & McCaul, 1987; Tam, Schmidt, et al., 1996; Weisner, 1990). At this point, we know very little about the extent to which health care, criminal justice, welfare, and mental health agencies routinely screen patients and clients for substance abuse problems and provide brief interventions or referrals to substance abuse treatment (Cherpitel, 1992; Fleming & Barry, 1991; Glaze & Coggan, 1987; Gureje, Obikoya, et al., 1992; King, 1986; Magruder-Habib, Fraker, et al., 1983). So far, no researchers have explored the implications for access of employing substance abuse treatment providers in health and social service agencies outside the specialty treatment sector (e.g., in primary health care settings or jails).

## THE FUTURE OF RESEARCH ON ACCESS AND NEED

Over the past two decades or so, substance abuse treatment systems have undergone vast changes affecting access. Treatment capacity and the number of clients have almost doubled, with most of the increase occurring in the private sector. Separate funding mechanisms in the public and private sectors have given rise to a two-tiered system, with different types of clients and services available to clients in governmental, as opposed to nonprofit and for-profit, private, programs. The rise of managed care in the private sector has led to a dramatic shift from residential to outpatient services, and to considerable decreases in length of stay. Public sentiment seems to have drifted toward a heightened awareness of crime and addiction, resulting in stricter penalties on alcohol- and drug-related crimes and, ultimately, in closer relations between the criminal justice and substance abuse treatment systems. Future developments in organization and financing are hard to predict. For instance, as managed care further penetrates the public sector, it may lead to yet more substantial changes in the types of services offered there, perhaps pressuring systems to emphasize more medically oriented services, as has been the case in the private sector. The future of research on access and need, to a considerable degree, will involve making sense of how these profound changes at the organizational and societal levels alter individuals' prospects of obtaining help for addictive disorders when they need it, and how these larger changes influence the pathways of social pressure and referral that lead to treatment.

In this chapter, we have touched upon a variety of these open questions and, based on existing research, have offered some hunches about where future research on these topics might lead. These have included the measurement problems with establishing the magnitude of need for services in defined populations, with disentangling need and demand for services, and with the conceptual difficulties involved in choosing among different definitions of need. We have emphasized the need to expand the frame of reference in substance abuse services research by studying organizations outside the specialty alcohol and drug systems, and by looking at environmental factors. Research bearing on questions of access and need has been biased toward studies of help-seeking at the individual level. Such studies have often drawn on a tacit model of voluntary treatment seeking that bears little relation to the realities of substance abuse treatment entry, which is usually subject to a high degree of coercion, the vagaries of professional gatekeeping, and financial barriers imposed by cost containment strategies. In the future, research on access and need will be required to frame questions more broadly, in ways that encompass multiple levels of explanation and examine effects that crosscut individual, organizational, and societal levels of analysis.

## ACKNOWLEDGMENTS

An earlier version of this chapter was prepared under contract with the U.S. National Institute on Alcohol Abuse and Alcoholism (NIAAA) for the Panel on Utilization and Cost, National Advisory Council's Subcommittee for Health Services Research. We wish to thank Richard Longabaugh and Jerry Spicer for helpful comments.

## REFERENCES

Aday, L., & Anderson, R. A. (1974). A framework for the study of access to medical care. *Health Services Research, 9*, 208–220.

Aday, L. A. (1972). *The utilization of health services: Indices and correlates.* Washington, DC: National Center for Health Services Research and Development.

Aday, L. A., Begley, C. E., et al. (1993). *Evaluating the medical care system: Effectiveness, efficiency, and equity.* Ann Arbor, MI: Health Administration Press.

Alterman, A. I., Droba, M., et al. (1992). Response to day hospital treatment by patients with cocaine and alcohol dependence. *Hospital and Community Psychiatry, 43*(9), 930–932.

Altman, L., & Goldstein, J. M. (1988). Impact of HMO model type on mental health service delivery. In S. Feldman & S. R. Blum (Eds.), *Administration in mental health* (Vol. 15, pp. 246–261). New York: Human Sciences Press.

American Psychiatric Association. (1994). *Diagnostic and statistical manual of mental disorders* (4th ed.). Washington, DC: American Psychiatric Press.

Ames, G. (1982). *Maternal alcoholism and family life: A cultural model of research and intervention.* PhD dissertation, University of California, San Francisco.

Ames, G. (1993). Research and strategies for the primary prevention of workplace alcohol problems. *Alcohol Health and Research World, 17*(1), 19–27.

Anderson, R. A., & Newman, J. P. (1973). Societal and individual determinants of medical utilization in the United States. *Milbank Memorial Fund Quarterly, 51,* 95–124.

Bailey, M. B., & Leach, B. (1965). *Alcoholics Anonymous: Pathways to recovery.* New York: National Council on Alcoholism.

Bannenberg, A. F., Raat, H., et al. (1992). Demand for alcohol treatment by problem drinkers. *Journal of Substance Abuse Treatment, 9*(1), 59–62.

Bardsley, P. E., & Beckman, L. J. (1988). The health belief model and entry into alcoholism treatment. *International Journal of the Addictions, 23*(1), 19–28.

Batten, H. L. (1993). *Drug services research survey: Phase I Final Report: Non-correctional facilities—Revised.* Waltham, MA: Institute for Health Policy, Brandeis University.

Beckman, L. J. (1975). Women alcoholics: A review of social and psychological studies. *Journal of Studies on Alcohol, 36,* 797–825.

Beckman, L. J., & Amaro, H. (1986). Personal and social difficulties faced by women and men entering alcoholism treatment. *Journal of Studies on Alcohol, 47*(2), 135–146.

Blum, T. C., Roman, P. M., et al. (1993). Alcohol consumption and work performance. *Journal of Studies on Alcohol, 54*(1), 61–70.

Borenstein, D. B. (1990). Managed care: A means of rationing psychiatric treatment. *Hospital and Community Psychiatry, 41*(10), 1095–1098.

Browne, B., Browne, R. F., et al. (1987). Effect of mandated drug, alcohol, and mental health benefits on group health insurance premiums. *Journal of the American Society of Chartered Life Underwriters & Chartered Financial Consultants, 41*(1), 74–78.

Caetano, R., & Kaskutas, L. A. (1995). Changes in drinking patterns among Whites, Blacks and Hispanics: 1984–1992. *Journal of Studies on Alcohol, 56*(5), 558–565.

Caetano, R., & Room, R. (1994). Alcohol dependence in the 1990 U.S. national alcohol survey: Operationalizing and comparing two nosological systems. *Drug and Alcohol Review, 13,* 257–267.

Cahalan, D., Cisin, I. H., et al. (1969). *American drinking practices: A national study of drinking behavior and attitudes.* New Brunswick, NJ: Rutgers Center of Alcohol Studies.

Chambliss, W. (1973, November/December). The saints and the roughnecks. *Society,* pp. 24–31.

Cherpitel, C. J. (1992). Drinking patterns and problems: A comparison of ER patients in an HMO and in the general population. *Alcoholism: Clinical and Experimental Research, 16*(6), 1104–1109.

Chopra, K., Preston, D., et al. (1979). The effect of constructive coercion on the rehabilitative process. *Journal of Occupational Medicine 21*(11), 749–752.

Clark, R. E., Dorwart, R. A., et al. (1994). Managing competition in public and private mental health agencies: Implications for services and policy. *Milbank Quarterly, 72*(4), 653–678.

Clark, R. E. &, Fox, T. S. (1993). A framework for evaluating the economic impact of case management. *Hospital and Community Psychiatry, 44*(5), 469–473.

Clayton, R. R. (1986). Multiple drug use: epidemiology, correlates, and consequences. In M. Galanter (Ed.), *Recent developments in alcoholism* (Vol. 4, pp. 7–38). New York: Plenum.

D'Aunno, T., Sutton, R. I., et al. (1991). Isomorphism and external support in conflicting institutional environments: A study of drug abuse treatment units. *Academy of Management Journal, 34,* 636–661.

England, M. J., & Vaccaro, V. A. (1991). New systems to manage mental health care. *Health Affairs, 10*(4), 129–137.

Farid, B., & Clarke, M. E. (1992). Characteristics of attenders to community based alcohol treatment centre with special reference to sex differences. *Drug and Alcohol Dependence, 30,* 33–36.

Feldstein, P. J., Wickizer, T. M., et al. (1988). Private cost containment: The effects of utilization review programs on health care use and expenditures. *New England Journal of Medicine, 318,* 1310–1314.

Finlay, D. G. (1975). Helping alcoholic clients: Some guidelines for social workers and other helping professionals. *Alcohol, Health and Research World, Summer Experimental Issue,* 20–23.

Fleming, M. F., & Barry, K. L. (1991). The effectiveness of alcoholism screening in an ambulatory care setting. *Journal of Studies on Alcohol, 52*(1), 33–36.

Freeman, M. A., & Trabin, T. (1994). *Managed behavioral healthcare: History, models, key issues, and future course.* Report prepared by Behavioral Health Alliance for the U.S. Department of Health and Human Services.

Freund, D. A., Rossiter, L. F., et al. (1989). Evaluation of the Medicaid competition demonstrations. *Health Care Financing Review, 11*(2), 77–81.

General Accounting Office. (1993). *Drug use measurement: Strengths, limitations, and recommendations for improvement.* Washington, DC: General Accounting Office.

Gerstein, D. R., & Harwood, H. J. (Eds.). (1990). *Treating drug problems: Vol. 1. A study of the evolution, effectiveness, and financing of public and private drug treatment systems.* Washington, DC: National Academy Press.

Glaze, L., & Coggan, P. (1987). Efficacy of an alcoholism self-report questionnaire in a residency clinic. *Journal of Family Practice, 25,* 60–64.

Gottheil, E., McLellan, A. T., et al. (1981). Reasonable and unreasonable methodological standards for the evaluation of alcoholism treatment. In E. Gottheil, A. T. McLellan, & K. A. Druley (Eds.), *Matching patient needs and treatment methods in alcoholism and drug abuse* (pp. 371–389). Springfield, IL: Charles C Thomas.

Gottheil, E., McLellan, A. T., et al. (1992). Length of stay, patient severity and treatment outcome: Sample data from the field of alcoholism. *Journal of Studies on Alcohol, 53*(1), 69–75.

Greenley, J. R., & Mechanic, D. (1976). Social selection in seeking help for psychological problems. *Journal of Health and Social Behavior, 17*, 249–262.

Gureje, O., Obikoya, B., et al. (1992). Alcohol abuse and dependence in an urban primary care clinic in Nigeria. *Drug and Alcohol Dependence, 30*, 163–167.

Harrison, L. D. (1992). Trends in illicit drug use in the United States: Conflicting results from national surveys. *International Journal of the Addictions, 27*(7), 817–847.

Harwood, R. (forthcoming). How many people are in need of treatment? *National Institute of Drug Abuse Monograph: Proceedings of Planning Meeting: Health Services Research II, Bethesda, MD, Jan. 31–Feb. 1, 1994.* Washington, DC: National Institute of Drug Abuse.

Hayashida, M., Alterman, A. I., et al. (1989). Comparative effectiveness and costs of inpatient and outpatient detoxification of patients with mild-to-moderate alcohol withdrawal syndrome. *New England Journal of Medicine, 320*(6), 358–365.

Helzer, J. E., Burnam, A., et al. (1991). Alcohol use and dependence. In L. N. Robins & D. Regier (Eds.), *Psychiatric disorders in America: The Epidemiologic Catchment Area study* (pp. 81–116). New York: Free Press.

Helzer, J. E., & Pryzbeck, T. R. (1988). The co-occurrence of alcoholism with other psychiatric disorders in the general population and its impact on treatment. *Journal of Studies on Alcohol, 49*, 219–224.

Hingson, R., Mangione, T., et al. (1982). Seeking help for drinking problems: A study in the Boston metropolitan area. *Journal of Studies on Alcohol, 43*, 273–288.

Hingson, R., Scotch, N., et al. (1980). Recognizing and seeking help for drinking problems. *Journal of Studies on Alcohol, 41*, 1102–1117.

Hoffman, N. G., & Harrison, P. A. (1986). *CATOR 1986 report: Findings two years after treatment.* St. Paul, MN: CATOR.

Horwitz, A. (1977). Social networks and pathways to psychiatric treatment. *Social Forces, 56*(1), 86–105.

Hubbard, R. L. (1990). Treating combined alcohol and drug abuse in community-based programs. In M. Galanter (Ed.), *Recent developments in alcoholism* (Vol. 8, pp. 273–284). New York: Plenum.

Hubbard, R. L., Marsden, M. E., et al. (1989). *Drug abuse treatment: A national study of treatment effectiveness.* Chapel Hill: University of North Carolina Press.

Institute of Medicine. (1990). *Broadening the base of treatment for alcohol problems.* Washington, DC: National Academy Press.

Intagliata, J. (1982). Improving the quality of community care for the chronically mentally disabled: The role of case management. *Schizophrenia Bulletin, 8*, 655–674.

Jackson, J. K. (1954). The adjustment of the family to the crisis of alcoholism. *Quarterly Journal of Studies on Alcohol, 15*, 562–585.

Jackson, J. K., & Kogan, K. L. (1963). The search for solutions: Help-seeking patterns of families of active and inactive alcoholics. *Quarterly Journal of Studies on Alcohol, 24*, 449–472.

Jacob, O. (1985). *Public and private sector issues on alcohol and other drug abuse: A special report with recommendations.* Rockville, MD: U.S. Department of Health and Human Services, Public Health Service.

Janes, C. R., & Ames, G. M. (1993). The workplace. In M. Galanter (Ed.), *Ten years of progress: Social and cultural perspectives, physiology and biochemistry, clinical pathology, trends in treatment* (Vol. 11, pp. 124–138). New York: Plenum.

Jordan, C. M., & Oei, T. P. S. (1989). Help-seeking behavior in problem drinkers: A review. *British Journal of Addiction, 84,* 979–988.

Keeler, E. B., Manning, W. G., et al. (1988). The demand for episodes of mental health services. *Journal of Health Economics, 7,* 369–392.

King, M. (1986). At risk drinking among several practice attendees: Validation of the CAGE questionnaires. *Psychological Medicine, 16,* 213–217.

Kitsuse, J. (1962). Societal reaction to deviant behavior: Problems of theory and methods. *Social Problems, 9,* 247–256.

Lehman, A. F. (1987). Capitation payment and mental health care: A review of the opportunities and risks. *Hospital and Community Psychiatry, 38*(1), 31–38.

Lemert, E. (1972). *Human deviance, social problems and social control.* Englewood Cliffs, NJ: Prentice-Hall.

Lesswing, N. J., & Dougherty, R. J. (1993). Psychopathology in alcohol- and cocaine-dependent patients: A comparison of findings from psychological testing. *Journal of Substance Abuse Treatment, 10*(1), 53–58.

Leukefeld, C. G., & Tims, F. R. (1993). Drug abuse treatment in prisons and jails. *Journal of Substance Abuse Treatment, 10*(1), 77–84.

Levin, B. L., Glasser, J. H., et al. (1984). Changing patterns in mental health service coverage within health maintenance organizations. *American Journal of Public Health, 74*(5), 453–458.

Lindbeck, V. L. (1972). The woman alcoholic: A review of the literature. *International Journal of the Addictions, 7,* 567–580.

Lipsky, M. (1980). *Street-level bureaucracy: Dilemmas of the individual in public services.* New York: Russell Sage Foundation.

Lo, A., & Woodward, A. (1993). An evaluation of freestanding alcoholism treatment for Medicare recipients. *Addiction, 88,* 53–67.

Magruder-Habib, K., Hubbard, R. L., et al. (1992). Effects of drug misuse treatment on symptoms of depression and suicide. *International Journal of the Addictions, 27*(9), 1035–1065.

Magruder-Habib, K. M., Fraker, G. G., et al. (1983). Correspondence of clinicians' judgments with the Michigan Alcoholism Screening Test in determining alcoholism in Veterans Administration outpatients. *Journal of Studies on Alcohol, 44,* 872–884.

Mattson, M. E., Allen, J. P., et al. (1994). A chronological review of empirical studies matching alcoholic clients to treatment. *Journal of Studies on Alcohol, 12,* 16–29.

Mauer, M. (1992). *Americans behind bars: One year later.* Washington, DC: Sentencing Project.

McGuire, T. G., Dickey, B., et al. (1987). Differences in resource use and cost among facilities treating alcohol, drug abuse, and mental disorders: Implications for design of a prospective payment system. *American Journal of Psychiatry, 144*(5), 616–620.

McKinlay, J. B. (1972). Some approaches and problems in the study of the use of services—an overview. *Journal of Health and Social Behavior, 13,* 115–152.

McLellan, A. T., Alterman, A. I., et al. (1993). Psychosocial services in substance abuse treatment?: A dose ranging study of psychosocial services. *Journal of American Medical Association, 269*(15), 1953–1959.

McLellan, A. T., Alterman, A. I., et al. (1994). Similarity of outcome predictors across opiate, cocaine and alcohol treatments: Role of treatment services. *Journal of Consulting and Clinical Psychology, 62*(6), 1141–1158.

McLellan, A. T., Grissom, G., et al. (1993). Substance abuse treatment in the private setting: Are some programs more effective than others? *Journal of Substance Abuse Treatment, 27,* 561–570.

McLellan, A. T., Luborsky, L., et al. (1983a). Predicting response to alcohol and drug abuse treatments: Role of psychiatric severity. *Archives of General Psychiatry, 40,* 620–625.

McLellan, A. T., Luborsky, L., et al. (1983b). Increased effectiveness of substance abuse treatment: A prospective study of patient–treatment "matching." *Journal of Nervous and Mental Disease, 171*(10), 597–605.

Mechanic, D. (1975). Sociocultural and social-psychological factors affecting personal responses to psychological disorder. *Journal of Health and Social Behavior, 16,* 393–404.

Mechanic, D. (1976). Sex, illness, illness behavior, and the use of health services. *Journal of Human Stress, 2,* 29–40.

Mechanic, D. (1979). Correlates of physician utilization: Why do major multivariate studies of physician utilization find trivial psychosocial and organizational effects? *Journal of Health and Social Behavior, 20,* 387–397.

Mechanic, D., Schlesinger, M., et al. (1995). Management of mental health and substance abuse services: state of the art and early results. *Milbank Quarterly, 73*(1), 19–56.

Mendel, W. M., & Rapport, S. (1969). Determinants of the decision for psychiatric hospitalization. *Archives of General Psychiatry, 20,* 321–328.

Mezochow, J., Miller, S., et al. (1987). The impact of cost containment on alcohol and drug treatment. *Hospital and Community Psychiatry, 38*(5), 506–510.

Midanik, L. T., & Clark, W. B. (1994). The demographic distribution of U.S. drinking patterns in 1990: Descriptions and trends from 1984. *American Journal of Public Health, 84*(8), 1218–1222.

Mitchell, J. B., Dickey, B., et al. (1987). Bringing psychiatric patients into the Medicare prospective payment system: Alternatives to DRGs. *American Journal of Psychiatry, 144,* 610–615.

Morgan, P., & Weisner, C. (1991). *Contracting out the welfare state: Alcohol treatment in the United States.* Berkeley, CA: Alcohol Research Group.

Morgenstern, J., & McCrady, B. S. (1992). Curative factors in alcohol and drug treatment: Behavioral and disease model perspectives. *British Journal of Addiction, 87,* 901–912.

Norton, R., & Noble, J. (1987). Combined alcohol and other drug use and abuse: a status report. *Alcohol Health & Research World, 11*(4), 78–81.

Polich, J., & Orvis, B. (1979). *Alcohol problems: Patterns and prevalence in the U.S. Air Force.* Santa Monica, CA: Rand Corporation.

Price, R. H., & D'Aunno, T. (1992). The organization and impact of outpatient drug abuse treatment services. In R. R. Watson (Ed.), *Drug and alcohol abuse reviews: Vol. 3. Treatment of drug and alcohol abuse* (pp. 37–60). Clifton, NJ: Humana Press.

Regier, D. A., & Farmer, M. E. et al. (1990). Comorbidity of mental disorders with alcohol and other drug abuse: Results from the Epidemiologic Catchment Area (ECA) study. *Journal of the American Medical Association, 264*(19), 2511–2518.

Regier, D. A., Narrow, W. E., et al. (1993). The de facto U.S. mental and addictive disorders service system: Epidemiologic Catchment Area prospective 1-year prevalence rates of disorders and services. *Archives of General Psychiatry, 50*(2), 85–94.

Ridgely, M. S., Goldman, H. H., et al. (1990). Barriers to the care of persons with dual diagnoses: Organizational and financing issues. *Schizophrenia Bulletin, 16*(1), 123–132.

Rogowski, J. A. (1992). Insurance coverage for drug abuse. *Health Affairs, 11*(3), 137–148.

Roman, P. (1988). Growth and transformation in workplace alcoholism programming. In M. Galanter (Ed.), *Recent developments in alcoholism* (Vol. 6, pp. 131–158). New York: Plenum.

Room, R. (1977). Measurement and distribution of drinking patterns and problems in general populations. In G. Edwards, M. M. Gross, M. Keller, J. Moser, & R. Room (Eds.), *Alcohol-related disabilities* (pp. 61–87). Geneva: World Health Organization.

Room, R. (1978). Governing images of alcohol and drug problems: The structure, sources and sequels of conceptualizations of intractable problems. *Sociology,* Berkeley: University of California.

Room, R. (1980). Treatment-seeking populations and larger realities. In G. Edwards & M. Grant (Eds.), *Alcoholism treatment in transition* (pp. 205–224). London, Croom Helm.

Room, R., Graves, K., et al. (1995). Trends in public opinion about alcohol policy initiatives in Ontario and the U.S.: 1989–91." *Drug and Alcohol Review, 14,* 35–47.

Room, R., Greenfield, T., et al. (1991). "People who might have liked you to drink less: Changing responses to drinking by U.S. family members and friends, 1979–1990. *Contemporary Drug Problems 18*(4), 573–595.

Ross, H. E. (1989). Alcohol and drug abuse in treated alcoholics: A comparison of men and women. *Alcoholism: Clinical and Experimental Research, 13*(6), 810.

Rushing, W. A. (1972). Individual resources, societal reaction, and hospital commitment. *American Journal of Sociology, 77,* 511–526.

Scheff, T. (1964). The societal reaction to deviance: Ascriptive elements in the psychiatric screening of mental patients in a Midwestern state. *Social Problems, 11,* 401–413.

Schlesinger, M., Bentkover, J., et al. (1987). The privatization of health care and physician's perceptions of access to hospital services. *Milbank Quarterly, 65*(1), 25–58.

Schmidt, L., & Weisner, C. (1993a). Developments in alcoholism treatment: a ten year review. In M. Galanter (Ed.), *Recent developments in alcoholism* (Vol. 11, pp. 369–396). New York: Plenum.

Schmidt, L., & Weisner, C. (1993b, October 18–22). *"Spare people" in the public sector human services.* Paper presented at the International Conference on Alcohol and Drug Treatment Systems Research, Kettil Bruun Society for Social and Epidemiological Research on Alcohol, Toronto, Canada.

Schmidt, L., & Weisner, C. (1995). The emergence of problem-drinking women as a special population in need of treatment. In M. Galanter (Ed.), *Recent developments in alcoholism* (Vol. 12, pp. 309–326). New York: Plenum.

Schmidt, L., Weisner, C., et al. (1994). Substance abuse and the course of welfare dependency. *American Journal of Public Health, 88*(11), 1616–1622.

Schmidt, L. A. (1995). The role of problem drinking in psychiatric admissions. *Addiction, 90*(3), 375–390.

Scott, R. (1987). *Organizations: Rational, natural and open systems.* Englewood Cliffs, NJ: Prentice-Hall.

Stitzer, M. L., & McCaul, M. E. (1987). Criminal justice interventions with drug and alcohol abusers: The role of compulsory treatment. In E. K. Morris & C. J. Braukmann (Eds.), *Behavioral approaches to crime and delinquency* (pp. 331–360). New York: Plenum.

Strumwasser, I., Patanjpe, M., et al. (1991). Appropriateness of psychiatric and substance abuse hospitalization. *Medical Care, 29*(8 suppl.), AS77–AS90.

Tam, T., Schmidt, L., et al. (1996). Patterns in the institutional encounters of problem drinkers in a community human services network. *Addiction, 91*(5), 657–669.

Thom, B. (1986). Sex differences in help-seeking for alcohol problems: 1. The barriers to help-seeking. *British Journal of Addiction, 81,* 777–788.

Tischler, G. L. (1990). Utilization management of mental health services by private third parties. *American Journal of Psychiatry, 147*(8), 967–973.

U.S. Bureau of Justice Statistics. (1991). *Prisoners in 1991.* Washington, DC: U.S. Department of Justice.

U.S. National Institute on Drug Abuse. (1990). *Prevalence of drug use in the DC metropolitan area household population, 1990.* Washington, DC: U.S. Health and Human Services.

Vannicelli, M. (1984). Barriers to the treatment of alcoholic women. *Substance and Alcohol Actions/Misuse, 5,* 29–37.

Walsh, D. C., Hingson, R. W., et al. (1991). A randomized trial of treatment options for alcohol-abusing workers. *New England Journal of Medicine, 325*(11), 775–782.

Weisner, C. (1985). A case study of the transition from alcohol treatment to environmental concerns. In N. Giesbrecht & A. E. Cox (Eds.), *Prevention: Alcohol and the environment: Issues, constituencies, and strategies* (pp. 143–150). Toronto: Addiction Research Foundation.

Weisner, C. (1990). Coercion in alcohol treatment. In Institute of Medicine, *Broadening the base of treatment for alcohol problems: Report of a study by a committee of the Institute of Medicine* (pp. 579–609). Washington, DC: National Academy of Sciences Press.

Weisner, C. (1990). The role of alcohol-related problematic events in treatment entry. *Drug and Alcohol Dependence, 26*(2), 93–102.

Weisner, C. (1992). The merging of alcohol and drug treatment: A policy review. *Journal of Public Health Policy, 13*(1), 66–80.

Weisner, C., Greenfield, T., et al. (1995). Trends in the treatment of alcohol problems in the U.S. general population, 1979 through 1990. *American Journal of Public Health, 85*(1), 55–60.

Weisner, C., & Midanik, L. (1993, June 19–24). *The relationship of drinking patterns to drug use: Findings from the 1984 and 1990 national alcohol surveys.* Paper presented at the annual meeting of the Research Society on Alcoholism, San Antonio, TX.

Weisner, C., & Room, R. (1984). Financing and ideology in alcohol treatment. *Social Problems, 32*(2), 167–188.

Weisner, C., & Schmidt, L. (1992). Gender disparities in treatment for alcohol problems. *Journal of the American Medical Association, 268*(14), 1872–1876.

Weisner, C., & Schmidt, L. (1993). Alcohol and drug problems among diverse health and social service populations. *American Journal of Public Health, 83*(6), 824–829.

Weisner, C., Schmidt, L., et al. (1995). Assessing bias in community-based prevalence estimates: Towards an unduplicated count of problem drinkers and drug users. *Addiction, 90*(3), 391–406.

Weisner, C., & Schmidt, L. A. (1995). Expanding the frame of health services research in the drug abuse field. *Health Services Research, 30*(5), 707–727.

Wells, K. B., Hosek, S. D., et al. (1992). The effects of preferred provider options in fee-for-service plans on use of outpatient mental health services by three employee groups. *Medical Care, 30*(5), 412–427.

Wheeler, J. R. C., Fadel, H., et al. (1992). Ownership and performance of outpatient substance abuse treatment centers. *American Journal of Public Health, 82*(5), 711–718.

Wilde, W. A. (1968). Decision-making in a psychiatric screening agency. *Journal of Health and Social Behavior, 9*, 215–221.

Wilsnack, S. C., & Beckman, L. J. (Eds.). (1984). *Alcohol problems in women.* New York: Guilford Press.

Wilsnack, S. C., Klassen, A. D., et al. (1991). Predicting onset and chronicity of women's problem drinking: A five-year longitudinal analysis. *American Journal of Public Health, 81*(3), 305–318.

Wiseman, J. (1980). The "home treatment": The first step in trying to cope with an alcoholic husband. *Family Relations, 29*, 541–549.

Wolfe, H. L., & Sorenson, J. L. (1989). Dual diagnosis patients in the urban psychiatric emergency room. *Journal of Psychoactive Drugs, 21*(2), 169–175.

Woody, G. E., McLellan, A. T., et al. (1984). Psychiatric severity as a predictor of benefits from psychotherapy. *American Journal of Psychiatry, 141*, 1171–1176.

Woody, G. E., McLellan, A. T., et al. (1991). Addressing psychiatric comorbidity. *NIDA Research Monograph, 106*, 152–166.

World Health Organization. (1993). *International classification of diseases and related health problems* (10th ed.). Geneva: Author.

Yahr, H. T. (1988). A national comparison of public and private sector alcoholism treatment delivery system characteristics. *Journal of Studies on Alcohol, 49*, 233–239.

# 4

## Resolving Alcohol and Drug Problems: Influences on Addictive Behavior Change and Help-Seeking Processes

JALIE A. TUCKER
MICHELE PUKISH KING

Traditional views of substance abuse that are guided by a disease or addiction model have inextricably tied the recovery process to participation in formal intensive treatment or mutual help groups like Alcoholics or Narcotics Anonymous. Willingness to seek help is viewed as a necessary first step in a process of recovery that is preceded by denial and "hitting bottom," and entering treatment requires acceptance of the social label of alcoholic or addict, with its lifelong proscription against substance use. Conversely, refusing to seek help is viewed as evidence of denial and a lack of motivation to change that must be broken down, typically through confrontation, until the need for help is recognized. As discussed in this chapter, substantial scientific evidence questions this conventional view of recovery and the essential role of help-seeking in promoting it. This work indicates that (1) there are multiple pathways to problem resolution, which can occur with or without interventions; (2) certain behavior change processes and environmental contexts are common to successful resolutions achieved through the different pathways; (3) seeking help from formal treatment or mutual help groups is an uncommon resolution pathway; and (4) patterns of help-seeking are influenced by social processes and the nature of substance-related problems, more so than by denial or a lack of motivation for change.

A basic orienting assumption of the chapter is that the variables influencing the addictive behavior change process are not wholly redundant with those influencing the help-seeking process. This follows from the facts that help-seeking is uncommon and that interventions are neither a necessary nor a sufficient condition for behavior change. Although this distinction is not widely recognized because conventional views tie help-seeking and recovery together, separating them is essential to understanding both processes and their potential interaction (Tucker & Gladsjo, 1993). Studying how substance-related problems are resolved apart from the effects of interventions will reveal the natural behavior patterns involved in successful change and will inform the development of improved interventions to facilitate the natural forces that support it. Studying influences on help-seeking will aid the development of more appealing interventions for the majority of persons with addictive disorders who avoid or delay seeking assistance.

The chapter first discusses patterns and processes involved in addictive behavior change and then considers help-seeking patterns and processes, and discusses evidence obtained from treated and untreated samples. Both literatures have focused more on treated substance abusers and have neglected the much larger population of untreated persons with problems, a fact that, in the context of the alcohol literature, Room (1977) referred to as the "two worlds of alcohol problems." The lack of integration of knowledge obtained from substance abusers with different help-seeking experiences is a serious limitation. As noted by Mechanic (1978), we "risk confusing etiology with social and psychological processes leading to care unless the relationship between treated and untreated cases is clearly known" (p. 270). By considering together evidence on behavior change and help-seeking processes obtained from substance abusers with different help-seeking experiences, we seek to integrate knowledge across the two worldviews and have adopted a broad perspective on the addictive behavior change process that is not tied exclusively to participation in interventions. It is one that we believe is conducive to advancing understanding of the change process and the role that interventions can play in promoting it.

# PATTERNS AND PROCESSES
# IN ADDICTIVE BEHAVIOR CHANGE

## Treatment-Assisted Behavior Change

Most of what is known about addictive behavior change comes from studies of treated substance abusers, particularly from treatment outcome evaluations. As summarized here, this work has revealed the limited effect that a single course of treatment often has in promoting sustained behavior change. Although this generalization is discouraging, the lengthy follow-up assessments included in this research have made important positive contributions by illuminating previously unappreciated features of the patterns and processes involved in addictive behavior change. These features may prove important for devising improved interventions and merit investigation using substance abusers with a wider range of help-seeking experiences.

- Most interventions produce some short-term benefits for many clients (e.g., reduced substance use, improvements in related life problems), but by the end of the first year after treatment, the great majority of clients have engaged in some substance use, and many have resumed pretreatment levels of abuse (e.g., Finney & Moos, 1991; Hubbard & Marsden, 1986; Moos, Finney, & Cronkite, 1990; Tucker, Vuchinich, & Harris, 1985; Watson & Pucel, 1985).
- Outcomes do not vary substantially with the type or intensity of treatment received, or with the goals of treatment (e.g., McLellan et al., 1994; Project MATCH Research Group, 1997; Sanchez-Craig, Annis, Bornet, & MacDonald, 1984; Sobell & Sobell, 1987).
- Long-term outcomes are highly variable and encompass abstinence, nonproblem substance use, and substance misuse, often by the same individuals at different points in time (e.g., Finney & Moos, 1991; Marlatt, Curry, & Gordon, 1988; Miller, 1996; Polich, Armor, & Braiker, 1981; Rychtarik, Foy, Scott, Lokey, & Prue, 1987; Simpson & Sells, 1982; Vaillant, 1983; Watson & Pucel, 1985; Yates & Norris, 1981).
- Outcomes have a stronger relationship with client resources and environmental circumstances during the posttreatment period than with treatment-specific or most client characteristics (e.g., Humphreys, Moos, & Cohen, 1997; Moos et al., 1990; Polich et al., 1981; Tucker, Vuchinich, & Gladsjo, 1990/1991).

For example, Project MATCH, the largest comparative alcoholism treatment evaluation ever conducted, found similar 1-year outcomes across the study's three treatment conditions (12-step facilitation, cognitive-behavioral, and motivational enhancement therapy). Studies of drug treatment outcomes have similarly found few differences across treatment modalities (e.g., McLellan et al., 1994). Moreover, the commonly observed variability in individuals' substance use from one follow-up point to the next has been related to changing environmental circumstances (reviewed by Tucker et al., 1990/1991). Positive outcomes have been associated with fewer negative events and with greater client resources during the post-treatment interval (e.g., Kosten, Rounsaville, & Kleber, 1986; Moos et al., 1990; Polich et al., 1981), whereas relapses have been associated with greater negative events and emotions (e.g., Hore, 1971; Marlatt & Gordon, 1980; Shiffman, 1982; Vuchinich & Tucker, 1996a).

These findings point to the importance of better understanding the variability in addictive behavior patterns and processes over time, and how that variability relates to the surrounding contexts (cf. Miller, 1996). As discussed next, natural resolutions achieved without interventions offer an opportunity to study the temporal course, patterns, and processes involved in successful change in the absence of interventions when the influence of extratreatment contextual variables on behavior is most likely to be detected. Though previously understudied, this information is crucial to devising interventions to facilitate the naturally occurring change process and timing their delivery when individuals are receptive and in need of them.

## Natural Resolutions without Interventions

Information about natural resolutions has been gathered from three sources (reviewed by Mariezcurrena, 1994; Smart, 1975/1976; Sobell, Sobell, & Toneatto, 1992; Stall & Biernacki, 1986): (1) treatment outcome evaluations that included control groups of untreated or minimally treated substance abusers (e.g., Edwards et al., 1977; Kendell & Staton, 1966; Robson, Paulus, & Clark, 1965; Timko, Finney, Moos, & Moos, 1995), (2) large sample surveys of alcohol and drug use practices and problems that included untreated substance abusers (e.g., Armor & Meshkoff, 1983; Hingson, Mangione, Meyers, & Scotch, 1982; Sobell, Cunningham, & Sobell, 1996; Weisner, 1987), and (3) smaller sample, process-oriented studies that focused on behavior change attempts by untreated substance abusers (e.g., Graeven & Graeven, 1983; King & Tucker, 1998; Klingemann, 1991; Tucker, Vuchinich, & Gladsjo, 1994; Tucker, Vuchinich, & Pukish, 1995).

The first two types of research were instrumental in drawing attention to the fact that problem resolution can occur in the absence of interventions. In the case of treatment outcome studies, however, the phenomenon was viewed as a nuisance variable that could obscure detection of the effects of treatment and thus required statistical control (Eysenck, 1952). In the treatment literature, such "spontaneous remission" was of little interest in its own right, a fact that has probably contributed to its neglect until the limitations of treatment-produced behavior change were widely documented. For this reason, we and others (e.g., Sobell et al., 1992) prefer the term "natural resolution," which connotes interest in understanding the variables that support this naturally occurring process (cf. Vaillant, 1983).

Survey research has had a more salutary effect on the development of knowledge about natural resolutions and related topics. Surveys have revealed the help-seeking problem and the occurrence of natural resolutions, provided data on rates and patterns of addictive behavior change over the lifespan, and pointed to the influence of the environmental context on resolution patterns, which is consistent with treatment outcome research. Although resolution rates vary according to how remission is defined and measured (Roizen, Cahalan, & Shanks, 1978; Room, 1977), natural resolutions appear to be more common than treatment-assisted ones and are more likely to involve moderation outcomes, at least in the case of resolving alcohol problems (e.g., Armor & Meshkoff, 1983; Sobell, Cunningham, & Sobell, 1996).

For example, survey research has revealed consistent trends in resolution patterns related to age and gender. Alcohol and drug use is highest in adolescence and early adulthood and then declines with age (e.g., Cahalan & Room, 1974; Clark & Midanik, 1982; Hilton, 1987; Williams & Debakey, 1992), and many substance abusers "mature out" of drug misuse by mid-life (e.g., Cahalan & Room, 1974; Henley & Adams, 1973; Singh & Williams, 1983; Snow, 1973; White & Bates, 1995; cf. Winick, 1964), often without treatment. At all ages, men use and abuse alcohol and other drugs at higher rates than women (Cahalan & Room, 1974; Clark & Midanik, 1982; Hilton, 1987; Raveis & Kandel, 1987; Williams & Debakey, 1992). These age- and gender-related trends are robust and have been observed across studies that varied with respect to participant ethnicity, study location, and sampling procedures (e.g., Caetano & Kaskutas, 1995; Cahalan & Room, 1974; Clark & Midanik, 1982; Drew, 1968; Polich & Kaelber, 1985; Roizen, 1987; Sobell, Cunningham, & Sobell, 1996).

Surveys also have implicated the environmental context as important in the resolution process (e.g., Kandel & Logan, 1984; Raveis & Kandel, 1987; Room, 1989). For example, a prospective study by Robins and colleagues (e.g., Robins, Helzer, & Davis, 1975) of heroin abuse among Vietnam veterans before and after they returned stateside is a landmark in the natural resolution literature, demonstrating both the phenomenon and the role of the environment in problem development and its resolution. Very high remission rates were observed after military discharge among veterans who had used heroin and other drugs in Vietnam, and remission generally occurred without treatment. The results, summarized by Robins (1993), presaged later findings in the natural resolution and help-seeking literatures, and cannot be discounted as an anomaly related to the Vietnam experience: "Narcotic use and narcotic addiction were extremely common in Vietnam (although not as common as use of alcohol and marijuana); [drug] availability was the main explanation; . . . addiction was rare and brief after return, even when men continued to use narcotics; [but] veterans re-addicted *and entering treatment* had as high a relapse rate as civilian [treated heroin addicts]" (p. 1046).

Thus, there is congruence between survey research and treatment outcome studies regarding the occurrence of natural resolutions and the role that environmental variables play in promoting resolutions achieved with and without interventions. The Robins data also hint that treatment-seeking populations may have more severe problems than those who do not seek treatment, a theme that will be developed later in the chapter. But first, it is important to explicate how contextual variables support resolution by considering process-oriented studies of behavior change, most of which were conducted using untreated substance abusers.

## Environmental Contexts Surrounding the Resolution Process

Bailey and Stewart (1967) reported one of the earliest investigations of the life circumstances surrounding natural resolutions, in this case, among former problem drinkers who had maintained nonproblem, moderation drinking for over 2 years when assessed. Commonly cited influences on the initiation and maintenance of behavior change were health problems, a change in occupation, and increased marital satisfaction. Later research identified similar factors in natural resolutions of alcohol (e.g., Goodwin, Crane, & Guze, 1971; Humphreys, Moos, & Finney, 1995; Klingemann, 1991; Knupfer, 1972; Saunders & Kershaw, 1979; Stall, 1983; Tuchfeld, 1981; Tucker et al., 1994, 1995) and other drug (e.g., Jorquez, 1983; Perri, Richards, & Schultheis, 1977; Robins, Helzer, & Davis, 1975; Schasre, 1966; Waldorf, 1983; Waldorf & Biernacki, 1979) problems. These and other studies are summarized in several reviews that reached similar conclusions (Mariezcurrena, 1994; Smart, 1975/1976; Sobell et al., 1992; Stall & Biernacki, 1986). For example, in a review of studies of natural resolutions of alcohol, opiate, or tobacco abuse, Stall and Biernacki found that factors important to behavior change fell into life event categories of physical health, intimate relations, finances, and social relationships. Idiosyncratic "significant accidents" (e.g., religious experiences, escape from arrest or injury) also were cited with some frequency.

A limitation of many studies is that the assessment of environmental circumstances often was limited to the period immediately preceding the initiation of behavior change (e.g., the onset of sustained abstinence), which precludes the study of factors important for maintenance. Given the ubiquity of unsuccessful quit attempts among substance abusers, this suggests that many encounter circumstances that motivate resolution, but fewer encounter circumstances that maintain it. More recent studies have thus extended the assessment interval to include a several year period surrounding the typically circumscribed act of stopping alcohol (e.g., Humphreys et al., 1995; King & Tucker, 1998; Tucker et al., 1994) or other drug (e.g., Klingemann, 1991) abuse. Several retrospective studies that included lengthy assessment intervals surrounding the onset of stable natural resolutions (e.g., King & Tucker, 1998; Klingemann, 1991; Tucker et al., 1994, 1995) found that negative events decreased from the pre- through the postresolution period, that positive events increased after initial behavior change, or both.

Similar postresolution improvements have been observed in two prospective studies of natural resolutions (Humphreys et al., 1995; Tucker & Vuchinich, 1997a). These prospective replications suggest that the patterns of events found to surround resolutions in the retrospective studies bear real-time relationships with the behavior change process and are not inaccurate retrospective reconstructions. Humpreys et al. found that minimally assisted problem drinkers who achieved stable abstinence or moderation drinking over a 3-year follow-up reported postresolution improvements in occupational, financial, health, and psychological functioning. Tucker and Vuchinich found significant increases in positive events from the preresolution year through the first postresolution year among problem drinkers who had maintained abstinence or moderation drinking for a year or more. Collectively, these studies suggest that negative events motivate resolution attempts and that positive events help maintain behavior change. They also argue for taking a temporally extended perspective on the contexts that support addictive behavior change, with emphasis on the maintenance interval.

A key remaining issue is the extent to which a core set of contextual changes influences resolutions achieved by substance abusers with different help-seeking experiences and the unique contributions that interventions may make in promoting change. A retrospective study by Tucker et al. (1995) investigated this issue using former problem drinkers who had different help-seeking histories (no assistance, AA participation only, or treatment plus AA) and who had maintained stable abstinence for 2 years or more. Events were assessed retrospectively during the 2 years before and 2 years after the initiation of abstinence. As shown in Figure 4.1 and consistent with earlier natural resolution studies (e.g., Klingemann, 1991; Tucker et al., 1994), negative events decreased and positive events increased across the 4-year interval, with positive changes being most pronounced during the first year of abstinence. Moreover, it was during the first year of abstinence that interventions were found to contribute to the

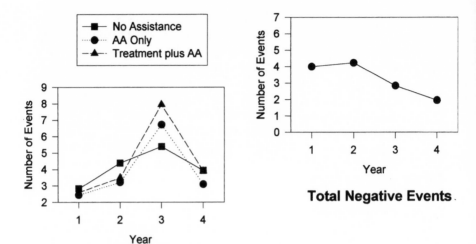

**Total Negative Events**

**Total Positive Events**

**FIGURE 4.1.** Event occurrences surrounding resolution among former problem drinkers with different help-seeking experiences. Participants initiated stable abstinence at the start of year 3 of the 4-year assessment interval. Data are from Tucker, Vuchinich, and Pukish (1995).

resolution process. The interaction with help-seeking status observed for positive events showed that receipt of an intervention, especially formal treatment, facilitated positive postresolution changes. These positive events primarily reflected improvements in social functioning and health habits (e.g., exercise and eating habits, quitting smoking).

These findings were subsequently replicated and extended by Tucker and Vuchinich (1997b), who included the three resolved groups of Tucker et al. (1995) and also included control groups of nonresolved problem drinkers, one for each help-seeking group. The results replicated Tucker et al. (1995) for the resolved participants and further showed that the pattern of positive and negative events was uniquely associated with the resolution process; that is, over a comparable period that matched the drinking status groups on the length of recall, the nonresolved participants reported increased negative events and no change over time in positive events.

Taken together, these studies suggest that, whether treatment-assisted or not, the addictive behavior change process often evolves over several years that bracket the discrete act of quitting substance use and is surrounded by a common molar environmental context. The first conclusion is consistent with Prochaska and DiClemente's (1986; Prochaska, DiClemente, & Norcross, 1992) long-term view of the behavior change process, although they do not focus on environmental variables. Interventions appear to facilitate more circumscribed positive, postresolution changes, and these help-seeking differences overlay the more general contextual changes found to surround resolutions achieved through any one of several pathways.

In drawing attention to the role of the molar environmental context in the addictive behavior change process, these findings may appear to conflict with the numerous accounts (e.g., Ludwig, 1985; Prochaska et al., 1992; Sobell, Sobell, Toneatto, & Leo, 1993; Velicer, DiClemente, Prochaska, & Brandenburg, 1985) that characterize the process primarily in terms of cognitive or other internal state changes (e.g., decisional balance, cognitive appraisal) that are hypothesized to occur in response to the environmental variables emphasized in this chapter. This is more a matter of conceptual preference than one that can be resolved fully through empirical means, and we prefer to view the perspectives as representing different levels of analysis of the same behavioral process.

What is important to recognize, however, is that the perspectives suggest somewhat different methodological approaches to investigating addictive behavior change. The cognitive-behavioral perspective typically relies on the substance abuser to identify the relevant variables (e.g., internal state changes), often without measuring the surrounding environmental contexts, which are viewed as important only to the extent that they affect the relevant internal states. This approach risks obtaining reports that largely reflect attributional processes and may obscure relevant controlling variables that operate outside of awareness or over longer periods of time (cf. Nisbett & Wilson, 1977). The molar behavioral perspective (e.g., Vuchinich & Tucker, 1996b; see Chapter 7, this volume) points to the importance of objectively characterizing the environmental contexts surrounding behavior change, while also assessing the lay epistemology (e.g., causal attributions) of the substance abuser. This allows identification of areas of convergence and divergence between the two levels of analysis, both of which are probably important for understanding and promoting behavior change.

## Resolutions that Involve Substance Use without Problems

U.S. drug policies and the U.S. treatment industry have adopted abstinence as the singular goal of interventions, but this proscription against substance use is at odds with outcomes of both natural and intervention-assisted resolutions. Evidence of sustained, nonproblem substance use following problem use has been well documented using both treated and untreated samples for a range of substances, including alcohol (e.g., Armor &

Meshkoff, 1983; King & Tucker, in press; Polich et al., 1981; Roizen et al., 1978; Sobell et al., 1992), opiates (e.g., Harding, Zinberg, Stelmark, & Berry, 1980; Nurco, Cisin, & Balter, 1981; Robins et al., 1975; Zinberg & Jacobson, 1976), cocaine (e.g., Murphy, Reinarman, & Waldorf, 1989), and marijuana (e.g., Lasagna, 1986). Even in abstinence-oriented treatment programs, moderation outcomes reliably occur in a subset of clients (e.g., Simpson & Sells, 1982; Sobell & Sobell, 1987; Taylor, Helzer, & Robins, 1986), though debate continues over their frequency of occurrence, in part because of differences in how nonproblem substance use has been defined.[1] Moreover, pharmacotherapies that involve methadone maintenance or nicotine replacement are aimed at facilitating less harmful or nonproblem substance use. Such prescribed drug substitutions are intended for short-term use as an aid in transitioning toward abstinence, but, in practice, they often are used for many years, sometimes in combination with limited use of the illicit drug (e.g., Bianchi, Maremmani, Meloni, & Tagliamonte, 1992).

The alcohol literature (e.g., Armor & Meshkoff, 1983; Sobell et al., 1996) further suggests that moderation outcomes may be relatively more common among natural than treatment-assisted resolutions. For example, in a prospective follow-up of treated and untreated problem drinkers, Armor and Meshkoff (1983) found that the percentage of good outcomes, defined as including both abstinence and moderation drinking, was similar across help-seeking groups. However, among the subset of participants with good outcomes, abstinence was more common among treated participants, and moderation was more common among untreated participants. Thus, exposure to abstinence-oriented treatment facilitated the occurrence of abstinent outcomes but did not improve overall success rates.

Probably because alcohol is a widely used legal drug, it is within the alcohol literature that moderation outcomes have been most vigorously debated and researched. Although describing the "controlled drinking controversy" is beyond the scope of this chapter (for summaries, see Marlatt, 1983; Miller, 1983), suffice it to say that proponents and critics agree that "too many reasonably good studies have noted a return to moderate drinking to conclude it never happens" (Taylor et al., 1986, p. 120). Most of what is known about moderation outcomes comes from treatment evaluation studies involving problem drinkers. In a review of 22 such studies, Miller (1983) concluded:

> Successful controlled drinkers are generally found to be younger (under 40), nonaddictive individuals with fewer life problems related to alcohol and less than 10 years of problem drinking history. Those who succeed in moderation also tend not to regard themselves as alcoholics and to not subscribe to the disease model of alcoholism. Individuals

who successfully attain and maintain abstinence have been found to be precisely opposite on all of these dimensions. (p. 22)

In a more recent review of treatment studies, Rosenberg (1993) similarly concluded that high problem severity is a contraindication for moderation but noted that severity is a multidimensional construct and that individual dimensions differ in their ability to predict drinking outcomes. Moreover, even at high levels of severity, some alcoholics can sustain stable moderation, a finding also observed in natural resolution samples (e.g., Armor & Meshkoff, 1983; King & Tucker, in press; Sobell et al., 1992).

Another qualification of such "dependence hypothesis" accounts of drinking outcomes concerns the role of patient expectations and beliefs in promoting abstinence or moderation. In a widely cited study of treated problem drinkers, Orford and Keddie (1986) found no significant relationship between pretreatment dependence levels and successful moderation or abstinent outcomes. Outcomes were instead related to clients' initial beliefs about appropriate drinking goals, the beliefs of the treatment personnel, and the compatibility of the two, thus supporting what they termed a "persuasion hypothesis." Other studies with treated (e.g., Miller, Leckman, Delaney, & Tinkcom, 1992) and untreated (e.g., King & Tucker, in press) problem drinkers similarly found that those who achieved moderation were likely to reject labels such as "alcoholic" or "problem drinker" and to view alcohol problems as a bad habit more so than as a disease. Furthermore, some studies (e.g., Booth, Dale, & Ansari, 1984; Orford & Keddie, 1986; Sanchez-Craig et al., 1984; cf. Sobell & Sobell, 1987) found that allowing clients to choose their drinking goals had positive effects on treatment outcomes. These findings argue for greater flexibility in goal setting and for client involvement in the process (see Miller & Rollnick's, 1991, approach to this issue).

## Transitioning toward Less Harmful Substance Use

Because nonproblem substance use must be entertained in an expanded perspective on addictive behavior change (see Chapters 1 and 2, this volume), we believe that it is important to move beyond debate over whether such outcomes occur (they do) and can be sustained (they can) to inquiring how they occur and examining the variables that promote or contraindicate them. Research on these issues is in its infancy, but understanding how transitions from substance misuse to nonproblem use or abstinence occur is fundamental to improving interventions to facilitate the natural forces that promote resolution. Understanding them also is central to implementing effective harm reduction programs that support an incremental, "step-down" approach to habit change (e.g., Heather, Wodak, Nadelmann, & O'Hare, 1993; Marlatt, 1998; Marlatt & Tapert, 1993). In contrast to abstinence-oriented programs, harm reduction programs recognize that drug use and drug-related problems are somewhat independent dimensions, and any change that reduces the harm or risk of harm associated with drug use is encouraged, even if it falls short of abstinence. As discussed below, such incremental changes occur naturally among many substance abusers, often in the absence of interventions.

Several studies have examined how abstinent or moderation outcomes are achieved following alcohol abuse (e.g., King & Tucker, in press; Knupfer, 1972; Miller & Page, 1991; Rychtarik et al., 1987; Sobell et al., 1992; Tucker et al., 1994, 1995; cf. Miller, 1996). This work has shown that considerable variability exists in the number of quit attempts that may precede stable resolutions and that many attempts involve trials of controlled, moderate use, even if abstinence is the eventual stable outcome. Nevertheless, in studies that investigated how problem drinkers achieved stable abstinence (e.g., Sobell et al., 1992; Tucker et al., 1994, 1995), most participants initiated abstinence abruptly over a day or so ("cold turkey"), while a minority gradually reduced consumption over months or years until enduring abstinence was achieved. These variable cessation patterns were observed in both intervention-assisted and natural resolutions (e.g., Tucker et al., 1995) and, among treated samples, abstinence often was initiated prior to help-seeking (e.g., Maisto, Sobell, Sobell, Lei, & Sykora, 1988; Tucker, 1995). The latter finding suggests that interventions often function to consolidate behavior changes that were motivated by extratherapeutic influences.

With respect to moderation outcomes, one or both of the following pathways have typically been observed (e.g., King & Tucker, in press; Knupfer, 1972; Miller & Page, 1991; Rychtarik et al., 1987; Sobell et al., 1992): (1) abstaining for a sustained interval (months to years) and then resuming limited, nonproblem drinking, or (2) cutting down gradually over several months or years until stable moderation is achieved. In addition, Sobell et al. (1992) and King and Tucker (in press) observed that problem drinkers who achieved stable moderation reported making changes in their drinking practices as part of their resolution. Changing to a less preferred alcoholic beverage, limiting the number of drinks per occasion, changing drinking companions, and drinking in different locations or under different circumstances were common.

A literature also exists on the strategies that drug abusers use to control or stop substance use (e.g., Blackwell, 1983; Crawford, Washington, & Senay, 1983; Remien et al., 1995; Waldorf, 1983; White & Bates, 1995). Much of this work was conducted in the ethnographic tradition of extensively observing drug abusers in their usual drug-taking social environments (e.g., Lambert, Ashery, & Needle, 1995) and contrasts with the focus of the alcohol literature on identifying predictors of treatment outcomes. Common strategies used to control drug use include limiting or titrating the amount of drug administered; limiting the location and times of use; prioritizing obligations to family, work, and school in relation to drug use; and budgeting ahead the amount of money to be spent on drugs. In the case of stopping drug use, frequently reported strategies include moving to another location, breaking company with other substance users, self-medicating with drugs other than the drug of abuse to overcome withdrawal symptoms, and seeking support from family and friends.

The naturalistic studies of controlled substance use, particularly opiates, conducted by Zinberg (e.g., 1984) and colleagues (e.g., Harding et al., 1980; Zinberg, Harding, & Winkeller, 1977; Zinberg & Jacobsen, 1976) provide especially compelling evidence for the social nature of influences on controlled illicit drug use. A major conclusion of this work is that the development and maintenance of controlled substance use depends on participation in a peer user group that models controlled, nonproblem use and exposes members to drug-taking rituals, social sanctions, and norms that support controlled use and discourage harmful use. In a similar vein, Maloff, Becker, Fonaroff, and Rodin (1979) identified five informal sociocultural controls that influence the use of alcohol, tobacco, other drugs, and food: (1) cultural "recipes" that describe what substances should be used in what amounts to achieve desired and accepted effects; (2) learning to use through association with "teachers" who transmit information about what, when, how, where, and with whom to use; exposure to (3) sumptuary rules that specify who is eligible to use particular substances and for what purposes and to (4) social sanctions that reinforce appropriate use of substances; and (5) everyday social relations that make it expedient for people to use in some ways and inconvenient to use in others.

These findings are informative about how social controls develop to reduce the harmful effects of drug use, and they have intervention implications. First, the data suggest that a zero tolerance approach aimed at eliminating drug availability and all drug use will retard the development and operation of natural social controls that reduce drug-related problems. Second, if substance abusers are isolated together from mainstream social groups (as they often are in U.S. intervention programs), they are likely to remain at risk for uncontrolled drug use until they can be integrated into a peer user group that teaches and socially reinforces patterns of use that minimize drug-related harms.

Another finding with intervention implications is that reducing or eliminating use of one drug is sometimes followed by increased use of another, often less harmful drug for a time before use of that drug is stopped as well (e.g., Waldorf, 1983; Wille, 1983). Wille (1983), for example, reported that some heroin addicts who eventually became drug free had a transitional period of a year or more when they used other drugs such alcohol, marijuana, tranquilizers, hypnotics, or antidepressants. A short-term analysis of the behavior change process would regard the other drug use as a negative outcome, rather than as a "step down" in the risks of harm associated with substance use undertaken as part of a lengthy resolution process. Marijuana, in particular, appears to function as a substitute or "reverse" gateway drug when individuals try to stop using more harmful drugs such as opiates or alcohol (Marlatt, 1998; Waldorf, 1983). Whether or not marijuana use is eventually eliminated, switching to it under these circumstances is a form of harm reduction.

Studying these kinds of extended drug use patterns may reveal much about the genesis, maintenance, and resolution of polydrug abuse and may help illuminate the optimal sequencing of drug cessation when multiple drug classes are involved. Research on sequencing is in the incipient stages but has received some recent empirical attention with respect to quitting alcohol abuse and smoking. In a longitudinal study of smoking cessation in relation to stable resolutions of alcohol problems (Sobell, Sobell, & Kozlowski, 1996), 48.6% of participants resolved their alcohol problems first, 40.5% quit smoking first, and the rest had more or less concurrent resolutions within a year or less of one another. The findings indicate that there is variability in the temporal sequencing of dual resolutions, but it is noteworthy that among participants with more severe alcohol and smoking habits, resolution from alcohol abuse tended to occur first.

## Summary

Research on drug use transitions indicates that variability exists in the changes that substance abusers make while attempting to resolve their problem or to use drugs in a less harmful way. Some changes are abrupt, but many involve more gradual changes in complex patterns of substance use and related behaviors over longer intervals. Such incremental changes are different from the abrupt behavior changes required upon entry into abstinence-oriented treatment programs. Existing treatments are thus ill prepared to facilitate many of the naturally occurring changes common to the resolution process and do not easily accommodate the fact that the often lengthy change process may involve periods of nonabstinence and drug use substitutions of a nonprescribed and prescribed nature. The poor correspondence between the needs and natural behavior patterns of substance abusers and what current treatments offer probably has contributed to the help-seeking problem, which is discussed next.

# HELP-SEEKING PATTERNS AND PROCESSES

The research discussed in preceding sections has advanced understanding of the addictive behavior change process but leaves unaddressed the broader issue of why substance abusers elect different pathways to problem resolution and why so many avoid using existing helping resources. This section summarizes research on help-seeking, which is reviewed elsewhere (Hartnoll, 1992; Jordan & Oei, 1989; Marlatt, Tucker, Donovan, & Vuchinich, 1997). Research on help-seeking is a recent development and has developed apart from research on resolution processes, but it is essential to increasing the scope and appeal of services (Onken, Blaine, & Boren, 1997). Chapter 3, this volume, also discusses these issues from a public health perspective.

## Patterns of Help-Seeking

Large sample surveys of the help-seeking patterns of substance abusers (e.g., Hingson, Scotch, Day, & Culbert, 1980; Narrow, Regier, Rae, Manderscheid, & Locke, 1993; Price, Cottler, & Robins, 1991; Regier, Narrow, Rae, Manderscheid, Locke, & Goodwin, 1993; Room, 1989; Weisner, Greenfield, & Room, 1995) have consistently found that only a small minority participate in formal or informal interventions (ranging from about 10% to 20% across studies). Among the minority who seek help, only about half of the services used come from the professional sector and, within that sector, care is diffused through the mental health, medical, and human services systems (Narrow et al., 1993; Regier et al., 1993). Few affected individuals receive help from specialty programs or professionals equipped to treat substance use disorders.

Outside of the professional sector, many persons seek help from family and friends or participate in mutual help groups guided by the 12-step principles of Alcoholics Anonymous (Narrow et al., 1993; Regier et al., 1993; Room, 1989; Weisner et al., 1995). Currently, such groups are the only widely available, community-based alternative to formal treatment, but they are not universally appealing (George & Tucker, 1996; Tucker, 1995). Mutual help groups that offer alternative perspectives on addictive behavior change are now emerging at the grassroots level (e.g., Rational Recovery, Women for Sobriety, Secular Organization for Sobriety, Moderation Management), but they are not yet widely available.

These findings strongly suggest that the relevant segments of the U.S. health and mental health services system, including both formal and informal helping resources, do not have wide appeal for the health care consumer with an alcohol or drug problem. When help-seeking does occur, it typically is late in problem development (e.g., Bucholz, Homan, & Helzer,

1992; Schuckit, Anthenelli, Bucholz, Hesselbrock, & Tipp, 1995), often follows the experience of multiple negative consequences and events (e.g., Brooke, Fudala, & Johnson, 1992; Power, Hartnoll, & Chalmers, 1992; Weisner, 1990a, 1990b), may involve coercive elements (e.g., De Leon, 1988; Pringle, 1982; Stitzer & McCaul, 1987), and often follows what is probably a less stigmatizing contact with a health care professional (e.g., Bucholz et al., 1992; Price et al., 1991).

Research has further shown that avoiding or delaying entry into interventions usually is not due to a denial process or failing to recognize that a problem exists but has more to do with concerns about available treatments (Marlatt et al., 1997; Pringle, 1982). Contrary to traditional wisdom about why so few substance abusers seek help, recognition of substance abuse often occurs early in problem development and is associated with the emergence of heavy (e.g., near daily) substance use (e.g., Hingson et al., 1980, 1982; Skinner, Glaser, & Annis, 1982; Tucker & Simpson, 1998). Help-seeking is nevertheless often delayed. The following section summarizes evidence pertinent to understanding why this is the case.

## Help-Seeking Processes

As reviewed by Marlatt et al. (1997), most studies have evaluated associations between help-seeking status (treated vs. untreated) and demographic, substance use, psychosocial, and health variables. This research has revealed relationships of variable strength that generally point away from an account of help-seeking based on relatively static individual characteristics (e.g., demographics, habitual drug use patterns) or structural barriers to treatment (e.g., geographic distance) toward one that emphasizes the dynamic nature of help-seeking within the surrounding social contexts.

Variables found to have modest or inconsistent relationships with help-seeking status include demographic characteristics, with the exception of gender; that is, women substance abusers are proportionately underrepresented in help-seeking samples (e.g., Schober & Annis, 1996; Weisner, 1993; Weisner et al., 1995). Heavy substance use by itself also is not a good predictor of help-seeking, nor are structural variables such as treatment cost, access, or distance to treatment facilities (e.g., Cunningham, Sobell, Sobell, Agrawal, & Toneatto, 1993; Tucker, 1995). Even when treatment is accessible and low cost, there often are social impediments to its use (e.g., George & Tucker, 1996; Room, 1989).

Variables that have a stronger relationship with help-seeking are largely social in nature. Greater help-seeking is associated with greater psychosocial problems, especially interpersonal problems, related to substance use. Research has repeatedly suggested that dealing with these problems is a primary motive for help-seeking, more so than wanting to reduce substance use (e.g., Graeven & Graeven, 1983; Pringle, 1982; Rounsaville & Kleber, 1985; Thom, 1986; Tucker, 1995). For example, two individuals can use drugs in the same amounts and with the same frequency, but it is the one who is also experiencing psychosocial problems who will be more likely to seek help. However, most interventions focus primarily, if not exclusively, on reducing drug use and often fail to address, or to address quickly enough, the life–health problems that bring many clients into treatment. This emphasis has likely contributed to the low rates of help-seeking among substance abusers and to the difficulties in retaining them in treatment.

A related influence on help-seeking patterns is how individuals' social networks respond to their need to curtail drug use and to seek help. Few substance abusers seek help without first having received social network feedback about their drug problem (e.g., Gainey, Peterson, Wells, Hawkins, & Catalano, 1995; George & Tucker, 1996; Room, 1989). For example, in a study of problem drinkers (George & Tucker, 1996), those who entered formal treatment had received consistent social messages to stop drinking and to seek help, and this consistency seemed important to surmount the stigma and inconvenience of formal treatment. Those who participated only in AA had social networks who had responded inconsistently to their drinking problems. This suggests that the alternative social network provided by mutual help groups, along with the consistent support they provide for problem resolution, is an important part of their appeal.

Other barriers to help-seeking reflect the stigma associated with substance use disorders and its treatment (Fink & Tasman, 1992) and the perceived limitations of available interventions. Cunningham et al. (1993), for example, found that alcohol and drug abusers who entered treatment did so in spite of embarrassment, concerns about privacy, and the stigma associated with treatment. Such barriers were even more pronounced among untreated substance abusers, many of whom wanted to handle the problem on their own. Other studies have variously found that substance abusers are critical of current treatments, lack information about treatment options, or believe that certain interventions (e.g., methadone maintenance) will make their addiction worse (e.g., Klingemann, 1991; Rounsaville & Kleber, 1985). Furthermore, many individuals with substance-related problems reject labels such as alcoholic or drug addict (e.g., King & Tucker, in press; Sobell et al., 1992), the acceptance of which is an early requirement of 12-step interventions, or they find other aspects of 12-step programs (e.g., the group format and testimony requirement) to be unappealing (e.g., George & Tucker, 1996).

## Implications for Promoting Help-Seeking

Research on help-seeking indicates that current interventions are stigmatizing and that social factors play an important role in promoting or discouraging their use. As discussed in Chapter 1, this volume, and by others (e.g., Des Jarlais, 1995; Marlatt, 1998), the use of stigma as a behavior control tactic is an American approach that has been increasingly questioned in countries that have pursued harm reduction policies and programs. In the United States, short of dissolving the stigma of substance abuse and its treatment (which seems highly unlikely, at least in the short run), solving the help-seeking problem will require the development of low-threshold interventions that do not require passage through gatekeeper institutions such as the health care system, which identify and label substance abusers. As discussed throughout this book, traditional treatments are most suitable for persons with severe problems and need to be supplemented with a range of intervention options that better match the heterogeneous needs and problems of substance abusers. These expanded alternatives should include interventions that are community-based, less intensive in scope, and problem-specific (Institute of Medicine, 1990).

The informal social network merits attention as a means of promoting help-seeking and behavior change. Research on how to involve network members in constructive ways in the help-seeking and behavior change process is in the incipient stages but points away from the controversial confrontational methods used to coerce clients into treatment (Miller, Benefield, & Tonigan, 1993). A promising alternative approach reported by Sisson and Azrin (1986) involved behavioral interventions with the family members (primarily wives) of alcoholics that reduced physical abuse directed toward them and promoted entry into treatment by their alcoholic spouses. Peer counseling approaches among adolescents and young adults is another application that makes use of the social network. Such approaches seem to be more effective in preventing drug problems in youths compared to the ubiquitous DARE program implemented by adult police officers (Ennet, Tobler, Ringwalt, & Flewelling, 1994).

Intervention opportunities also exist for medical personnel, since contact with them often precedes entry into substance-focused treatments. However, this typically occurs later in problem development relative to negative social consequences (e.g., Bucholz et al., 1992). Similar opportunities also exist in the legal system, but they are complicated by the conflicting nature of viewing substance abuse as a behavior problem worthy of treatment versus one that should result in punitive legal consequences.

Finally, like the addictive behavior change process, the process of seeking help often unfolds over a long period of time, and individual help-seeking episodes that seem to have no immediate effect on behavior may be part of a more temporally extended behavior pattern that eventually leads to stable resolution. In some cases, treatment may be sought not to initiate behavior change, but to maintain it (Tucker, 1995) and, in other cases, seeking one form of help may serve as a gateway to receiving another. For example, some participants in a community-based needle-exchange program went on to seek medical or drug abuse treatment through this low-threshold intervention (Carvell & Hart, 1990).

## CONCLUSIONS

The research summarized here argues for adopting a lengthy temporal view of the addictive behavior change process that does not tie problem resolution to interventions and for recognizing that help-seeking and behavior change processes, while related, are influenced by somewhat different variable classes. The major relationships are summarized in Table 4.1 and highlight the importance of studying behavior change processes among substance abusers with different help-seeking experiences.

As summarized in Table 4.2, research on help-seeking and behavior change supports revisions in several assumptions of 12-step and disease model views of addiction and recovery (cf. Pattison, Sobell, & Sobell, 1977). This work questions dominant views about the critical role of intensive treatment in the resolution process and instead reveals considerable variability in the pathways that result in stable resolutions, including with respect to help-seeking patterns and the behavior change process. Both literatures point to the need for greater emphasis on understanding the social environmental contexts that surround and influence help-seeking and behavior change processes.

**TABLE 4.1. Variable Classes Associated with Help-Seeking and Behavior Change Processes in Individuals with Alcohol and Drug Problems**

|  | Modest association | Stronger association |
|---|---|---|
| Help-seeking | Demographics<br>Habitual substance use<br>Treatment access and cost | Substance-related psychosocial problems<br>Social network responses |
| Behavior change | Receipt of treatment<br>Treatment characteristics<br>Most client characteristics | Environmental contexts surrounding behavior change attempts |

**TABLE 4.2. 12-Step and Disease Model Perspectives on Addiction and Recovery Compared with Research Findings on Help-Seeking and Behavior Change Processes**

| 12-step/disease model | Research findings |
| --- | --- |
| Development of addiction and recovery from it follow a singular course, and lifelong abstinence is essential. | Problem development and the processes and outcomes involved in problem resolution vary across individuals. |
| Largely unalterable biological factors are the main controlling variables of addiction. | Changeable environmental contexts influence the initiation, maintenance, and resolution of addictive behaviors. |
| Accepting the need for treatment and external help is a required initial step in the recovery process. | Resolution can occur through several pathways, and interventions are neither a necessary nor a sufficient condition for its occurrence. |
| Entering treatment for any purpose other than giving up substance use is a form of denial, and eliminating substance use will eliminate all related life problems. | The functional value of interventions varies across individuals, and dealing with life problems associated with substance use often motivates help-seeking. |
| Avoiding or delaying help-seeking reflects a denial process and a lack of intrinsic motivation to change. | Social forces influence help-seeking patterns and processes, and dominant intervention approaches in the United States are stigmatizing. |

Because research on addictive behavior change has largely developed apart from research on help-seeking, many questions remain about how the two processes may interact over time and how different interventions might facilitate positive change at different points in the resolution process and move individuals toward less harmful substance use or abstinence. Related questions deserving of further empirical attention concern how transitions between substance abuse, nonproblem use, and abstinence occur; the environmental contexts that surround them; and the behavioral processes involved.

Investigating these issues entails research questions and methods that extend beyond the dominant, controlled clinical trial approach to investigating treatment-produced behavior change to include naturalistic, descriptive studies of change in substance abusers with a range of help-seeking patterns (cf. Lambert et al., 1995). As discussed in Chapter 1 of this volume, treatment outcome evaluations have contributed much to knowledge about addictive behavior change, but they have limitations related to their focus on treated samples and the artificial constraints they place on the help-seeking and treatment engagement process (Moos & Finney,

1983). Naturalistic studies of help-seeking and resolution processes and outcomes among substance abusers with different help-seeking experiences are needed to complement the large database generated from controlled clinical trials (Blacker & Mortimore, 1996; Seligman, 1995). The diverse literatures cited in this chapter, ranging from large sample surveys to controlled clinical trials to process-oriented naturalistic studies, show how knowledge culled through different research approaches championed by different disciplines can converge to contribute a rich perspective on complex behavior patterns. Collectively, these findings have contributed powerful evidence in support of the major themes articulated in this book and elsewhere (e.g., Institute of Medicine, 1990).

Increased knowledge about these issues will provide guidance in developing an expanded approach to interventions for addictive behaviors. Traditional formal treatments typically have been aimed at motivating and implementing active behavior change (i.e., initiating abstinence) (cf. Prochaska et al., 1992) and help is often curtailed soon after individuals achieve their initial goals. Focusing on such a brief phase of the often lengthy, complex, and variable addictive behavior change process is a serious limitation of dominant clinical treatment approaches to behavior change. Interventions that facilitate progress during other phases of the change process are clearly needed (see Chapters 5, 6, and 9, this volume), and how best to make them readily available when clients need them is a key issue for future research.

Expanding the continuum of change along which interventions operate is a common theme that runs through several recent intervention alternatives, including relapse prevention (e.g., Marlatt & Gordon, 1985), motivational interviewing (e.g., Miller & Rollnick, 1991), guided self-change (e.g., Sobell, Cunningham, Sobell, Agrawal, et al., 1996), harm reduction (e.g., Marlatt & Tapert, 1993), and stepped-care (e.g., Abrams, Emmons, Niaura, Goldstein, & Sherman, 1991) approaches. As discussed in the second part of this book, these innovations hold promise for reaching the underserved majority of substance abusers with less severe problems who avoid existing treatments, as well as those with more severe problems who are not ready to give up drug use, but want to reduce its harmful consequences.

## ACKNOWLEDGMENT

Preparation of this chapter was supported by Grant Nos. R01 AA08972 and K02 AA00209 to Jalie A. Tucker from the National Institute on Alcohol Abuse and Alcoholism.

## NOTE

1. Data-based guidelines are available for defining nonproblem alcohol consumption; for example, Sanchez-Craig, Wilkinson, and Davila (1995) provide sex-adjusted definitions of moderation drinking. They are generally lacking for other drug classes, probably because their illicit status will always render any use risky with respect to legal consequences. This does not preclude, however, the development of guidelines that reduce other risks (e.g., health, social, and vocational risks) to low levels.

## REFERENCES

Abrams, D. B., Emmons, K. M., Niaura, R., Goldstein, M. G., & Sherman, C. B. (1991). Tobacco dependence: An integration of individual and public health perspectives. In P. E. Nathan, B. S. McCrady, & W. Frankenstein (Eds.), *Annual review of addictions research and treatment* (Vol. 1, pp. 391–436). New York: Pergamon Press.

Armor, D. J., & Meshkoff, J. E. (1983). Remission among treated and untreated alcoholics. In N. K. Mello (Ed.), *Advances in substance abuse: Behavioral and biological research* (Vol. 3, pp. 239–269). Greenwich, CT: JAI Press.

Bailey, M. B., & Stewart, J. (1967). Normal drinking by persons reporting previous problem drinking. *Quarterly Journal of Studies on Alcohol, 28,* 305–315.

Bianchi, E., Maremmani, I., Meloni, D., & Tagliamonte, A. (1992). Controlled use of heroin in patients on methadone maintenance treatment. *Journal of Substance Abuse Treatment, 9,* 383–387.

Blacker, C. V. R., & Mortimore, C. (1996). Randomized controlled trials and naturalistic data: Time for a change? *Human Psychopharmacology, 11,* 353–363.

Blackwell, J. C. (1983). Drifting, controlling and overcoming: Opiate users who avoid becoming chronically dependent. *Journal of Drug Issues, 13,* 219–236.

Booth, P. G., Dale, B., & Ansari, J. (1984). Problem drinkers' goal choice and treatment outcome: A preliminary study. *Addictive Behaviors, 9,* 357–364.

Brooke, D., Fudala, P. J., & Johnson, R. E. (1992). Weighing the pros and cons: Help-seeking by drug misusers in Baltimore, USA. *Drug and Alcohol Dependence, 31,* 37–43.

Bucholz, K. K., Homan, S. M., & Helzer, J. E. (1992). When do alcoholics first discuss drinking problems? *Journal of Studies on Alcohol, 53,* 582–589.

Caetano, R., & Kaskutas, L. A. (1995). Changes in drinking patterns among whites, blacks, and Hispanics, 1984–1992. *Journal of Studies on Alcohol, 56,* 558–565.

Cahalan, D., & Room, R. (1974). *Problem-drinking among American men* (Monograph No. 7). New Brunswick, NJ: Rutgers Center of Alcohol Studies.

Carvell, A. M., & Hart, G. J. (1990). Help-seeking and referrals in a needle exchange: A comprehensive service to injecting drug users. *British Journal of Addiction, 85,* 235–240.

Clark, W. B., & Midanik, L. (1982). Alcohol use and alcohol problems among U.S. adults: Results of the 1979 national survey. In National Institute on Alcohol Abuse and Alcoholism (Ed.), *Alcohol consumption and related problems* (Alcohol and

Health Monograph No. 1, DHHS Publication No. ADM 82-1190). Washington, DC: Government Printing Office.

Crawford, G. A., Washington, M. C., & Senay, E. C. (1983). Careers with heroin. *International Journal of the Addictions, 18,* 701–715.

Cunningham, J. A., Sobell, L. C., Sobell, M. B., Agrawal, S., & Toneatto, T. (1993). Barriers to treatment: Why alcohol and drug abusers delay or never seek treatment. *Addictive Behaviors, 18,* 347–353.

De Leon, G. (1988). Legal pressure in therapeutic communities. *Journal of Drug Issues, 18,* 625–640.

Des Jarlais, D. C. (1995). Harm reduction: A framework for incorporating science into drug policy (editorial). *American Journal of Public Health, 85,* 10–12.

Drew, L. R. H. (1968). Alcoholism as a self-limiting disease. *Quarterly Journal of Studies on Alcohol, 29,* 956–967.

Edwards, G., Orford, J., Egert, S., Guthrie, S., Hawker, A., Hensman, C., Mitcheson, M., Oppenheimer, E., & Taylor, C. (1977). Alcoholism: A controlled trial of "treatment" and "advice." *Journal of Studies on Alcohol, 38,* 1004–1031.

Ennet, S. T., Tobler, N. S., Ringwalt, C. L., & Flewelling, R. L. (1994). How effective is drug abuse resistance education? A meta-analysis of Project DARE outcome evaluations. *American Journal of Public Health, 84,* 1394–1401.

Eysenck, H. (1952). The effects of psychotherapy: An evaluation. *Journal of Consulting Psychology, 16,* 319–324.

Fink, P. J., & Tasman, A. (Eds.). (1992). *Stigma and mental illness.* Washington, DC: American Psychiatric Association Press.

Finney, J. W., & Moos, R. H. (1991). The long-term course of treated alcoholism: I. Mortality, relapse, and remission rates and comparisons with community controls. *Journal of Studies on Alcohol, 52,* 44–54.

Gainey, R. R., Peterson, P. L., Wells, E. A., Hawkins, J. D., & Catalano, R. F. (1995). The social networks of cocaine users seeking treatment. *Addiction Research, 3,* 17–32.

George, A. A., & Tucker, J. A. (1996). Help-seeking by problem drinkers: Social contexts surrounding entry into alcohol treatment or Alcoholics Anonymous. *Journal of Studies on Alcohol, 57,* 449–457.

Goodwin, D. W., Crane, J. B., & Guze, S. B. (1971). Felons who drink: An eight-year follow-up. *Quarterly Journal of Studies on Alcohol, 32,* 136–147.

Graeven, D. B., & Graeven, K. A. (1983). Treated and untreated addicts: Factors associated with participation in treatment and cessation of heroin use. *Journal of Drug Issues, 13,* 207–236.

Harding, W. M., Zinberg, N. E., Stelmark, S. M., & Berry, M. (1980). Formerly-addicted-now-controlled opiate users. *International Journal of the Addictions, 15,* 47–60.

Hartnoll, R. (1992). Research and the help-seeking process. *British Journal of Addiction, 87,* 429–437.

Heather, N., Wodak, A., Nadelmann, E., & O'Hare, P. (1993). *Psychoactive drugs and harm reduction: From faith to science.* London: Whurr.

Henley, J. R., & Adams, L. D. (1973). Marijuana use in post college cohorts: Correlates of use, prevalence patterns and factors associated with cessation. *Social Problems, 20,* 514–520.

Hilton, M. E. (1987). Drinking patterns and drinking problems in 1984: Results from a general population survey. *Alcoholism: Clinical and Experimental Research, 11*, 167–175.

Hingson, R., Mangione, T., Meyers, A., & Scotch, N. (1982). Seeking help for alcohol problems: A study in the Boston metropolitan area. *Journal of Studies on Alcohol, 43*, 273–288.

Hingson, R., Scotch, N., Day, N., & Culbert, A. (1980). Recognizing and seeking help for drinking problems. *Journal of Studies on Alcohol, 41*, 1102–1117.

Hore, B. D. (1971). Life events and alcoholic relapse. *British Journal of Addiction, 6*, 25–37.

Hubbard, R. L., & Marsden, M. E. (1986). Relapse to use of heroin, cocaine and other drugs in the first year after treatment. *Relapse and recovery in drug abuse* (NIDA Research Monograph No. 72, pp. 247–253). Rockville, MD: National Institute on Drug Abuse.

Humphreys, K., Moos, R. H., & Cohen, C. (1997). Social and community resources and long-term recovery from treated and untreated alcoholism. *Journal of Studies on Alcohol, 58*, 231–238.

Humphreys, K., Moos, R. H., & Finney, J. W. (1995). Two pathways out of drinking problems without professional treatment. *Addictive Behaviors, 20*, 427–441.

Institute of Medicine. (1990). *Broadening the base of treatment for alcohol problems.* Washington, DC: National Academy Press.

Jordan, C. M., & Oei, T. P. (1989). Help-seeking behaviour in problem drinkers: A review. *British Journal of Addiction, 84*, 979–988.

Jorquez, J. (1983). The retirement phase of heroin using careers. *Journal of Drug Issues, 13*, 343–365.

Kandel, D. B., & Logan, J. A. (1984). Patterns of drug use from adolescence to young adulthood: I. Periods of risk for initiation, continued use and discontinuation. *American Journal of Public Health, 74*, 660–666.

Kendell, R. E., & Staton, M. L. (1966). The fate of untreated alcoholics. *Quarterly Journal of Studies on Alcohol, 27*, 30–41.

King, M. P., & Tucker, J. A. (1998). Natural resolution of alcohol problems without treatment: Environmental contexts surrounding the initiation and maintenance of stable abstinence or moderation drinking. *Addictive Behaviors, 23*, 537–541.

King, M. P., & Tucker, J. A. (in press). Behavior change patterns and strategies distinguishing moderation drinking and abstinence during the natural resolution of alcohol problems without treatment. *Psychology of Addictive Behaviors.*

Klingemann, H. K.-H. (1991). The motivation for change from problem alcohol and heroin use. *British Journal of Addiction, 86*, 727–744.

Knupfer, G. (1972). Ex-problem drinkers. In M. Roff, L. N. Robins, & M. Pollack (Eds.), *Life history research in psychopathology* (Vol. 2, pp. 256–280). Minneapolis: University of Minnesota Press.

Kosten, T. R., Rounsaville, B. J., & Kleber, H. D. (1986). A 2.5-year follow-up of depression, life crises, and treatment effects on abstinence among opioid addicts. *Archives of General Psychiatry, 43*, 733–738.

Lambert, E. Y., Ashery, R. S., & Needle, R. H. (1995). *Qualitative methods in drug abuse and HIV research* (NIDA Research Monograph No. 157). Rockville, MD: Department of Health and Human Services, National Institutes of Health.

Lasagna, L. (1986). Is the social use of marijuana dangerous or addicting? *Drugs and Society, 2*, 77–81.

Ludwig, A. M. (1985). Cognitive processes associated with "spontaneous" recovery from alcoholism. *Journal of Studies on Alcohol, 46,* 53–58.

Maisto, S. A., Sobell, L. C., Sobell, M. B., Lei, H., & Sykora, K. (1988). Profiles of drinking patterns before and after outpatient treatment for alcohol abuse. In T. Baker & D. Cannon (Eds.), *Assessment and treatment of addictive behaviors* (pp. 3–27). New York: Praeger.

Maloff, D., Becker, H. S., Fonaroff, A., & Rodin, J. (1979). Informal social controls and their influence on substance use, *Journal of Drug Issues, 9,* 161–184.

Mariezcurrena, R. (1994). Recovery from addictions without treatment: Literature review. *Scandinavian Journal of Behaviour Therapy, 23,* 131–154.

Marlatt, G. A. (1983). The controlled drinking controversy: A commentary. *American Psychologist, 38,* 1097–1110.

Marlatt, G. A. (Ed.). (1998). *Harm reduction: Pragmatic strategies for managing high-risk behaviors.* New York: Guilford Press.

Marlatt, G. A., Curry, S., & Gordon, J. R. (1988). A longitudinal analysis of unaided smoking cessation. *Journal of Consulting and Clinical Psychology, 56,* 715–720.

Marlatt, G. A., & Gordon, J. R. (1980). Determinants of relapse: Implications for the maintenance of behavioral change. In P. Davidson & S. Davidson (Eds.), *Behavioral medicine: Changing lifestyles* (pp. 410–452). New York: Brunner/Mazel.

Marlatt, G. A., & Gordon, J. R. (Eds.). (1985). *Relapse prevention: Maintenance strategies in the treatment of addictive behaviors.* New York: Guilford Press.

Marlatt, G. A., & Tapert, S. R. (1993). Harm reduction: Reducing the risks of addictive behaviors. In J. S. Baer, G. A. Marlatt, & R. McMahon (Eds.), *Addictive behaviors across the lifespan* (pp. 243–273). Newbury Park, CA: Sage.

Marlatt, G. A., Tucker, J. A., Donovan, D. M., & Vuchinich, R. E. (1997). Help-seeking by substance abusers: The role of harm reduction and behavioral-economic approaches to facilitate treatment entry and retention. In L. S. Onken, J. D. Blaine, & J. J. Boren (Eds.), *Beyond the therapeutic alliance: Keeping the drug dependent individual in treatment* (NIDA Research Monograph No. 165, pp. 44–84). Rockville, MD: Department of Health and Human Services, National Institutes of Health.

McLellan, A. T., Alterman, A. I., Metzger, D. S., Grissom, G. R., Woody, G. E., Luborsky, L., & O'Brien, C. P. (1994). Similarity of outcome predictors across opiate, cocaine, and alcohol treatments: Role of treatment services. *Journal of Consulting and Clinical Psychology, 62,* 1141–1158.

Mechanic, D. (1978). Sociocultural and social-psychological factors affecting personal responses to psychological disorder. *Journal of Health and Social Behavior, 6,* 393–404.

Miller, W. R. (1983). Controlled drinking: A history and critical review. *Journal of Studies on Alcohol, 44,* 68–83.

Miller, W. R. (1996). What is a relapse? Fifty ways to leave the wagon. *Addiction, 91*(Suppl.), S15–S27.

Miller, W. R., Benefield, R. G., & Tonigan, J. S. (1993). Enhancing motivation for change in problem drinking: A controlled comparison of two therapist styles. *Journal of Consulting and Clinical Psychology, 61,* 455–461.

Miller, W. R., Leckman, A. L., Delaney, H. D., & Tinkcom, M. (1992). Long-term follow-up of behavioral self-control training. *Journal of Studies on Alcohol, 53,* 249–261.

Miller, W. R., & Page, A. C. (1991). Warm turkey: Other routes to abstinence. *Journal of Substance Abuse Treatment, 8,* 227–232.

Miller, W. R., & Rollnick, S. (Eds.). (1991). *Motivational interviewing: Preparing people to change addictive behavior.* New York: Guilford Press.

Moos, R. H., & Finney, J. W. (1983). Expanding the scope of alcoholism treatment evaluation. *American Psychologist, 38,* 1036–1044.

Moos, R. H., Finney, J. W., & Cronkite, R. C. (1990). *Alcoholism treatment: Context, process, and outcome.* New York: Oxford University Press.

Murphy, S. B., Reinarman, C., & Waldorf, D. (1989). An eleven-year follow-up of a network of cocaine users. *British Journal of Addiction, 84,* 427–436.

Narrow, W. E., Regier, D. A., Rae, D. S., Manderscheid, R. W., & Locke, B. A. (1993). Use of services by persons with mental and addictive disorders. *Archives of General Psychiatry, 50,* 95–107.

Nisbett, R. E., & Wilson, T. D. (1977). Telling more than we can know. *Psychological Review, 84,* 231–259.

Nurco, D. N., Cisin, I. H., & Balter, M. B. (1981). Addict careers: III. Trends over time. *International Journal of Addictions, 16,* 1357–1363.

Orford, J., & Keddie, A. (1986). Abstinence or controlled drinking in clinical practice: A test of the dependence and persuasion hypothesis. *British Journal of Addiction, 81,* 495–504.

Onken, L. S., Blaine, J. D., & Boren, J. J. (Eds.). (1997). *Beyond the therapeutic alliance: Keeping the drug dependent individual in treatment* (NIDA Research Monograph No. 165, whole issue). Rockville, MD: Department of Health and Human Services, National Institutes of Health.

Pattison, E. M., Sobell, M. B., & Sobell, L. C. (Eds.). (1977). *Emerging concepts of alcohol dependence.* New York: Springer.

Perri, M., Richards, C., & Shultheis, F. (1977). Behavioral self-control and smoking cessation: A study of self-initiated attempts to reduce smoking. *Behavior Therapy, 8,* 360–365.

Polich, J. M., Armor, D. J., & Braiker, H. B. (1981). *The course of alcoholism: Four years after treatment.* Santa Monica, CA: RAND Corporation.

Polich, J. M., & Kaelber, C. T. (1985). Sample surveys and the epidemiology of alcoholism. In M. A. Schuckit (Ed.), *Alcohol patterns and problems* (pp. 43–77). New Brunswick, NJ: Rutgers University Press.

Power, R., Hartnoll, R., & Chalmers, C. (1992). The role of significant life events in discriminating help-seeking among illicit drug users. *International Journal of the Addictions, 27,* 1019–1034.

Price, R. K., Cottler, L. B., & Robins, L. N. (1991). Patterns of drug abuse treatment utilization in a general population. In L. Harris (Ed.), *Problems of drug dependence, 1990* (NIDA Research Monograph No. 105, pp. 466–467). Washington, DC: U.S. Government Printing Office.

Pringle, G. H. (1982). Impact of the criminal justice system on the substance abusers seeking professional help. *Journal of Drug Issues, 12,* 275–283.

Prochaska, J. O., & DiClemente, C. C. (1986). Towards a comprehensive model of change. In W. R. Miller & N. Heather (Eds.), *Treating addictive behaviors: Processes of change* (pp. 3–28). New York: Plenum.

Prochaska, J. O., DiClemente, C. C., & Norcross, J. C. (1992). In search of how people change: Applications to addictive behaviors. *American Psychologist, 47,* 1102–1114.

Project MATCH Research Group. (1997). Matching alcoholism treatment to client heterogeneity: Project MATCH posttreatment drinking outcomes. *Journal of Studies on Alcohol, 58,* 7–29.

Raveis, V. H., & Kandel, D. (1987). Changes in drug behavior from the middle to the late twenties: Initiation, persistence and cessation of use. *American Journal of Public Health, 77,* 607–611.

Regier, D. A., Narrow, W. E., Rae, D. S., Manderscheid, R. W., Locke, B. Z., & Goodwin, F. K. (1993). The de facto U.S. mental and addictive disorders service system. *Archives of General Psychiatry, 50,* 85–94.

Remien, R. H., Goetz, R., Rabkin, J. G., Williams, J. B. W., Bradburg, M., Ehrhardt, A. A., & Gorman, J. M. (1995). Remission of substance use disorders: Gay men in the first decade of AIDS. *Journal of Studies on Alcohol, 56,* 226–232.

Robins, L. N. (1993). Vietnam veterans' rapid recovery from heroin addiction: A fluke or normal expectation? *Addiction, 88,* 1041–1054.

Robins, L. N., Helzer, J. E., & Davis, D. H. (1975). Narcotic use in Southeast Asia and afterward. *Archives of General Psychiatry, 32,* 955–961.

Robson, R. A. H., Paulus, I., & Clarke, G. G. (1965). An evaluation of the effect of a clinic treatment program on the rehabilitation of alcoholic patients. *Quarterly Journal of Studies on Alcohol, 26,* 265–278.

Roizen, R. (1987). The great controlled-drinking controversy. In M. Galanter (Ed.), *Recent development in alcoholism* (Vol. 5, pp. 245–279). New York: Plenum.

Roizen, R., Cahalan, D., & Shanks, P. (1978). "Spontaneous remission" among untreated problem drinkers. In D. B. Kandel (Ed.), *Longitudinal research on drug use* (pp. 197–221). Washington, DC: Hemisphere.

Room, R. (1977). Measurement and distribution of drinking patterns and problems in general populations. In G. Edwards, M. M. Gross, M. Keller, J. Moser, & R. Room (Eds.), *Alcohol-related disabilities* (pp. 61–87). Geneva: World Health Organization.

Room, R. (1989). The U.S. general population's experiences of responding to alcohol problems. *British Journal of Addiction, 84,* 1291–1304.

Rosenberg, H. (1993). Prediction of controlled drinking by alcoholics and problem drinkers. *Psychological Bulletin, 113,* 129–139.

Rounsaville, B. J., & Kleber, H. D. (1985). Untreated opiate addicts. *Archives of General Psychiatry, 42,* 1072–1077.

Rychtarik, R. G., Foy, D. W., Scott, T., Lokey, L., & Prue, D. M. (1987). Five-six-year follow-up of broad-spectrum behavioral treatment for alcoholism: Effects of training controlled drinking skills. *Journal of Consulting and Clinical Psychology, 55,* 106–108.

Sanchez-Craig, M., Annis, H. M., Bornet, A. R., & MacDonald, K. R. (1984). Random assignment to abstinence and controlled drinking: Evaluation of a cognitive-behavioral program for problem drinkers. *Journal of Consulting and Clinical Psychology, 52,* 390–403.

Sanchez-Craig, M., Wilkinson, D. A., & Davila, R. (1995). Empirically based guidelines for moderate drinking: 1-year results from three studies with problem drinkers. *American Journal of Public Health, 85,* 823–828.

Saunders, W. M., & Kershaw, P. W. (1979). Spontaneous remission from alcoholism— A community study. *British Journal of Addiction, 74,* 251–265.

Schasre, R. (1966). Cessation patterns among neophyte heroin users. *International Journal of Addictions, 1,* 23–32.

Schober, R., & Annis, H. M. (1996). Barriers to help-seeking for change in drinking: A gender-focused review of the literature. *Addictive Behaviors, 21,* 81–92.

Schuckit, M. A., Anthenelli, R. M., Bucholtz, K. K., Hesselbrock, V. M., & Tipp, J. (1995). The time course of development of alcohol-related problems in men and women. *Journal of Studies on Alcohol, 56,* 218–225.

Seligman, M. E. P. (1995). The effectiveness of psychotherapy: The Consumer Reports study. *American Psychologist, 50,* 965–974.

Shiffman, S. (1982). Relapse following smoking cessation: A situational analysis. *Journal of Consulting and Clinical Psychology, 50,* 71–86.

Simpson, D. D., & Sells, S. B. (1982). Effectiveness of treatment for drug abuse: An overview of the DARP research program. *Advances in Alcohol and Drug Abuse, 2,* 7–29.

Sisson, R. W., & Azrin, N. H. (1986). Family-member involvement to initiate and promote treatment of problem drinkers. *Journal of Behavior Therapy and Experimental Psychiatry, 17,* 15–21.

Skinner, H. A., Glaser, F. B., & Annis, H. M. (1982). Crossing the threshold: Factors in self-identification as an alcoholic. *British Journal of Addiction, 77,* 51–64.

Smart, R. (1975/1976). Spontaneous recovery in alcoholics: A review and analysis of available research. *Drug and Alcohol Dependence, 1,* 277–285.

Snow, M. (1973). Maturing out of narcotic addiction in New York City. *International Journal of Addictions, 8,* 921–938.

Sobell, L. C., Cunningham, J. A., & Sobell, M. B. (1996). Recovery from alcohol problems with and without treatment: Prevalence in two population studies. *American Journal of Public Health, 86,* 966–972.

Sobell, L. C., Cunningham, J. A., Sobell, M. B., Agrawal, S., Gavin, D. R., Leo, G. I., & Singh, K. N. (1996). Fostering self-change among problem drinkers: A proactive community intervention. *Addictive Behaviors, 21,* 817–833.

Sobell, L. C., Sobell, M. B., & Kozlowski, L. T. (1995). Dual recoveries from alcohol and smoking problems. In J. B. Fertig & J. A. Allen (Eds.), *Alcohol and tobacco: From basic science to clinical practice* (NIAAA Research Monograph No. 30, pp. 207–224). Rockville, MD: National Institute on Alcohol Abuse and Alcoholism.

Sobell, L. C., Sobell, M. B., & Toneatto, T. (1992). Recovery from alcohol problems without treatment. In N. Heather, W. R. Miller, & J. Greeley (Eds.), *Self-control and addictive behaviors* (pp. 192–242). New York: Maxwell Macmillan.

Sobell, L. C., Sobell, M. B., Toneatto, T., & Leo, G. I. (1993). What triggers the resolution of alcohol problems without treatment? *Alcoholism: Clinical and Experimental Research, 17,* 217–224.

Sobell, M. B., & Sobell, L. C. (1987). Conceptual issues regarding goals in the treatment of alcohol problems. In M. B. Sobell & L. C. Sobell (Eds.), *Moderation as a goal or outcome of treatment for alcohol problems: A dialogue* (pp. 1–37). New York: Haworth Press.

Stall, R. (1983). An examination of spontaneous remission form problem drinking in the Bluegrass region of Kentucky. *Journal of Drug Issues, 13,* 191–206.

Stall, R., & Biernacki, P. (1986). Spontaneous remission from the problematic use of substances: An inductive model derived from a comparative analysis of the alcohol, opiate, tobacco, and food/obesity literatures. *International Journal of the Addictions, 21,* 1–23.

Stitzer, M. L., & McCaul, M. E. (1987). Criminal justice interventions with drug and alcohol abusers. In E. K. Morris & C. J. Braukmann (Eds.), *Behavioral approaches to crime and delinquency: A handbook of application, research, and concepts* (pp. 331–361). New York: Plenum.

Taylor, J. R., Helzer, J. E., & Robins, L. N. (1986). Moderate drinking in ex-alcoholics: Recent studies. *Journal of Studies on Alcohol, 47,* 115–121.

Thom, B. (1986). Sex differences in help-seeking for alcohol problems: 1. The barriers to help-seeking. *British Journal of Addiction, 81,* 777–202.

Timko, C., Finney, J. W., Moos, R. H., & Moos, B. S. (1995). Short-term treatment careers and outcomes of previously untreated alcoholics. *Journal of Studies on Alcohol, 56,* 597–610.

Tuchfeld, B. S. (1981). Spontaneous remission in alcoholics: Empirical observations and theoretical implications. *Journal of Studies on Alcohol, 42,* 626–641.

Tucker, J. A. (1995). Predictors of help-seeking and the temporal relationship of help to recovery among treated and untreated recovered problem drinkers. *Addiction, 90,* 805–809.

Tucker, J. A., & Gladsjo, J. A. (1993). Help-seeking and recovery by problem drinkers: Characteristics of drinkers who attended Alcoholics Anonymous or formal treatment or who recovered without assistance. *Addictive Behaviors, 18,* 529–542.

Tucker, J. A., & Simpson, C. (1998). *Temporal sequencing of alcohol-related problems, problem recognition, and help-seeking episodes.* Manuscript in preparation.

Tucker, J. A., & Vuchinich, R. E. (1997a). Unpublished data. Auburn University, Auburn, AL.

Tucker, J. A., & Vuchinich, R. E. (1997b). *Molar environmental contexts surrounding stable abstinent resolutions achieved by problem drinkers with different help-seeking experiences.* Manuscript in preparation.

Tucker, J. A., Vuchinich, R. E., & Gladsjo, J. A. (1990/1991). Environmental influences on relapse in substance use disorders. *International Journal of the Addictions, 25,* 1017–1050.

Tucker, J. A., Vuchinich, R. E., & Gladsjo, J. A. (1994). Environmental events surrounding natural recovery from alcohol-related problems. *Journal of Studies on Alcohol, 55,* 401–411.

Tucker, J. A., Vuchinich, R. E., & Harris, C. V. (1985). Determinants of substance abuse relapse. In M. Galizio & S. A. Maisto (Eds.), *Determinants of substance abuse: Biological, psychological and environmental factors* (pp. 383–421). New York: Plenum.

Tucker, J. A., Vuchinich, R. E., & Pukish, M. M. (1995). Molar environmental contexts surrounding recovery from alcohol problems by treated and untreated problem drinkers. *Experimental and Clinical Psychopharmacology, 3,* 195–204.

Vaillant, G. E. (1983). *The natural history of alcoholism.* Cambridge, MA: Harvard University Press.

Velicer, W. F., DiClemente, C. C., Prochaska, J. O., & Brandenberg, N. (1985). Decisional balance measure for assessing and predicting smoking status. *Journal of Personality and Social Psychology, 48,* 1279–1289.

Vuchinich, R. E., & Tucker, J. A. (1996a). Alcoholic relapse, life events, and behavioral theories of choice: A prospective analysis. *Experimental and Clinical Psychopharmacology, 4,* 19–28.

Vuchinich, R. E., & Tucker, J. A. (1996b). The molar context of alcohol abuse. In L.

Green & J. Kagel (Eds.), *Advances in behavioral economics: Vol. 3. Substance use and abuse* (pp. 133–162). Norwood, NJ: Ablex.

Waldorf, D. (1983). Natural recovery from opiate addiction: Some social-psychological processes of untreated recovery. *Journal of Drug Issues, 13,* 237–280.

Waldorf, D., & Biernacki, P. (1979). Natural recovery from opiate addictions: A review of the incidence literature. *Journal of Drug Issues, 9,* 282–289.

Watson, C. G., & Pucel, J. (1985). Consistency of posttreatment alcoholics' drinking patterns. *Journal of Consulting and Clinical Psychology, 53,* 679–683.

Weisner, C. (1987). The social ecology of alcohol treatment in the U.S. In M. Galanter (Ed.), *Recent developments in alcoholism* (Vol. 5, pp. 203–243). New York: Plenum.

Weisner, C. (1990a). The role of alcohol-related problematic events in treatment entry. *Drug and Alcohol Dependence, 26,* 93–102.

Weisner, C. (1990b). The alcohol treatment-seeking process from a problems perspective: Responses to events. *British Journal of Addiction, 85,* 561–569.

Weisner, C. (1993). Toward an alcohol treatment entry model: A comparison of problem drinkers in the general population and in treatment. *Alcoholism: Clinical and Experimental Research, 17,* 746–752.

Weisner, C., Greenfield, T., & Room, R. (1995). Trends in the treatment of alcohol problems in the U.S. general population, 1979 through 1990. *American Journal of Public Health, 85,* 55–60.

White, H. R., & Bates, M. E. (1995). Cessation from cocaine use. *Addiction, 90,* 947–957.

Wille, R. (1983). Processes of recovery form heroin dependence: Relationship to treatment, social changes and drug use. *Journal of Drug Issues, 13,* 333–342.

Williams, G. D., & Debakey, S. F. (1992). Change in levels of alcohol consumption: United States, 1983–1988. *British Journal of Addictions, 87,* 643–648.

Winick, C. (1964). The life cycle of the narcotic addict and of addiction. *Bulletin of Narcotics, 16,* 1–11.

Yates, F. E., & Norris, H. (1981). The use of treatment: An alternative approach to the evaluation of alcoholism services. *Behavioural Psychotherapy, 9,* 291–309.

Zinberg, N. E. (1984). *Drug, set, and setting: The basis for controlled intoxicant use.* New Haven, CT: Yale University Press.

Zinberg, N. E., Harding, W. M., & Winkeller, M. (1977). A study of social regulatory mechanisms in controlled illicit drug users. *Journal of Drug Issues, 7,* 117–133.

Zinberg, N. E., & Jacobson, R. C. (1976). The natural history of "chipping." *American Journal of Psychiatry, 133,* 37–40.

# 5

## Motivation for Behavior Change and Treatment among Substance Abusers

### DENNIS M. DONOVAN
### DAVID B. ROSENGREN

The costs associated with formal substance abuse treatment in conjunction with relatively high rates of attrition and poor treatment outcomes have led to an increased focus on the processes and mechanisms involved in self-change strategies, help-seeking behavior, treatment entry, and treatment retention (e.g., Onken, Blaine, & Boren, 1997; see Chapters 3 and 4, this volume). Substantial numbers of substance abusers have been able to resolve their substance use problems without seeking formal treatment (Blomqvist, 1996; Cunningham, Sobell, Sobell, & Kapur, 1995; Hasin & Grant, 1995; Sobell, Cunningham, & Sobell, 1996; Tucker, Vuchinich, & Pukish, 1995), while others utilize the resources available to them through self-help groups (e.g., Alcoholics Anonymous, Cocaine Anonymous). Those substance abusers who engage in formal treatment represent only a small subset of those with problems and of those who resolve their problems with alcohol or drugs. Gaining an understanding of the processes involved in self-change and treatment seeking should help inform "the treatment course of early cases, cases considered 'unmotivated,' and cases that don't match the preferred treatment courses" (Jordan & Oei, 1989, p. 979) and lead to more appropriate and rational allocations of resources to prevention and treatment (Blomqvist, 1996). This position also is consistent with the recommendation of the Institute of Medicine (1990) that increased attention be given to those individuals having substance abuse problems who are found outside of traditional treatment settings, suggesting an expansion of secondary preventive interventions to a broader range of individuals and thereby providing benefits to a larger segment of the population than is found in formal treatment.

The purpose of this present chapter is to discuss issues involved in the decision to change one's addictive behavior, to seek formal treatment, or both. A model of motivation is presented that attempts to incorporate a number of the elements found in the self-change and help-seeking processes described more fully in earlier chapters of this book (Chapters 3 and 4). It should be noted that this model, which focuses heavily on internal, cognitive processes, is only one of a number of possible explanatory models that can be applied to motivation and the process of change in addictive behaviors (e.g., Finney & Moos, 1995; Fiorentine & Anglin, 1994; Jordan & Oei, 1989; Weisner, 1993).

## MOTIVATION: WHAT IS IT?

"Motivation" is thought to play an important role in the decision to change one's substance use and/or to seek help. Saunders, Wilkinson, and Towers (1996) noted that, while important, there is little agreement on the actual nature of motivation. This construct has been defined in a number of ways and has been implicated at a number of levels in relation to addictive behaviors (e.g., Davidson, 1996; Miller, 1985, 1989; Saunders & Wilkinson, 1990; Saunders et al., 1996). Addictive behaviors have been described as "motivational" problems (e.g., Cox & Klinger, 1988; Heather, 1992), and a number of models concerning the role of motivation in help-seeking and treatment entry have been proposed (e.g., Finney & Moos, 1995; Grant, 1996; Jordan & Oei, 1989; Saunders, et al. 1996). Many of these models have been informed by studies of self-change and the natural recovery process (e.g., Bammer & Weekes, 1994; Klingemann, 1991, 1992, 1994; Sobell, Sobell, & Toneatto, 1992; Stall & Biernacki, 1986; Tucker & Gladsjo, 1993). Such studies reveal that change is typically not spontaneous, but rather a process that involves a number of steps, the first of which is the recognition of a problem and building up the motivation for the user "trying to cure himself" (Stall & Biernacki, 1986) and "resolving to stop" (Klingemann, 1991). Motivation may be viewed either as a predisposing element or as a mediating variable in the process of behavior change or help-seeking.

Not all in the substance abuse treatment field have viewed the natural recovery process positively. Many substance abuse professionals have discounted the claims of substance abusers who reportedly resolved their alcohol and drug problems in the absence of treatment, suggesting that these individuals clearly must not have been truly dependent on alcohol or drugs, that the apparent "change" can be attributed to a diagnostic failure, that they were in denial of their problem, or that their recovery was not "as complete" as those receiving treatment (Blomqvist, 1996; Chiauzzi & Liljegren, 1993). Similarly, Miller (1985), in an extensive review of the concept of motivation as it applies to substance abuse treatment entry and compliance, noted that in more traditional views of addictive behaviors, motivation was thought of as a relatively stable personality trait of the substance abuser. Within this perspective, "poor motivation" and "lack of interest" were equated with the use of defense mechanisms such as minimization, denial, rationalization, and resistance, and were considered to be nearly universal traits among substance abusers. Although such constructs are often cited by clinicians as explanatory factors for substance abusers' failure to enter and complete treatment, and for negative treatment outcomes, variations in the conceptualization and measurement of motivation and lack of empirical research make this claim difficult to assess (DeLeon, Melnick, Kressel, & Jainchill, 1994; Miller, 1985). Furthermore, available research provides only limited empirical support for motivation as a trait (Miller, 1985).

More recent research and clinical approaches with substance abusers have moved away from conceptualizing motivation as a character trait of the individual or as compliance (or noncompliance) with treatment requirements to an emphasis on the individual's problem awareness and readiness for change (Jordan & Oei, 1989; Klingemann, 1991; Miller, 1985, 1989; Prochaska, DiClemente, & Norcross, 1992). These more recent approaches to behavior change have suggested that "lack of motivation" represents a lack of awareness of problems or is a function of the interpersonal working relationship between the abuser and therapist; as such, each of these can be appropriate targets for intervention (e.g., Jordan & Oei, 1989; Miller, 1985, 1989; Miller & Rollnick, 1991). An important clinical implication of this revised approach to motivation is that it stresses the importance and necessity of interacting with the client "where he or she is" and assisting in a process to increase motivation for and readiness to change addictive behavior (Jordan & Oei, 1989; Marlatt, Tucker, Donovan, & Vuchinich, 1997). Such an approach, which also attempts to reduce the barriers to change, is consistent with the underlying assumptions of "harm reduction" (DeJarlais, 1995; Marlatt, 1996; Marlatt et al., 1997; Springer, 1991).

Another important recent development in the conceptualization of motivation is that it is viewed as a multidimensional construct having multiple determinants (e.g., DeLeon & Jainchill, 1986; DeLeon et al., 1994; Simpson & Joe, 1993). The fact that many substance abusers who perceive themselves as having a problem are able to change on their own without formal treatment, while others seek such help, suggests that there is a *motivation or readiness to change one's behavior* that is related to but different from a *motivation or readiness to seek help and enter treatment.* In this context, "lack of motivation" is viewed not as a trait, but rather as a possible lack of awareness of a problem, lack of a perceived need to change, lack of a perceived need to seek treatment, and/or lack of interest in available treatment options (Jordan & Oei, 1989; Simpson & Joe, 1993). Saunders et al. (1996) argued that individuals who continue to drink or use drugs rather than choosing to quit or seek help are not "unmotivated"; rather, their motivation to continue using is stronger than their motivation to stop, with the positive aspects of continued use perceived as outweighing the negative aspects of use. A resultant question is what needs to happen for this motivational balance to shift toward a belief that changing one's behavior is viewed more positively than continued drinking or drug use?

## MOTIVATION FOR BEHAVIOR CHANGE

As noted earlier, a dimension important in the recovery process appears to be the motivation to change one's substance use patterns. Motivation, in this context, has been defined as the reasons individuals choose to change their addictive behavior and the strength of their desire to do so (Curry, Wagner, & Grothaus, 1990). Similarly, Horvath (1993) defined motivation as consisting essentially of the individual strongly believing in both the desirability and the likelihood of change. As discussed here, a number of factors presumably contribute to this motivation to change.

Studies of the process of quitting alcohol or drug use in the absence of treatment suggest that developing a readiness to change is seldom a sudden event (Bammer & Weekes, 1994; Klingemann, 1991; Stall & Biernacki, 1986; Waldorf, 1983; see Chapter 4, this volume). The process more typically involves a chain of events that leads to a growing awareness of a problem, a decision to do something differently, followed by a transitional phase that involves developing change strategies and implementing them. "Critical events" or "triggers" that appear to precipitate a sudden change might better be viewed as the "straw that broke the camel's back," that is, as a gradual, cumulative build up of negative events capped off by an event that otherwise might not have been considered important, but that serves to initiate the change process (Jordan & Oei, 1989; Oppenheimer, Sheehan, & Taylor, 1988; Sobell, Sobell, Toneatto, & Leo, 1993).

The gradual aggravation of the negative effects of alcohol and drug use on the social and/or physical domains of the person's life describes the classic form of "hitting bottom" (Jellinek, 1952; Klingemann, 1991). While this traditional notion of "hitting bottom" and perceiving a loss of control over one's addictive behavior has often been reported as a reason for entertaining the need for change and has been thought to be a necessary component in recovery (Bammer & Weekes, 1994; Cunningham, Sobell, Sobell, & Gaskin, 1994; Klingemann, 1991), this represents only one of a number of patterns of events that lead to problem awareness or motivation. Klingemann (1991), for instance, suggests that the motivation to change may be prompted specifically by negative experiences and/or by qualitatively changed life perspectives or positive experiences. It further appears that the change process results from an interaction of environmental influences, including negative events and adverse consequences related to substance use, attitudinal changes, and a reorientation of one's behavior in relationship to substance use (Blomqvist, 1996).

At least two common themes are found across these multiple pathways to problem awareness. First, in each case, there appears to have been some actual or feared negative event or loss, or some actual or anticipated positive life change. Second, a cognitive reflection and appraisal process appears to be involved in moderating the impact of such events (Hartnoll, 1992). Although this is not universal among all individuals who quit problem substance use (Tuchfeld, 1981; Tucker et al., 1995) and the relative impact of the events themselves versus the individual's reaction to them is still open to some debate (Blomqvist, 1996), many individuals appraise negative life events as either significant personal losses or strong emotional conflicts between their current life situation and a desired situation or valued goals (Klingemann, 1991). It appears to be the functional meaning that the person attaches to such events, rather than the number or type of events experienced, that differentiates between individuals who resolved their substance abuse problems on their own and those who did not (Klingemann, 1994; Ludwig, 1985). Clearly, those events that are appraised by the individual as having the greatest perceived personal impact, regardless of the frequency of occurrence, will have the most bearing on motivating behavior change (Oppenheimer et al., 1988), although their relationship to help-seeking among substance abusers is more equivocal (Marlatt et al., 1997).

The appraisal process often takes the form of weighing the "pros and cons" of continuing to use drugs (Horvath, 1993; Powell, Bradley, & Gray, 1992; Powell et al., 1993); it also may involve an evaluation of the perceived benefits and consequences associated with reducing or stopping drug use fully (Cunningham et al., 1994; Cunningham, Sobell, Gavin, & Sobell, 1997; Klingemann, 1991; Rollnick, Morgan, & Heather, 1996; Solomon & Annis, 1989, 1990). Powell et al. (1992), for instance, found a number of components that defined both the pros and cons of continued opiate use. The "pros" of continued use included the perceived benefits of emotional relief or escape, positive lifestyle factors, pleasure and positive drug effects, relief from physical pain and withdrawal distress, and social and interpersonal benefits. On the downside, continued use was associated with "cons" such as a general negative perception of one's self and the drug scene, a poor or diminished quality of life, concern about criminal involvement, a sense of personal failure, and pressure from others. Sobell et al. (1993) and Cunningham et al. (1995) found that this cognitive appraisal or evaluation process of weighing of the pros and cons of continued use was the most commonly reported reason given by those who resolved their substance abuse problem without treatment. The decision to change one's drinking or drug use pattern thus appears to be motivated in part by the appraisal that the negative consequences of continued use outweigh its perceived benefits. Furthermore, Rollnick, et al. (1996) and Cunningham et al. (1997) have found that measures of outcome expectancies concerning the pros and cons of stopping use or reducing drinking were related to treatment outcomes.

A variable class related to the pros and cons of use and potentially contributing to the change process is substance-related outcome expectancies (e.g., Brown, 1993; Goldman, Brown, & Christiansen, 1987; Oei & Baldwin, 1994). Initial work in this area focused on the perceived positive outcomes that individuals anticipate from alcohol and drug use, including physiological, emotional, behavioral, and interpersonal effects. More recently, interest has increased in the role of negative, substance-related outcome expectancies as a source of motivation in behavior change (e.g., McMahon & Jones, 1993). In particular, it is suggested that the negative experiences and aversive consequences associated with substance use are translated into negative expectancies concerning the anticipated effects of continued use. Much like the "pros" associated with substance use, the positive expectancies are presumed to motivate continued substance use and to reflect the possible reasons for using; the negative expectancies, similar to the "cons," are thought to serve as a disincentive for continued use and to reflect the reasons for restraining or stopping use (McMahon & Jones, 1993).

Components of both positive and negative expectancies have been found to predict relapse among alcohol abusers following treatment, with relapses being associated with positive expectancies and longer periods of abstinence or moderation being associated with negative expectancies (Jones & McMahon, 1994) . Also, McMahon and Jones (1996) found that measures of alcohol abusers' negative expectancies about alcohol consumption and their readiness to change their drinking were both predictive of the time to relapse following treatment. Individuals who held more negative alcohol-related outcome expectancies or those who were assessed as being in more advanced stages of readiness to change (each presumed to reflect higher levels of motivation to stop drinking) had a significantly longer time between treatment and taking a first drink than did those who held fewer negative expectancies or who were at less advanced stages of readiness to change (McMahon & Jones, 1996). Interestingly, the measures of readiness to change and negative outcome expectancies were relatively independent, suggesting that these two constructs may reflect somewhat different aspects of, and make independent contributions to, the motivation to change drinking behavior.

While similarities exist across alcohol and drug abusers in factors found to contribute to the development of problem awareness and readiness to change process (e.g., Abellanas & McLellan, 1993; Blomqvist, 1996; Klingemann, 1991; Stall & Biernacki, 1986), there also appears to be some degree of specificity of factors as a function of the drug of abuse. Klingemann (1991), for instance, found that cognitive appraisal and consciousness-raising components were more notable among heroin addicts than among alcoholics, and decisions to change among heroin addicts were influenced relatively more by social factors. There also are reports of a minority of substance abusers who have successfully reduced or resolved their problem, usually gradually, without having made an initial deliberate decision to change; instead, the commitment to maintain the change appears to have developed during or after its occurrence (e.g., King & Tucker, in press; Waldorf, 1983).

Based upon the apparent process and pattern of change associated with natural recovery from substance abuse problems, a number of authors have suggested a sequential or stage process. Tuchfeld (1981), for instance, suggested multiple steps in the recovery process: problem recognition, disengagement, initial changes in substance use behaviors, and sustained resolution or maintenance. Similarly, Klingemann (1991, 1992) suggested three primary stages: motivation, action, and maintenance. With some exceptions and qualifications (see Chapter 6, this volume), the stages of motivation and self-change found in the natural recovery process are broadly consistent with the theoretical model of change developed by Prochaska and DiClemente (DiClemente, 1991; Prochaska & DiClemente, 1986; Prochaska et al., 1992), which includes the stages of precontemplation, contemplation, preparation, and action. In the precontemplation stage, the person may not be aware of a problem or that change is needed or desirable. Based on increased self-evaluation, the individual gains awareness of a problem during the contemplation stage but has not yet committed to change; this consideration of behavior change may or may not lead to a commitment to change and preparation to do so. In the action stage, the individual initiates behavior change with or without the assistance of external interventions (Prochaska et al., 1992).

The relationship of the stages of readiness to change to alcohol or drug treatment entry has not been investigated adequately (Carney & Kivlahan, 1995; DiClemente & Hughes, 1990; Isenhart, 1994). Initial work in this area, such as that of Rollnick et al. (1996), found a positive relationship between treatment outcome expectancies (e.g., the belief that treatment will or will not result in positive and desired outcomes), evaluations of the perceived costs and benefits of reducing or stopping drinking, and the stage of readiness to change. Individuals in the preparation stage had more positive expectations about treatment than did those in the contemplation stage, who in turn had more positive expectations than those in the precontemplation stage. Prochaska et al. (1994) similarly found that progression through the stages of readiness to change involved an increasing awareness of the advantages of behavior change and decreasing concern about the disadvantages.

Based on the research on natural recovery, Figure 5.1 depicts the relationship of the appraisal process to the decision to change substance use behavior. Although more hypothetical, the figure also depicts the suggested influence of interpersonal and psychological functioning, social resources, and available coping skills. It is assumed that individuals who are able to translate their primary appraisal of increased problem awareness into a motivation to change and who successfully implement self-change strategies, have a number of social and personal resources, including social support for reducing or discontinuing alcohol and drug use, interpersonal skills, and affective, cognitive, and behavioral coping skills that they

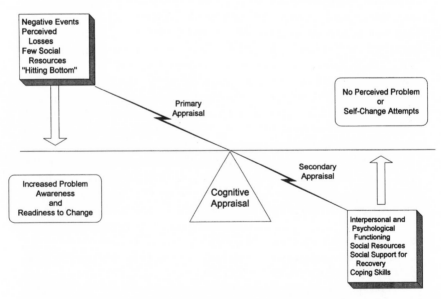

**FIGURE 5.1.** Relationship between cognitive appraisal, social resources, and problem perception: Factors in motivation to change without formal treatment.

can employ to initiate and maintain their change efforts (Blomqvist, 1996; Brennan, Moos, & Mertens, 1994; Finney & Moos, 1995; Klingemann, 1992).

## MOTIVATION FOR SEEKING HELP

Those individuals who continue to view their alcohol or drug use as a problem, who have a desire to change but who have failed in their attempts at self change, are likely to look for other avenues of help. However, as discussed in Chapters 3 and 4 of this volume, this does not necessarily imply that they will seek formal treatment. For example, Klingemann (1994) indicated that seeking treatment represents only one possible option that an individual may consider as potentially helpful. Hasin (1994) found that fewer than 10% of alcohol abusers had sought any type of help in their attempt to resolve their drinking-related problems. Of the available alternatives for help, the ranking from most to least frequently employed were physicians or medical care providers; Alcoholics Anonymous (AA) or alcohol treatment; priest, minister, or rabbi; general hospitals; and health/mental health programs. Twice the percentage of participants sought help from AA compared to professional alcohol treatment programs. This finding is consistent with those of Burton and Williamson (1995) and Hasin and Grant (1995), who found that self-help approaches such as AA were more common as an initial choice among substance abusers than was formal treatment. Also, gender differences are often found with respect to help-seeking, with men being more likely to approach alcohol treatment and women being more likely to seek help initially from medical professionals (Schober & Annis, 1996).

It further appears that help-seeking is related to greater severity of psychological, interpersonal, social, and physical problems associated with substance use (e.g., Marlatt et al., 1997), and the nature of the perceived problems may partially determine which type of is assistance pursued. Thom (1987) found that nearly three-fourths of the men and one-fourth of the women who entered specialized alcohol treatment identified problems related to alcohol abuse as their primary problem in need of change, and that gender differences existed in the types of problems motivating treatment entry. Men were more likely to identify alcohol as the source of the problems in their life (e.g., legal, financial, family, and work-related difficulties), whereas women were more likely to view their problems in terms of health and mental health concerns, and as involving the experience of stressful events and negative emotional states such as anxiety and depression. This difference in problem perception may contribute to women's greater likelihood of seeking help in nonspecialized health and mental health settings rather than in alcohol treatment programs compared to men (Schober & Annis, 1996; Weisner & Schmidt, 1992).

## MOTIVATION FOR TREATMENT ENTRY AND ENGAGEMENT

Individuals appear to seek formal substance abuse treatment only after attempts at self-change, self-help, and other forms of help have failed (Jordan & Oei, 1989). For example, Finney and Moos (1995) have suggested that treatment entry represents a response on the part of the individual after other resources and responses have failed to resolve a problem situation. As such, those who seek professional treatment represent a subset of the population of substance abusers with problems. This implies that readiness to change, while related, is different from the motivation or readiness to engage in treatment (Simpson & Joe, 1993). This process is presented heuristically in Figure 5.2.

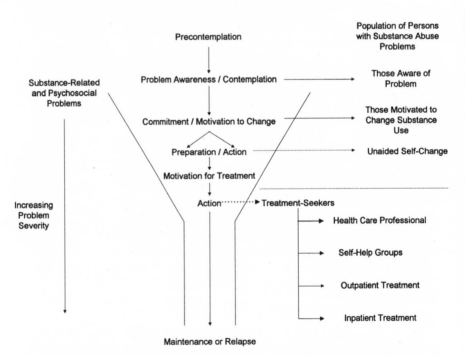

**FIGURE 5.2.** The subset of substance abusers who enter treatment: Relationships between problem severity, problem awareness, motivation for change, and help-seeking.

Miller (1985) has focused on motivation as an increased probability that the individual will seek, enter, and comply with treatment. DeLeon and Jainchill (1986) further suggested that motivation for substance abuse treatment is multidimensional and includes how clients perceive intrinsic pressures, external pressures, readiness for treatment, and the suitability of the treatment program. This differentiated view of treatment seeking is consistent with that presented by Jordan and Oei (1989), who suggested that the point at which the individual seeks some form of treatment represents a stage in a complex process that involves the interaction of internal and external influences that are affecting the individual at that point in time. In addition to such influences, the structure of the treatment system and the individual's perceptions of the accessibility, suitability, and efficacy of treatment also play major roles in determining the appraisal of the relative usefulness of treatment as an option (Jordan & Oei, 1989; Klingemann, 1994; McCaughrin & Howard, 1996; Pfeiffer, Feurlein, & Brenke-Schulte, 1991; Simpson & Joe, 1993).

## Locus of Motivation

Most clinical and research attention has been given to the relative strength of motivation, addressing the question about how motivated an individual is to change alcohol or drug use behaviors or to enter treatment. However, as noted earlier, DeLeon and Jainchill (1986) suggested that both intrinsic and extrinsic pressures contribute to the motivational matrix. Similarly, Ryan, Plant, and O'Malley (1995) suggested that another important dimension, which appears to cut across readiness for both change and treatment, is the *locus of motivation*. This variable addresses the question of the attributed source of the motivation and the reason(s) an individual is seeking to change behavior patterns or to enter treatment; that is, to what extent is the motivation attributable to internal/intrinsic factors or to external/extrinsic pressures?

Many, if not most, individuals seek treatment in response to some form of external pressure from their spouse or significant other, other family members, physicians, employers, and/or the legal system. Hasin (1994) found that such external social pressures, especially among highly dependent individuals, were significantly related to help-seeking in a population sample of current and former problem drinkers. Nevertheless, the reasons alcohol and drug abusers give for wanting to quit substance use or to enter treatment often reflect internal as well as external sources of motivation, typically in some combination rather than in a mutually exclusive manner. As an example, Murphy and Bentall (1992) found three primary factors in a measure of motivation to withdraw from heroin. The first was a "private affairs motivation" factor, which included items that reflected intrinsic reasons for giving up heroin such as "I am worried about my state of health" and "I will not have a good future if I continue to use heroin." The second factor, labeled "external constraints motivation," was composed of items suggestive of the role of extrinsic factors in decisions to withdraw from heroin (e.g., "I am afraid of getting into trouble with the police if I continue"). The final factor focused on the negative effects of heroin use per se as a motivator for discontinuing use (e.g., "Using heroin is dangerous" and "I no longer like using it"). Similarly, DeLeon and colleagues (DeLeon & Jainchill, 1986; DeLeon et al., 1994) differentiated between what they described as "circumstances," or extrinsic pressures, and "motivation," or intrinsic pressures. The former category included external factors such as losses (e.g., of family support, job, and children) and/or fears (e.g., fear of jail, health problems, accidental death from overdose) that led individuals to seek treatment. "Motivation," in this research, reflected inner reasons for seeking change or treatment, including both negative (e.g., tired of drug use and its associated lifestyle) and positive (e.g., hope for a new lifestyle, betterment on a personal or interpersonal level) factors.

Curry and colleagues (Curry et al., 1990; McBride et al., 1994) also have derived and investigated scales evaluating these two aspects of locus of motivation. Their intrinsic factors included health concerns and self-control; the extrinsic factors included social influence to stop use and legal concerns. McBride et al. (1994) investigated the intrinsic and extrinsic motivation for tobacco, marijuana, and cocaine users to quit, and found that the pattern of endorsement of each of these subfactors differed across the substances of abuse. Marijuana and cocaine abusers expressed less health-related concern than did tobacco smokers. Cocaine abusers were more strongly influenced by social pressure to stop than were the other two groups. Legal concerns were found to be the least motivating factor among the four subscales for both marijuana and cocaine abusers.

In a similar study using alcoholics, Ryan et al. (1995) measured internal and external motivation for treatment and found increased severity of substance-related problems to be associated with a greater degree of internal motivation. Ryan et al. suggested that such internalized motivation incorporates a personal commitment to change and a desire to change based in part on guilt and anxiety over one's substance use. Internalized motivation was negatively related to external pressures and positively related to interpersonal help-seeking (e.g., a motivation and willingness to share problems and relate to others during the course of treatment) and to the level of confidence one had in positive treatment effects. Those individuals characterized as internally motivated also were rated by clinicians, who were blind to the assessment scores, as more positively motivated and more engaged in treatment than were those who were classified as more externally motivated.

Locus of motivation may contribute to the type of treatment sought. Murphy and Bentall (1992), for instance, found that individuals who entered inpatient detoxification units to assist them in withdrawing from heroin had higher scores on both intrinsic and extrinsic measures of motivation than did those who attended outpatient community drug teams. Among the clients who were treated in an outpatient setting, those who primarily received psychosocial counseling had relatively higher scores on intrinsic motivation, whereas those who primarily received methadone treatment had higher scores on the extrinsic motivation factor.

The locus of motivation also may affect treatment engagement and retention. For example, in Ryan et al.'s (1995) research, the level of internal motivation at treatment intake predicted greater patient involvement and retention in an 8-week outpatient alcoholism treatment program. Clients were subsequently classified into one of four groups based on their level of internal and external motivation at intake. Clients high in *both* internal and external motivation showed the best attendance and treatment retention, while those low in internal motivation, regardless of their level of external motivation, had the poorest outcomes. Ryan et al. observed that while some sources of motivation appear external to an outside observer, the functional meaning of the external events that lead one to seek treatment may, in fact, have been incorporated as internal motivation. They further suggested that treatment may serve to help shift individuals' perception of causality from external to internal, as well as to move them along the stages of change.

The possibility of treatment shifting the locus of causality is supported by a qualitative analysis of responses given by methadone maintenance clients who had successfully completed a relapse prevention group to which they had been mandated because of continued cocaine use (Lovejoy et al., 1995). One of the main themes in the clients' perceived personal change was a shift from extrinsic to intrinsic motivation for treatment and increased motivation to stop using. Nearly two-thirds of the clients who completed the program indicated that they had been resistant and highly ambivalent at the start. Over half reported that while they had wanted to cut down on their drug use when they had entered the program, they initially had little faith that the program could help them, or felt that the staff did not really care about them. The great majority of clients (88%) reported becoming increasingly motivated for treatment over time, with growing attachment to their therapists being a major factor in this process. Another influential factor was the consistent positive regard that they received from their therapists, even when their attendance was sporadic or when they continued to use cocaine. Many clients indicated that they might otherwise have dropped out of treatment for fear of being punished or shamed for their noncompliance. Finally, patients reported becoming increasingly motivated to stop using cocaine, primarily because they had become more aware of the negative consequences of cocaine use and had more confidence in their ability to cut down or abstain. Lovejoy et al. (1995) suggested that, from a stages of change perspective, most clients likely entered the program in the precontemplation or contemplation stages, and the course of treatment appeared helpful in moving them through the preparation stage to the action stage. The progression of readiness to change appears to have been paralleled by a shift from little or no intrinsic motivation for treatment to clients' active use of treatment to implement positive changes in their cocaine use and other problem areas.

Finally, the utility of motivational measures in predicting behavior change outcomes is more equivocal and underresearched. McBride et al. (1994) found that the relative ratio of intrinsic to extrinsic motivation did not predict abstinence from marijuana or cocaine at a 3-month follow-up. However, DeLeon and colleagues (DeLeon & Jainchill, 1986; DeLeon et al., 1994) found that items derived from an intrinsic motivation scale predicted short-term retention in a therapeutic community setting, whereas no items from an external circumstances scale were predictive. However, measures of perceived need, readiness for treatment, and treatment suitability were found to be equally predictive, suggesting that these different measures may all reflect the same underlying construct to some considerable degree. The results suggest, nevertheless, that motivation should be conceptualized and assessed as a multivariate construct.

## Mandated Treatment

These findings about the possible shift in locus of causality and the progression across stages of readiness are particularly heartening for those who work with individuals mandated to treatment by the court or other agencies. It is commonly assumed that substance abusers in general, and especially those who are coerced into treatment, particularly by the courts for some substance-related offense, are not motivated for treatment, are less likely to comply with treatment recommendations, are more likely to drop out of treatment, and have poorer overall outcomes. Such individuals are often viewed by treatment staff as merely "putting in their time," with little likelihood of clinical benefit. This conventional wisdom is predicated on the belief that substance abusers cannot be helped until they "want to change" and that they have to be intrinsically motivated at the point of treatment entry if they are to engage in, comply with, and benefit from treatment (Hartnoll, 1992).

Fortunately, this does not appear to be the case (see reviews by DeLeon, 1988; Stitzer & McCaul, 1987). In addition to the apparent shift from an external to an internal locus of motivation, Wells-Parker (1994) noted that, on closer examination, it may be difficult to distinguish those who enter treatment voluntarily from those who are coerced or mandated with respect to treatment process or outcome measures. A number of studies have found relatively few differences between individuals who were and were not mandated into treatment with respect to program compliance and treatment outcomes (Brecht, Anglin, & Wang, 1993; DeLeon, 1988; Stitzer & McCaul, 1987). Brecht et al. (1993), for example, classified clients in methadone maintenance programs as having low, moderate, or high levels of legal coercion as a factor in their treatment entry. Few differences were found between the three groups at follow-up; all had shown substantial improvement in levels of narcotics use, criminal activities, and most other measures of social function. Brecht et al. concluded that legal coercion is a valid motivation for treatment entry, in that coerced and noncoerced clients responded in similar ways, regardless of gender or ethnicity. Similarly, over an 18-month follow-up, Watson, Brown, Tilleskjor, Jacobs, and Lucel (1988) found no differences in measures of control over drinking, number of drinking days, and intoxication between alcoholics who were coerced into treatment by commitment or pressure from others and alcoholics who had volunteered for treatment.

When differences have been found, they often favor the mandated clients. Mark (1988), for instance, evaluated the effect of being mandated to treatment among attrition-prone ethnic minority group members. Patients who met the criteria for success, namely, 6 months of uninterrupted treatment in an outpatient program plus maintenance of abstinence over the 6 months, were significantly more likely to have been sent to treatment by a coercive referral source (e.g., family, job, court, welfare, or child protective agencies). Approximately one-third of patients who were referred by intervention agents who could withhold rewards (e.g., welfare checks, return to job and a source of income, return to family) for noncompliance were retained in treatment, in contrast to less than one-fifth of the patients who were self-referred or referred by noncoercive agents (e.g., friend, social agency, or medical facility). Clearly, such contingencies appear to be powerful motivators of treatment engagement.

Finally, Krampen (1989) found that drinking outcomes for up to 1 year posttreatment were related to the reasons given for alcoholism treatment entry. Participants who remained abstinent were significantly more likely to report that their work, marriage, and driver's license were threatened by continuing to drink. In contrast, drinking during the follow-up period was associated with having lost a job, having had a spouse leave, or having had one's driver's license revoked because of drinking. These results further suggest that some external pressure is necessary for individuals to seek treatment and/or stop drinking. However, the prognosis appears less favorable for those individuals who have already experienced a loss in one of these areas. Thus, the greater the likelihood of losing a valued outcome due to continued substance use (i.e., a contingency still exists), the better the clinical and psychosocial outcomes among clients who have been mandated or coerced into treatment (Mark, 1988).

## Client Factors Contributing to the Decision to Seek Treatment

As noted previously, a number of internal and external factors, often in interaction, contribute to the decision to seek substance abuse treatment. The conceptual distinction between readiness for change and readiness to seek help or treatment participation has been supported by two lines of research. First, Tucker and Gladsjo (1993) and Tucker (1995) have focused on separating variables associated with drinking outcome status (e.g., drinking abusively or drinking problem resolved) from those associated with help-seeking status, which is basic to this distinction as it pertains to longer term outcomes. As summarized in Chapter 4 of this volume, successful behavior change is associated with positive environmental changes and with greater personal resources during the maintenance period, whereas help-seeking is associated with greater substance-related psychosocial problems prior to attempts at behavior change.

Second, results of recent studies evaluating measures of motivation among substance abusers provides another line of support. DeLeon and Jainchill (1986) and DeLeon et al. (1994) developed and evaluated measures to assess the reasons why opiate addicts sought treatment, their level of motivation, their perceived need for treatment compared to other options, and the perceived appropriateness or suitability of the treatment option chosen. While these scales are somewhat conceptually and statistically related, they provided an assessment of several domains important to understanding decisions to seek care. In a related study, Simpson and Joe (1993) used three measures that assess awareness of a drug problem, desire for help, and readiness for treatment. The scales were conceptualized as assessing the progressive levels of change associated with the Prochaska and DiClemente's (1986) stages of change model, moving from precontemplation through contemplation and determination to action. While a second-order factor defined as "general motivation" was found, the three scales appeared to represent relatively independent domains.

Overall, substance abusers who have a greater awareness of their problem, desire for help, and treatment readiness are more likely to enter treatment and less likely to drop out of treatment prematurely (DeLeon et al., 1994; Simpson & Joe, 1993). Moreover, there appears to be a critical threshold above which substance abusers who experience problems choose to change, and a second critical threshold above which they decide to seek treatment as the avenue for change. Just as one weighs the "pros" and "cons" of continuing or discontinuing drug use as a component in developing motivation to change (Cunningham et al., 1994), a similar appraisal process appears to be involved in decisions to seek or not to seek treatment. Varney et al. (1995) suggested that the decision by a substance abuser to seek help involves weighing the likelihood and value of the consequences of continuing to drink or use drugs against the anticipated positive consequences of seeking treatment. The individual presumably is likely to seek treatment if the anticipated positive consequences of treatment are perceived as both likely to occur and as more beneficial than the consequences of not seeking treatment (or continuing to use drugs). As described by Hartnoll (1992, p. 431), "The decision to take, or not to take, the action of seeking help is mediated by perceptions and interpretations on the part of the drug user and important others regarding the significance of a person's drug use and its consequences, regarding the nature and availability of different options for the future, and regarding the perceived need for, and value (and costs) of seeking help."

A number of personal characteristics appear more common in individuals who seek formal treatment compared to those who resolve their problems on their own or who seek help from self-help groups like AA. These are reviewed in Chapter 4 of this volume and in Marlatt et al. (1997), and, to a large extent, as suggested by Hartnoll (1992), are related to the negative consequences of substance use, as viewed either by the individual or by significant others. Those who seek formal treatment, when compared to those who resolved their problems on their own or through participation in self-help groups, can be characterized as (1) being more dependent on the target substance, based on objective diagnostic criteria; (2) perceiving themselves as dependent; (3) possibly using substances more frequently and at higher quantities; (4) having more negative consequences related to their substance use; (5) experiencing greater difficulties and expressing a greater need for help in a wide range of life areas (e.g., physical health, psychological status, social and interpersonal relationships, finances, legal status, living arrangements); (6) often having fewer social resources and poorer psychosocial function; (7) rating their lives as being out of control; and (8) having higher social pressure to seek treatment (e.g., Brennan et al., 1994; Burton & Williamson, 1995; George & Tucker, 1996; Hartnoll, 1992; Hasin & Grant, 1995; Marlatt et al., 1997; Oppenheimer et al., 1988; Power, Hartnoll, & Chalmers, 1992a, 1992b; Timko, Finney, Moos, Moos, & Steinbaum, 1993; Tucker, 1995; Tucker & Gladsjo, 1993; Varney et al., 1995).

It appears that abusers often wait until they have experienced multiple and more severe substance-related negative consequences and are unable to manage important aspects of their lives before seeking treatment (Burton & Williamson, 1995; Oppenheimer et al, 1988). As noted earlier, Ryan et al. (1995) found that greater problem severity was associated with higher levels of internalized motivation and interpersonal help-seeking. Similarly, Burton and Williamson (1995) found that the greater the number of negative consequences experienced, the greater the likelihood of entering treatment. Only 3.8% of those drinkers who experienced one negative consequence entered treatment, but the percentage entering treatment increased to 41.6% among those who had six negative consequences. Hasin (1994) found that severity of dependence and external social pressure, particularly in combination, were highly related to help-seeking in a population sample of current and former drinkers. Each additional source of external pressure increased the odds of treatment by a factor of about 60% when compared to the odds without the addition of the extra source. Thus, treatment entry may be motivated less by the individual's interest in stopping substance use, per se, than by their perception of the negative consequences of use and a desire to resolve problems with significant others (Tucker & Gladsjo, 1993; Varney et al., 1995).

## PROGRAMMATIC FACTORS INFLUENCING TREATMENT SEEKING

### Treatment Availability and Perceived Efficacy

Another important factor in the help-seeking process is the substance abuser's level of awareness and evaluation of available treatment services. Hartnoll (1992) suggested that an individual's cognitions, motivation, and decision making are influenced by knowledge of treatment alternatives, perceptions of their relative usefulness, and the relative costs (financial and psychological) of seeking treatment. While lack of such objective information may contribute to individuals not seeking treatment, this appears to be a relatively small factor in comparison with other potential influences (Carroll & Rounsaville, 1992; Cunningham, Sobell, Sobell, Agrawal, & Toneatto, 1993; Klingemann, 1991). Overall, the pattern of findings suggests that most substance abusers have some knowledge about available community resources if they were to choose to pursue treatment.

A potentially more important factor contributing to individuals delaying or never seeking treatment appears to reflect negative views of treatment and its effectiveness. Klingemann (1991), for example, found that those who recovered from alcohol or drug problems without treatment were indifferent to or openly critical of treatment. Although aware of available treatment alternatives, about half of the informed respondents criticized professional treatment, refused it for emotional reasons, or chose not to consider such treatment as a matter of principle. These views reflected their sense that they wanted, and that it was possible, to handle their problems on their own; that they would feel embarrassed or have their pride hurt by entering treatment; that there would be a negative stigma attached to them if they were to enter treatment; that treatment would be filled with moral lectures and pressure; that they would have difficulty sharing their problems with others; that treatment was irrelevant to their self-change plans; and that treatment was of questionable effectiveness, either in general or for the individual specifically (Cunningham et al., 1993; Klingemann, 1991; Lovaglia & Matano, 1994; Tucker, 1995).

Within this context, individuals may have high motivation to change but hold negative views about treatment and its efficacy, or feel that there is a mismatch between a particular treatment modality and their needs from and expectations of treatment (DeLeon et al., 1994). When compared to other alternatives, such as self-change or getting help from other sources (such as friends and family or through geographical relocation), treatment is not considered a viable option at the time of decision making. Thus, the perceived personal and psychological costs of treatment, per se, may be sufficiently steep to deter many substance abusers from seeking help.

In contrast, a positive appraisal of treatment and its efficacy is associated with treatment seeking and entry. Jordan and Oei (1989) noted the importance of individuals' beliefs about treatment being effective and deciding that treatment can help as being important influences on their seeking treatment. Similarly, Simpson and Joe (1993) suggested that increased motivation for treatment may be associated with expectations for treatment success. This relationship was demonstrated by Pfeiffer et al. (1991), who found that alcoholics who entered treatment were significantly more positive about the general consequences of starting treatment, considered their problem to be more harmful and uncontrollable, had more prior episodes of seeking help, were noticeably more conscious of negative consequences to themselves and others caused by their substance abuse, and were more positive in their expectations of treatment success. The results of a multivariate discriminate analysis indicated that the most important factor distinguishing between those who either did or did not enter treatment was their expectation of treatment success.

## Perceived Barriers to Treatment

A number of other real or perceived physical or psychological barriers may moderate the relationship between the motivation to change and readiness for treatment. Schober and Annis (1996) defined "barriers" as the reasons people have for not utilizing specialized addiction treatment services or not modifying their alcohol- or drug-related problem behaviors. Barriers, and the individual's appraisal of them, are thought to affect the decision-making process by inhibiting the motivation to change substance abuse behaviors (Schober & Annis, 1996) and by contributing to delaying or not seeking treatment (Brooke, Fudala, & Johnson, 1992; Cunningham et al., 1993; George & Tucker, 1996; Oppenheimer et al., 1988; Sheehan, Oppenheimer, & Taylor, 1986; Tucker, 1995). While the cognitive appraisal process may increase an individual's motivation to change, perceived barriers may lead to a rejection of treatment as a viable alternative (Cunningham et al., 1994). Some of these barriers may be more gender-specific (Allen, 1994; Allen & Dixon, 1994; Schutz, Rapti, Vlahov, & Anthony, 1994; Schober & Annis, 1996; Smith, 1992; Thom, 1987), such as concerns about treatment costs and how these will be covered, the need to be away from significant others and the normal social roles of parent or partner, needs for child care while in treatment, and concerns about being away from work (Allen & Dixon, 1994). Although endorsed less frequently than other reasons, a number of such perceived barriers to treatment, when endorsed, were rated as having a relatively high degree of impact on the decision to delay seeking treatment (Cunningham et al., 1993).

The pattern of findings related to the characteristics of those who seek treatment, as well as the possible processes involved in the decision to do so, leads to a heuristic depiction of the factors contributing to treatment seeking, presented in Figure 5.3. Not only do self-changers want to and feel as if they can manage their own problems, they have been described as adopting a wide variety of change strategies and implementing a plan and specific steps to control or discontinue their substance use (Hartnoll, 1992; Klingemann, 1991). Not viewing self-change as a viable option, or having been unsuccessful in prior attempts, a substance abuser may view treatment as one or, potentially, as the only, avenue for change (DeLeon & Jainchill, 1986; DeLeon et al., 1994). Those in treatment often report that they have a greater number of, or more pressing, concerns and express a greater need for help in a variety of life areas when compared to self-changers. Simpson and Joe (1993), for instance, found that a greater desire and perceived need for help were significantly related to entrance into and short-term retention in methadone maintenance. Those who enter treatment, in addition to experiencing more difficult problems, may have fewer social and interpersonal resources and reduced problem solving abilities, or their social networks may strongly support behavior change and treatment entry (e.g., George & Tucker, 1996). Conceivably, this balance of perceived need for help, despite the deterrent effects of perceived barriers and the strong desire for help in the absence of other

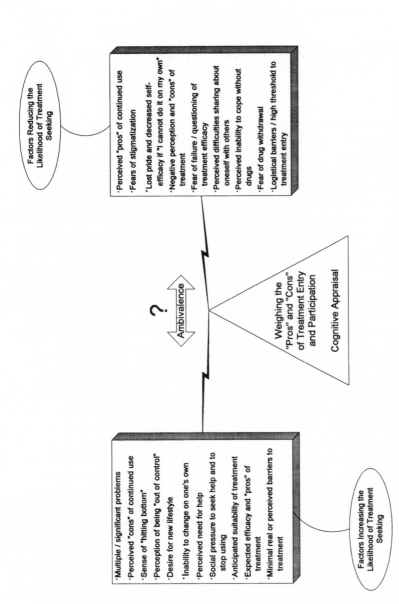

**Factors Reducing the Likelihood of Treatment Seeking**

- Perceived "pros" of continued use
- Fears of stigmatization
- Lost pride and decreased self-efficacy if "I cannot do it on my own"
- Negative perception and "cons" of treatment
- Fear of failure / questioning of treatment efficacy
- Perceived difficulties sharing about oneself with others
- Perceived inability to cope without drugs
- Fear of drug withdrawal
- Logistical barriers / high threshold to treatment entry

?

Ambivalence

Weighing the "Pros" and "Cons" of Treatment Entry and Participation

Cognitive Appraisal

**Factors Increasing the Likelihood of Treatment Seeking**

- Multiple / significant problems
- Perceived "cons" of continued use
- Sense of "hitting bottom"
- Perception of being "out of control"
- Desire for new lifestyle
- Inability to change on one's own
- Perceived need for help
- Social pressure to seek help and to stop using
- Anticipated suitability of treatment
- Expected efficacy and "pros" of treatment
- Minimal real or perceived barriers to treatment

**FIGURE 5.3.** Balancing the "pros" and "cons" of treatment entry and participation: Moving from readiness to change to readiness for treatment.

avenues to assume personal control, translates readiness for change into readiness for treatment.

## FUTURE DIRECTIONS AND IMPLICATIONS FOR ADDICTIONS RESEARCH, POLICY, AND PROGRAM DEVELOPMENT

Clearly, motivation or readiness to change, to seek help, and to seek treatment represent important components of the change process for many substance abusers. However, it is important to keep in mind that motivation represents only one class of variables that enters into the behavior change process and that influences the process and outcome of treatment. For example, Simpson and Joe (1993) pointed out that while motivation contributes unique variance to the prediction of treatment outcomes, it should be considered in the broader context of, and in conjunction with, several background, psychological, peer, social, and expectation variables. Similarly, Schober and Annis (1996) conceptualized addictive behavior change as a process mediated by several interacting factors, including (1) a person's background characteristics, such as gender and substance abuse history; (2) stage of change or motivation to produce positive behavior change; and (3) a decision-making process involving health beliefs and appraisals, such as outcome and self-efficacy expectancies, reasons for change, and barriers to change.

The concept of motivation is becoming more refined and differentiated, but there are a number of areas in need of further research. First, it is important that work continue on the development and validation of measures of motivation for change and for treatment and that this research be generalized across a range of drugs and alternatives to treatment (e.g., Rollnick et al., 1996; Cunningham et al., 1997; DeLeon et al., 1994).

Second, although many clinicians and researchers continue to consider motivation, at least in their assessment models, as a static variable (Murphy & Bentall, 1992), motivation appears to be a dynamic process that will vary across time and be moderated by a number of intrinsic and extrinsic factors (McBride et al., 1994; Miller, 1985; Prochaska et al., 1992). It is thus recommended that future research investigate the extent and structure of clients' motivation across time (Murphy & Bentall, 1992; Schober & Annis, 1996). Further work is needed to explore the relationship between motivation or readiness for change and motivation to seek treatment, as well variables that may moderate this relationship.

Third, considerable research has investigated the relationship between the role of expectancies concerning alcohol's effects and their influence on drinking behavior and treatment outcome (e.g., Goldman et al., 1987). However, corresponding work on the role of drug-effect expectancies has lagged behind work in the alcohol abuse area (Brown, 1993; Schafer & Brown, 1991). The relationship between positive and negative alcohol- and drug-related expectancies and indices of readiness to change needs to be explored further (e.g., McMahon & Jones, 1996). Weighing the positive expectancies ("pros") against anticipated or experienced proximal and distal negative outcomes ("cons") may be an important component in the process that leads an individual to perceive a need for behavior change and/or for treatment entry (e.g., Cunningham et al., 1994; Powell et al., 1992, 1993).

Fourth, Burton and Williamson (1995), among others, have noted that approximately 90% of individuals who have suffered a negative consequence from alcohol do not seek treatment. It is only after they experience multiple consequences that they seek help. These authors stress that in order to determine factors that contribute to this decision, it will be important to include both those who receive treatment and those who do not (cf. Tucker & Gladsjo, 1993). Recent advances in methodology, such as the inclusion of groups who have or have not resolved their substance use problems, and groups who did so on their own or through self-help groups, or through formal treatment (e.g., Sobell et al., 1993; Tucker & Gladsjo, 1993; Tucker et al., 1995), have allowed investigation of factors that influence help-seeking and recovery, while preventing erroneous conclusions about the relationship between recovery and a number of variable classes, including but not limited to help-seeking status (Sobell et al., 1993). Burton and Williamson (1995) also suggested that in addition to exploring substance abusers' reasons for seeking treatment or not, future studies should investigate whether, and how, the severity of associated harm influences the likelihood of seeking treatment.

Fifth, the motivations that substance abusers have for seeking help, including the intrinsic versus extrinsic locus of their motivation, are often assumed to influence the course and outcome of treatment (DeLeon et al., 1994; Murphy & Bentall, 1992). This assumption, however, has not been evaluated adequately (Simpson & Joe, 1993; Oppenheimer et al., 1988). Thus, relationships between level and type of motivation, specific reasons for and locus of seeking treatment, and treatment retention and treatment outcomes need to be investigated more fully (Cunningham et al., 1994; DeLeon et al., 1994; Murphy & Bentall, 1992; Oppenheimer et al., 1988).

Finally, although many individuals with alcohol and drug problems are able to change their substance use patterns without outside help, this begs the question of why current interventions are so unappealing to the great majority of substance abusers. In order to be more successful in attracting those who have need for treatment, it is important to understand the reasons for their delaying or not seeking help (Cunningham et al., 1993). This will require continued research on the real and perceived disincentives to help-seeking. Schober and Annis (1996) suggested a number of pertinent questions for future research, including: (1) male-female comparisons to identify possible gender differences in barriers to treatment and behavior change; (2) the relationship of gender to client and program barriers and help-seeking across health care service settings; (3) the impact of barriers to treatment on substance abusers who are in different stages of the change process; (4) the extent to which the behavioral effects of barriers may be moderated by other process factors during change, such as pros and cons analysis, self-efficacy, outcome expectancies, alcohol- and drug-effect expectancies; (5) whether any changes in perceived barriers occur from the time of treatment entry to completion; and (6) well-controlled clinical trials to evaluate the effects of treatment services that address the predominant needs of substance abusers.

More generally, the findings on help-seeking and treatment barriers have several policy and programmatic implications (Cunningham et al., 1993). This research suggests that treatment seeking will be facilitated if treatment is nonthreatening, has a low threshold for entry, "meets the individual where he or she is" with respect to both the degree of readiness to change and the physical location of services, and has no or minimal stigma attached to it. These program characteristics are consistent with the philosophy of harm reduction (Marlatt, 1996; Marlatt et al., 1997) and will require changes in the type of services available, as well as in how and where they are offered (Cunningham et al., 1993).

For example, needle exchange programs, developed within the framework of harm reduction or minimization (e.g., Brettle, 1991), represent a prototype of an approach that attempts to reduce barriers to help-seeking. The exchanges are typically located where there is a high density of intravenous (IV) drug users. They provide clean needles and equipment or instructions on how to clean equipment in order to reduce needle sharing among IV drug users and thus reduce the likelihood of their spreading HIV infection. Although not explicitly intended to move drug users toward drug treatment, needle exchange programs bring services to otherwise unreached populations of drug abusers (Grund et al., 1992) and serve as a conduit to drug treatment entry for some participants (Clark & Corbett, 1993). In addition to reducing barriers to receiving help, such programs can provide counseling and preventive health and drug education that may facilitate consideration of treatment as an option (Brettle, 1991) and can promote utilization of medical and psychosocial services (Carvell & Hart, 1990).

Many possible barriers to help-seeking are structural in nature and are under the control of treatment agencies, such as the availability of treatment slots and the length of time clients have to wait for intake appointments and admission to treatment. Structural changes must be entertained to increase help-seeking, and there are also strategies that can be employed if it is not possible to increase treatment access. These include providing intake appointments as soon as possible after an individual contacts an agency, even if entry into treatment has to be delayed (Stark, Campbell, & Brinkerhoff, 1990; Festinger, Lamb, Kountz, Kirby, & Marlowe, 1995), making appointment reminder calls (Gariti et al., 1995), and providing supportive services during the period when an individual has to wait between intake and admission to treatment (e.g., Brekke, 1989; Olkin & Lemle, 1984; Ravndal & Vaglum, 1992). Such changes have been shown to increase the likelihood that substance abusers who make initial contact with an agency will follow through and enter treatment.

Entering treatment does not necessarily imply, however, that an individual will become successfully engaged. Finney and Moos (1995) argued that seeking and entering treatment are only two stages of a complex, multifaceted treatment selection process. Once a decision to enter treatment is made, the treatment selection process involves the choice of or assignment to any number of intervention alternatives and the selection or receipt of varying amounts of treatment. Because many substance abusers remain in treatment for only brief periods before dropping out, developing and evaluating interventions to increase their motivation for and likelihood of continuing in treatment is a priority (Marlatt et al., 1997). These might involve motivational enhancement interventions conducted at the beginning of treatment (Allsop & Saunders, 1991; Bien, Miller, & Boroughs, 1993; Brown & Miller, 1993; Miller & Rollnick, 1991); role induction techniques that provide information to prepare participants for the treatment experience, demystify it, and provide clear expectations about the process (e.g., Stark & Kane, 1985; Zweben & Li, 1981); and case management services that provide help with the multiple other problems associated with substance abuse (e.g., Bokos, Mejita, Mickenberg, & Monks, 1992; Graham & Timney, 1990; Lidz, Bux, Platt, & Iguchi, 1992; Willenbring, Ridgely, Stinchfield, & Rose, 1991).

Understanding what motivates the addictive behavior change process, as well as the nature of impediments to it, is fundamental to developing interventions to help facilitate help seeking and successful behavior change (Cunningham et al., 1995; Schober & Annis, 1996). Empirically informed interventions designed to increase individuals' readiness to change and to facilitate the treatment entry process will be an important part of this expanded intervention initiative. As DeLeon et al. (1994, p. 510) pointed out, "External life pressures (circumstances) can influence inner reasons to change (motivation) which are necessary precursors to actually seeking treatment (readiness), and electing [a particular type of] treatment (suitability) subsumes both motivation and readiness." While the multiple and interacting factors associated with behavior change and help-seeking are receiving some much-deserved attention, research and practice in this area is in its infancy.

## ACKNOWLEDGMENT

Preparation of this chapter was supported by Grant No. R01-DA0875 from the National Institute on Drug Abuse and Collaborative Agreement No. U10-AA08436 from the National Institute on Alcohol Abuse and Alcoholism.

## REFERENCES

Abellanas, L., & McLellan, A. T. (1993). "Stages of change" by drug problem in concurrent opioid, cocaine, and cigarette users. *Journal of Psychoactive Drugs, 25,* 307–313.

Allen, K. (1994). Development of an instrument to identify barriers to treatment for addicted women, from their perspective. *International Journal of the Addictions, 29,* 429–444.

Allen, K., & Dixon, M. (1994). Psychometric assessment of the Allen Barriers to Treatment Instrument. *International Journal of the Addictions, 29,* 545–563.

Allsop, S., & Saunders, B. (1991). Reinforcing robust resolutions: Motivation in relapse prevention with severely dependent problem drinkers. In W. R. Miller & S. Rollnick, *Motivational interviewing: Preparing people to change addictive behavior* (pp. 236–247). New York: Guilford Press.

Bammer, G., & Weekes, S. (1994). Becoming an ex-user: Insights into the process and implications for treatment policy. *Drug and Alcohol Reviews, 13,* 285–292.

Bien, T. H., Miller, W. R., & Boroughs, J. M. (1993). Motivational interviewing with alcohol outpatients. *Behavioural and Cognitive Psychotherapy, 21,* 347–356.

Blomqvist, J. (1996). Paths to recovery from substance misuse: Change of lifestyle and the role of treatment. *Substance Use and Misuse, 31,* 1807–1852.

Bokos, P. J., Mejita, C. L., Mickenberg, J. H., & Monks, R. L. (1992). Case management: An alternative approach to working with intravenous drug users. In R. S. Ashery (Ed.), *Progress and issues in case management* (NIDA Research Monograph No. 127, pp. 92–111). Rockville, MD: National Institute on Drug Abuse.

Brecht, M. L., Anglin, M. D., & Wang, J. C. (1993). Treatment effectiveness for legally coerced versus voluntary methadone maintenance clients. *American Journal of Drug and Alcohol Abuse, 19,* 89–106.

Brekke, J. S. (1989). The use of orientation groups to engage hard-to-reach clients: Model, method, and evaluation. *Social Work with Groups, 12,* 75–88.

Brennan, P. L., Moos, R. H., & Mertens, J. R. (1994). Personal and environmental risk factors as predictors of alcohol use, depression, and treatment-seeking: A longitudinal analysis of late-life problem drinkers. *Journal of Substance Abuse, 6,* 191–208.

Brettle, R. P. (1991). HIV and harm reduction for injection drug users. *AIDS, 5*, 125–136.

Brooke, D., Fudala, P. J., & Johnson, R. E. (1992). Weighing up the pros and cons: Help-seeking by drug misusers in Baltimore, USA. *Drug and Alcohol Dependence, 31*, 37–43.

Brown, J. M., & Miller, W. R. (1993). Impact of motivational interviewing on participation and outcome in residential alcoholism treatment. *Psychology of Addictive Behaviors, 7*, 211–218.

Brown, S. A. (1993). Drug effect expectancies and addictive behavior change. Special Section: Motivation and addictive behaviors. *Experimental and Clinical Psychopharmacology, 1*, 55–67.

Burton, T. L., & Williamson, D. L. (1995). Harmful effects of drinking and the use and perceived effectiveness of treatment. *Journal of Studies on Alcohol, 56*, 611–615.

Carney, M. M., & Kivlahan, D. R. (1995). Motivational subtypes among veterans seeking substance abuse treatment: Profiles based on stagers of change. *Psychology of Addictive Behaviors, 9*, 135–142.

Carroll, K. M., & Rounsaville, B. J. (1992). Contrast of treatment-seeking and untreated cocaine abusers. *Archives of General Psychiatry, 49*, 464–471.

Carvell, A. M., & Hart, G. J. (1990). Help-seeking and referrals in a needle exchange: A comprehensive service to injecting drug users. *British Journal of Addiction, 85*, 235–240.

Chiauzzi, E. J., & Liljegren, S. (1993). Taboo topics in addiction treatment: An empirical review of clinical folklore. *Journal of Substance Abuse Treatment, 10*, 303–316.

Clark, H. W., & Corbett, J. M. (1993). Needle exchange programs and social policy. *Journal of Mental Health Administration, 20*, 66–71.

Cox, W. M., & Klinger, E. (1988). A motivational model of alcohol use [Special Issue: Models of addiction]. *Journal of Abnormal Psychology, 97*, 168–180.

Cunningham, J. A., Sobell, L. C., Gavin, D. R., & Sobell, M. B. (1997). Assessing motivation for change: Preliminary development and evaluation of a scale measuring the costs and benefits of changing alcohol or drug use. *Psychology of Addictive Behaviors, 11*, 107–114.

Cunningham, J. A., Sobell, L. C., Sobell, M. B., Agrawal, S., & Toneatto, T. (1993). Barriers to treatment: Why alcohol and drug abusers delay or never seek treatment. *Addictive Behaviors, 18*, 347–353.

Cunningham, J. A., Sobell, L. C., Sobell, M. B., & Gaskin, J. (1994). Alcohol and drug abusers' reasons for seeking treatment. *Addictive Behaviors, 19*(6), 691–696.

Cunningham, J. A., Sobell, L. C., Sobell, M. B., & Kapur, G. (1995). Resolution from alcohol problems with and without treatment: Reasons for change. *Journal of Substance Abuse, 7*, 365–372.

Curry, S. J., Wagner, E. H., & Grothaus, L. C. (1990). Intrinsic and extrinsic motivation for smoking cessation. *Journal of Consulting and Clinical Psychology, 58*, 310–316.

Davidson, R. (1996). Motivational issues in the treatment of addictive behaviour. In G. Edwards & C. Dare (Eds.), *Psychotherapy, psychological treatments and the addictions* (pp. 173–188). Cambridge, UK: Cambridge University Press.

DeJarlis, D. C. (1995). Harm reduction: A framework for incorporating science into drug policy [Editorial]. *American Journal of Public Health, 85*, 10–12.

DeLeon, G. (1988). Legal pressure in therapeutic communities. *Journal of Drug Issues*, *18*, 625–640.

DeLeon, G., & Jainchill, N. (1986). Circumstance, motivation, readiness and suitability as correlates of treatment tenure. *Journal of Psychoactive Drugs*, *18*, 203–208.

DeLeon, G., Melnick, G., Kressel, D., & Jainchill, N. (1994). Circumstances, motivation, readiness, and suitability (the CMRS Scales): Predicting retention in therapeutic community treatment. *American Journal of Drug and Alcohol Abuse*, *20*, 495–514.

DiClemente, C. C. (1991). Motivational interviewing and stages of change. In W. R. Miller & S. Rollnick, *Motivational interviewing: Preparing people to change addictive behavior* (pp. 191–202). New York: Guilford Press.

DiClemente, C. C., & Hughes, S. O. (1990). Stages of change profiles in outpatient alcoholism treatment. *Journal of Substance Abuse*, *2*, 217–235.

Festinger, D. S., Lamb, R. J., Kountz, M. R., Kirby, K. C., & Marlowe, D. (1995). Pretreatment dropout as a function of treatment delay and client variables. *Addictive Behaviors*, *20*, 111–115.

Finney, J. W., & Moos, R. H. (1995). Entering treatment for alcohol abuse: A stress and coping model. *Addiction*, *90*, 1223–1240.

Fiorentine, R., & Anglin, M. D. (1994). Perceiving need for drug treatment: A look at eight hypotheses. *International Journal of the Addictions*, *29*, 1835–1854.

Gariti, P., Alterman, A. I., Holub-Beyer, E., Volpicelli, J. R., Prentice, N., & O'Brien, C. P. (1995). Effects of an appointment reminder call on patient show rates. *Journal of Substance Abuse Treatment*, *12*, 207–212.

George, A. A., & Tucker, J. A. (1996). Help-seeking by problem drinkers: Social contexts surrounding entry into alcohol treatment or Alcoholics Anonymous. *Journal of Studies on Alcohol*, *57*, 449–457.

Goldman, M. S., Brown, S. A., & Christiansen, B. A. (1987). Expectancy theory: Thinking about drinking. In H. T. Blane & K. E. Leonard (Eds.), *Psychological theories of drinking and alcoholism* (pp. 181–226). New York: Guilford Press.

Graham, K., & Timney, C. B. (1990). Case management in addictions treatment. *Journal of Substance Abuse Treatment*, *7*, 181–188.

Grant, B. F. (1996). Toward an alcohol treatment model: A comparison of treated and untreated respondents with DSM-IV alcohol use disorders in the general population. *Alcoholism: Clinical and Experimental Research*, *20*, 372–378.

Grund, J. P. C., Blanken, P., Adriaans, N. F., Kaplan, C. D, Barendregt, C., & Meeuwsen, M. (1992). Reaching the unreached: Targeting hidden IDU populations with clean needles via unknown user groups. *Journal of Psychoactive Drugs*, *24*, 41–47.

Hartnoll, R. (1992). Research and the help-seeking process. *British Journal of Addiction*, *87*, 429–437.

Hasin, D. S. (1994). Treatment/self-help for alcohol related problems: Relationship to social pressure and alcohol dependence. *Journal of Studies on Alcohol*, *55*, 660–666.

Hasin, D. S., & Grant, B. F. (1995). AA and other help seeking for alcohol problems: Former drinkers in the U. S. general population. *Journal of Substance Abuse*, *7*, 281–292.

Heather, N. (1992). Addictive disorders are essentially motivational problems. *British Journal of Addiction*, *87*, 828–830.

Horvath, A. T. (1993). Enhancing motivation for treatment of addictive behavior: Guidelines for the psychotherapist. *Psychotherapy, 30,* 473–480.

Institute of Medicine. (1990). *Broadening the base of treatment for alcohol problems.* Washington, DC: National Academy Press.

Isenhart, C. E. (1994). Motivational subtypes in an inpatient sample of substance abusers. *Addictive Behaviors, 19,* 463–475.

Jellinek, E. M. (1952). Phases of alcohol addiction. *Quarterly Journal of Studies on Alcohol, 13,* 673–684.

Jones, B. T., & McMahon, J. (1994). Negative and positive alcohol expectancies as predictors of abstinence after discharge from a residential treatment program: A one-month and three-month follow-up study in men. *Journal of Studies on Alcohol, 55,* 543–548.

Jordan, C. M., & Oei, T. P. S. (1989). Help-seeking behaviour in problem drinkers: A review. *British Journal of Addiction, 84,* 979–988.

King, M. P., & Tucker, J. A. (in press). Behavior change patterns and strategies distinguishing moderation drinking and abstinence during the natural resolution of alcohol problems without treatment. *Psychology of Addictive Behaviors.*

Klingemann, H. K. -H. (1991). The motivation for change from problem alcohol and heroin use. *British Journal of Addiction, 86,* 727–744.

Klingemann, H. K-H. (1992). Coping and maintenance strategies of spontaneous remitters from problem use of alcohol and heroin in Switzerland. *International Journal of the Addictions, 27,* 1359–1388.

Klingemann, H. K-H. (1994). Environmental influences which promote or impede change in substance behaviour. In G. Edwards & M. Lader (Eds.), *Addiction: Processes of change* (pp. 131–161). Oxford, UK: Oxford University Press.

Krampen, G. (1989). Motivation in the treatment of alcoholism. *Addictive Behaviors, 14,* 197–200.

Lidz, V., Bux, D. A., Platt, J. J., & Iguchi, M. Y. (1992). Transitional case management: A service model for AIDS outreach project. In R. S. Ashery (Ed.), *Progress and issues in case management* (NIDA Research Monograph No. 127, DHHS Pub. No. (ADM) 92-1946, pp. 112–143). Washington, DC: Superintendent of Documents, U. S. Government Printing Office.

Lovaglia, M. J., & Matano, R. (1994). Predicting attrition from substance misuse treatment using the Inventory of Interpersonal Problems. *International Journal of the Addictions, 29,* 105–113.

Lovejoy, M., Rosenblum, A., Magura, S., Foote, J., Handelsman, L., & Stimmel, B. (1995). Patients' perspective on the process of change in substance abuse treatment. *Journal of Substance Abuse Treatment, 12,* 269–282.

Ludwig, A. M. (1985). Cognitive processes associated with "spontaneous" recovery from alcoholism. *Journal of Studies on Alcohol, 46,* 53–58.

Mark, F. O. (1988). Does coercion work? The role of referral source in motivating alcoholics in treatment. *Alcoholism Treatment Quarterly, 5,* 5–22.

Marlatt, G. A. (1996). Harm reduction: Come as you are. *Addictive Behaviors, 21,* 779–788.

Marlatt, G. A., Tucker, J. A., Donovan, D. M., & Vuchinich, R. E. (1997). Help-seeking by substance abusers: The role of harm reduction and behavioral-economic approaches to facilitate treatment entry and retention by substance abusers. In L. S.

Onken, J. D. Blaine, & J. J. Boren (Eds.), *Beyond the therapeutic alliance: Keeping the drug dependent individual in treatment* (NIDA Research Monograph No. 165, pp. 44–84). Rockville, MD: U.S. Department of Health and Human Services, Public Health Service, National Institutes of Health.

McBride, C. M., Curry, S. J., Stephens, R. S., Wells, E. A., Roffman, R. A., & Hawkins, J. D. (1994). Intrinsic and extrinsic motivation for change in cigarette smokers, marijuana smokers, and cocaine users. *Psychology of Addictive Behaviors, 8,* 243–250.

McCaughrin, W. C., & Howard, D. L. (1996). Variation in access to outpatient substance abuse treatment: Organizational factors and conceptual issues. *Journal of Substance Abuse, 8,* 403–415.

McMahon, J., & Jones, B. T. (1993). Negative expectancy in motivation. *Addiction Research, 1,* 145–155.

McMahon, J., & Jones, B. T. (1996). Post-treatment abstinence survivorship and motivation for recovery: The Readiness to Change (RCQ) and Negative Alcohol Expectancy (NAEQ) questionnaires. *Addiction Research, 4,* 161–176.

Miller, W. R. (1985). Motivation for treatment: A review with special emphasis on alcoholism. *Psychological Bulletin, 98,* 84–107.

Miller, W. R. (1989). Increasing motivation for change. In R. K. Hester & W. R. Miller (Eds.), *Handbook of alcoholism treatment approaches: Effective alternatives* (pp. 67–80). Elmsford, NY: Pergamon Press.

Miller, W. R., & Rollnick, S. (1991). *Motivational interviewing: Preparing people to change addictive behavior.* New York: Guilford Press.

Murphy, P. N., & Bentall, R. P. (1992). Motivation to withdraw from heroin: A factor analytic study. *British Journal of Addiction, 87,* 245–250.

Oei, T. P. S., & Baldwin, A. R. (1994). Expectancy theory: A two-process model of alcohol use and abuse. *Journal of Studies on Alcohol, 55,* 525–534.

Olkin, R., & Lemle, R. (1984). Increasing attendance in an outpatient alcoholism clinic: A comparison of two intake procedures. *Journal of Studies on Alcohol, 45,* 465–468.

Onken, L. S., Blaine, J. D., & Boren, J. J. (Eds.). (1997). *Beyond the therapeutic alliance: Keeping the drug dependent individual in treatment* (NIDA Research Monograph No. 165). Rockville, MD: National Institute on Drug Abuse, U. S. Department of Health and Human Services, Public Health Service, National Institutes of Health.

Oppenheimer, E., Sheehan, M., & Taylor, C. (1988). Letting the client speak: Drug misusers and the process of help seeking. *British Journal of Addiction, 83,* 635–647.

Pfeiffer, W., Feurlein, W., & Brenk-Schulte, E. (1991). The motivation of alcohol dependents to undergo treatment. *Drug and Alcohol Dependence, 29,* 87–95.

Powell, J., Bradley, B., & Gray, J. (1992). Classical conditioning and cognitive determinants of subjective craving for opiates: An investigation of their relative contributions. *British Journal of Addiction, 87,* 1133–1144.

Powell, J., Dawe, S., Richards, D., Gossop, M., Marks, I., Strang, J., & Gray, J. (1993). Can opiate addicts tell us about their relapse risk? Subjective predictors of clinical prognosis. *Addictive Behaviors, 18,* 473–490.

Power, R., Hartnoll, R., & Chalmers, C. (1992a). The role of significant life events in discriminating help-seeking among illicit drug users. *International Journal of the Addictions, 27,* 1019–1034.

Power, R., Hartnoll, R., & Chambers, C. (1992b). Help-seeking among illicit drug users: Some differences between a treatment and nontreatment sample. *International Journal of the Addictions, 27,* 887–904.

Prochaska, J. O., DiClemente, C. C., & Norcross, J. C. (1992). In search of how people change: Applications to addictive behaviors. *American Psychologist, 47,* 1102–1114.

Prochaska, J. O., Velicer, W. F., Rossi, J. S., Goldstein, M. G., Marcus, B. H., Rakowski, W., Fiore, C., Harlow, L. L., Redding, C. A., Rosenbloom, D., & Rossi, S. R. (1994). Stages of change and decisional balance for 12 problem behaviors. *Health Psychology, 13,* 39–46.

Prochaska, J. O., & DiClemente, C. C. (1986). Toward a comprehensive model of change. In W. R. Miller & N. Heather (Eds.), *Treating addictive behaviors: Processes of change* (pp. 3–27). New York: Plenum.

Ravndal, E., & Vaglum, P. (1992). Different intake procedures: The influence on treatment start and treatment response: A quasi-experimental study. *Journal of Substance Abuse Treatment, 9,* 53–58.

Rollnick, S., Morgan, M., & Heather, N. (1996). Development of a brief scale to measure outcome expectations of reduced consumption among excessive drinkers. *Addictive Behaviors, 21,* 377–387.

Ryan, R. M., Plant, R. W., & O'Malley, S. (1995). Initial motivations for alcohol treatment: Relations with patient characteristics, treatment involvement, and dropout. *Addictive Behaviors, 20,* 279–297.

Saunders, B., & Wilkinson, C. (1990). Motivation and addiction behaviour: A psychological perspective. *Drug and Alcohol Review, 9,* 133–142.

Saunders, B., Wilkinson, C., & Towers, T. (1996). Motivation and addictive behaviors: Theoretical perspectives. In F. Rotgers, D. S. Keller, & J. Morgenstern (Eds.), *Treating substance abuse: Theory and technique* (pp. 241–265). New York: Guilford Press.

Schafer, J., & Brown, S. A. (1991). Marijuana and cocaine effect expectancies and drug use patterns. *Journal of Consulting and Clinical Psychology, 59,* 558–565.

Schober, R., & Annis, H. M. (1996). Barriers to help-seeking for change in drinking: A gender-focused review of the literature. *Addictive Behaviors, 21,* 81–92.

Schutz, C. G., Rapiti, E., Vlahov, D., & Anthony, J. C. (1994). Suspected determinants of enrollment into detoxification and methadone maintenance treatment among injecting drug users. *Drug and Alcohol Dependence, 36,* 129–138.

Sheehan, M., Oppenheimer, E., & Taylor, C. (1986). Why drug users sought help from one London drug clinic. *British Journal of Addiction, 81,* 765–775.

Simpson, D. D., & Joe, G. W. (1993). Motivation as a predictor of early dropout from drug abuse treatment. *Psychotherapy, 30,* 357–368.

Smith, L. (1992). Help seeking in alcohol-dependent females. *Alcohol and Alcoholism, 27,* 3–9.

Sobell, L. C., Cunningham, J. A., & Sobell, M. B. (1996). Recovery from alcohol problems with and without treatment: Prevalence in two population surveys. *American Journal of Public Health, 86,* 966–972.

Sobell, L. C., Sobell, M. B., & Toneatto, T. (1992). Recovery from alcohol problems without treatment. In N. Heather, W. R. Miller, & J. Greely (Eds.), *Self-control and the addictive behaviours* (pp. 198–242). New York: Maxwell Macmillan.

Sobell, L. C., Sobell, M. B., Toneatto, T., & Leo, G. I. (1993). What triggers resolution of alcohol problems without treatment? *Alcoholism: Clinical and Experimental Research, 17,* 217–224.

Solomon, K. E., & Annis, H. M. (1989). Development of a scale to measure outcome expectancy in alcoholics. *Cognitive Research and Therapy, 13,* 409–420.

Solomon, K. E., & Annis, H. M. (1990). Outcome and efficacy expectancy in the prediction of post-treatment drinking behaviour. *British Journal of Addiction, 85,* 659–665.

Springer, E. (1991). Effective AIDS prevention with active drug users: The harm reduction model [Special Issue: Counseling chemically dependent people with HIV illness]. *Journal of Chemical Dependency Treatment, 4,* 141–157.

Stall, R., & Biernacki, P. (1986). Spontaneous remission from problematic use of substances: An inductive model derived from a comparative analysis of the alcohol, opiate tobacco, and food/obesity literatures. *International Journal of the Addictions, 21,* 1–23.

Stark, M. J., Campbell, B. K., & Brinkerhoff, C. V. (1990). "Hello, may we help you?" A study of attrition prevention at the time of the first phone contact with substance abusing clients. *American Journal of Alcohol Abuse, 16,* 67–76.

Stark, M. J., & Kane, B. J. (1985). General and specific role induction with substance-abusing clients. *International Journal of the Addictions, 20,* 1135–1141.

Stitzer, M. L., & McCaul, M. E. (1987). Criminal justice interventions with drug and alcohol abusers. In E. K. Morris & C. J. Braukmann (Eds.), *Behavioral approaches to crime and delinquency: A handbook of application, research, and concepts.* New York: Plenum.

Thom, B. (1987). Sex differences in help-seeking for alcohol problems—2. Entry into treatment. *British Journal of Addiction, 82,* 989–997.

Timko, C., Finney, J. W., Moos, R. H., Moos, B. S., & Steinbaum, D. P. (1993). The process of treatment selection among previously untreated help-seeking problem drinkers. *Journal of Substance Abuse, 5,* 203–220.

Tuchfeld, B. S. (1981). Spontaneous remissions in alcoholics: Empirical observations and theoretical implications. *Journal of Studies on Alcohol, 42,* 626–641.

Tucker, J. A. (1995). Predictors of help-seeking and the temporal relationship of help to recovery among treated and untreated problem drinkers. *Addictions, 90,* 805–809.

Tucker, J. A., & Gladsjo, J. A. (1993). Help-seeking and recovery by problem drinkers: Characteristics of drinkers who attended Alcoholics Anonymous or formal treatment or who recovered without assistance. *Addictive Behaviors, 18,* 529–542.

Tucker, J. A., Vuchinich, R. E., & Pukish, M. M. (1995). Molar environmental contexts surrounding recovery from alcohol problems by treated and untreated problem drinkers. *Experimental and Clinical Psychopharmacology, 3,* 195–204.

Varney, S. M., Rohsenow, D. J., Dey, A. N., Meyers, M. G., Zwick, W. R., & Monti, P. M. (1995). Factors associated with help seeking and perceived dependence among cocaine users. *American Journal of Drug and Alcohol Abuse, 21,* 81–91.

Waldorf, D. (1983). Natural recovery from opiate addiction: Some social-psychological processes of untreated recovery. *Journal of Drug Issues, 13,* 237–280.

Watson, C. G., Brown, K., Tilleskjor, C., Jacobs, L., & Lucel, J. (1988). The comparative recidivism rates of voluntary- and coerced-admission male alcoholics. *Journal
of Clinical Psychology, 44,* 573–581.

Weisner, C. (1993). Toward an alcohol treatment entry model: A comparison of problem drinkers in the general population and in treatment. *Alcoholism: Clinical and
Experimental Research, 17,* 746–752.

Weisner, C., & Schmidt, L. (1992). Gender disparities in treatment of alcohol problems. *Journal of the American Medical Association, 268,* 1872–1876.

Wells-Parker, E. (1994). Mandated treatment: Lessons from research with drinking and
driving offenders. *Alcohol Health and Research World, 18,* 302–306.

Willenbring, M., Ridgely, M. S., Stinchfield, R., & Rose, M. (1991). *Application of case
management in alcohol and drug dependence: Matching techniques and populations* (DHHS
Publication No. (ADM) 91-1766). Rockville, MD: National Institute on Alcohol
Abuse and Alcoholism.

Zweben, A., & Li, S. (1981). The efficacy of role induction in preventing early dropout
from outpatient treatment of drug dependency. *American Journal of Drug and Alcohol
Abuse, 8,* 171–183.

# 6

## Critical Perspectives
## on the Transtheoretical Model
## and Stages of Change

JAY JOSEPH
CURTIS BRESLIN
HARVEY SKINNER

The transtheoretical model advanced by James Prochaska, Carlo Di-Clemente, and colleagues proposes a new and integrative way of looking at behavior change. It has captured broad interest in research and practice. Much of the explosion in popularity the model has enjoyed can be attributed to its advantages, including the following:

1. *Extended scope.* The stages of change concept has shifted the emphasis from behavior change (action stage) to encompass the majority of individuals who are either unsure (contemplation) or are not currently thinking about change (precontemplation).
2. *Broadened time perspective.* The model and supporting research underscore that a number of attempts or iterations through the stages of change cycle is often needed before a long-term behavioral goal is achieved.
3. *Matching.* The model proposes that different processes are most relevant at different points along the readiness for change continuum and provides a guide for practitioners on how to adapt their approach to enhance motivation for change.
4. *Multidimensional outcomes.* The model emphasizes that evaluation should not only focus on behavioral change as a criterion or out-

come measure, but also include more comprehensive criteria regarding movement along the readiness for change continuum. The model emphasizes the value of including motivational measures, such as self-efficacy and decisional balance (pros and cons of change).

5. *Heuristic value.* The model is intuitively appealing because of its apparent simplicity. Like other stage models, for example, Piaget's (1926) stages of cognitive development, the stages of change framework provides a visually compelling metaphor. It has facilitated the incorporation of motivation enhancement and behavioral change concepts in professional education.

Despite its success and the fact that the model has been in existence in one form or another for nearly two decades, the number of commentaries on its strengths and weaknesses remains small (Bandura, 1995; Davidson, 1992a, 1992b; Farkas, Pierce, Gilpin, et al., 1996; Heather, 1992; Stockwell, 1992; Sutton, 1996). This chapter takes a step in filling the gap in the literature by providing a balanced critique of the model. Our aim is to underscore the important contributions of the model, while at the same time to clarify its limitations and aspects in need of further development and research.

We begin with a description of the key constructs of the model as they currently stand. A more detailed description can be found in Prochaska, DiClemente, and Norcross (1992). This is followed by an outline of the development of the model in the Historical Perspective section, a survey of publications related to the model in Research to Date, and a critical analysis of the model in the Evaluation section.

## OVERVIEW OF THE MODEL

The transtheoretical model brings together various theoretical constructs in an effort to describe the process of change in human behavior. The stages of change, processes of change, decisional balance, and self-efficacy are intertwined and interactive constructs that describe behavior change and characteristics of the change process (Prochaska, DiClemente, Velicer, Ginpil, & Norcross, 1985). The levels of change describe the content or domain that is being changed (Prochaska & DiClemente, 1984).

The stages of change serve to classify people according to their progression through the change process. Five stages have been identified (precontemplation, contemplation, preparation, action, and maintenance) initially through smoking cessation studies (DiClemente & Prochaska, 1982; Prochaska & DiClemente, 1983). These stages are proposed to extend to other types of behavior problems such as alcohol abuse (DiClemente & Hughes, 1990), weight control (Kirschenbaum et al., 1992), and condom use (Grimley, Riley, Bellis, & Prochaska, 1993). The stages of change construct is defined as follows (Prochaska, DiClemente, & Norcross, 1992):

- *Precontemplation*: no intention to take action within the next 6 months.
- *Contemplation*: intends to take action within the next 6 months.
- *Preparation*: intends to take action within the next 30 days and has taken some behavioral steps in this direction.
- *Action*: has changed overt behavior for less than 6 months.
- *Maintenance*: has changed overt behavior for more than 6 months.

A sixth stage (termination) in which individuals have no temptation and 100% self-efficacy applies to some behaviors but is not appropriate for others (Prochaska, Redding, & Evers, 1997). The stages are measured either through a categorization algorithm based on four of five questionnaire items or through a multiple-scale questionnaire, such as the University of Rhode Island Change Assessment (URICA) scale (McConnaughy, Prochaska, & Velicer, 1983) or the Stage of Change Readiness and Treatment Eagerness Scale (SOCRATES; Isenhart, 1994), which produces scale scores on dimensions corresponding to the stages.

Movement through the stages is not necessarily a straight path from precontemplation to maintenance. The pattern of successful change is conceptualized typically to be spiral, with relapse to an earlier stage and (re)cycling through the stages occurring before long-term maintenance is reached. The specific patterns of movement through the stages have been variously characterized as stable, progressive, or unstable (Prochaska, Velicer, Guadagnoli, Rossi, & DiClemente, 1991) and as stable, progressive, regressive, or recycling (Prochaska, DiClemente, & Norcross, 1992).

The 10 processes of change are assumed to represent elements underlying 24 systems of psychotherapy (Prochaska, 1984). They are intended to encompass activities that individuals commonly engage in to modify behavior, emotions, thoughts, or relationships related to the targeted behavior (Hotz, 1995). The processes are assumed to be common to self-change and to change that occurs within a formal treatment program (Sutton, 1996). The experiential processes are cognitive and/or affective in nature, whereas the behavioral processes are more action related (Prochaska et al., 1991). The processes as currently organized are described in Table 6.1 (Glanz, Lewis, & Rimer, 1997; Prochaska, DiClemente, & Norcross, 1992; Prochaska, Redding, & Evers, 1997). These 10 processes are typically measured through a 40-item Likert scale questionnaire (Prochaska, Velicer, DiClemente, & Fava, 1988) that solicits information from the

**TABLE 6.1. The Processes of Change**

| Process | Description |
|---|---|
| Experiential processes | |
| Consciousness raising | Finding and learning new facts, ideas, and tips that support health behavior change |
| Self-reevaluation | Realizing that the target behavior change is an important part of one's identity as a person |
| Environmental reevaluation | Realizing the negative impact of unhealthy behavior or the positive impact of healthy behavior on one's proximal social and physical environment |
| Dramatic relief | Experiencing negative emotions (fear, anxiety, worry) that go along with unhealthy or risky behavior |
| Self-liberation | Making a firm commitment to change |
| Behavioral processes | |
| Helping relationships | Seeking and using social resources to support healthy behavior change |
| Contingency management | Increasing rewards for positive behavior change and decreasing rewards of unhealthy behaviors |
| Counterconditioning | Substituting healthier alternative behaviors and cognitions for unhealthy behaviors |
| Stimulus control | Removing reminders or cues to engage in unhealthy behavior and adding cues or reminders to engage in healthy behavior |
| Social liberation | Realizing that the social norms are changing in the direction of supporting healthy behavior |

respondent on the frequency of use of each specific item (from $1 = Never$ to $5 = Repeatedly$).

Prochaska and DiClemente have asserted that the processes are related to stages of change (DiClemente & Prochaska, 1982; Prochaska & DiClemente, 1983), in that certain processes are associated with earlier stages of change, and others are associated with later stages of change. Perz, DiClemente, and Carbonari (1996) take this further and have suggested that optimal patterns of process use are related to movement from one stage to another. This suggests that different processes should be emphasized at different stages to encourage movement through the stages of change.

The related construct of decisional balance, derived from Janis and Mann's (1977) decision-making model, seeks to measure the relative importance an individual places on the advantages (pros) and disadvantages (cons) of engaging in the target behavior. According to the model, if the cons outweigh the pros, then motivation for behavior change will likely be low. Similarly, if the pros outweigh the cons, motivation for behavior change will likely be high. Prochaska, Velicer, Rossi, et al. (1994) suggested that the balance between pros and cons varies with an individual's stage of change. The decisional balance construct is typically measured using a 24-item Likert scale questionnaire that assesses the importance of each item in making a decision to change a specified behavior (from 1 = *Not important* to 5 = *Extremely important*).

Self-efficacy, another related concept, originally developed by Bandura (1977), is an individual's confidence in being able to change his or her behavior. The underlying assumption is that a person's perceived ability to change will mediate future attempts to change behavior. As with the processes of change and decisional balance, self-efficacy is postulated to vary with the stage of change. Self-efficacy is also thought to be of utility in predicting movement through the stages. Measurement of self-efficacy within the context of the transtheoretical model has been done using a 31-item Likert scale that measures an individual's perceived confidence in being able to change a behavior (DiClemente, Prochaska, & Gilbertini, 1985).

## HISTORICAL PERSPECTIVE

The transtheoretical model can be traced back to a comparative analysis of psychotherapy done in the late 1970s by Prochaska. He was trying to make sense of the overwhelming variety of conceptualizations and procedures that defined psychotherapy. Although it was neither the first attempt to compare psychotherapies (Luborksy, Singer, & Luborsky, 1975), nor the first to suggest that different forms of psychotherapy have major common elements (Rosenweig, 1936), the analysis was set apart from earlier work by its scope. It was comprehensive in that 18 therapy systems were examined among 300 therapy outcome studies (DiClemente & Prochaska, 1982). Prochaska also articulated a distinction between content (a therapy's theory of personality) and process (method of therapy), and attempted to distill the essential therapeutic processes underlying all of the examined therapy systems. Under the assumption that effective therapies share common processes (Prochaska et al., 1988), Prochaska (1979) reduced the multitude of therapy systems to five basic processes of change. Each of these five processes could be considered both at an experiential level (the level of the individual's experience) and at an environmental level (the level of the individual's environment), giving rise to 10 specific processes of change (DiClemente & Prochaska, 1982).

Dissatisfied that these 10 processes were an exhaustive list, Prochaska and DiClemente (1984) used their subsequent work with smokers (self-changers in particular) as a basis for testing three additional hypothesized processes of change, for a total of 13. A principal components factor analysis performed on two separate samples identified a set of 10 independent processes (factors) that were derived from the original set (Prochaska et al., 1988).

Thus, the transtheoretical model has its roots in a comparative analysis of different systems of psychotherapy, which was modified and refined on the basis of smoking cessation studies and gave rise to 10 processes of change. The stages of change construct, which currently occupies a pivotal role in the transtheoretical model, was added to the model after the processes of change. It first appeared as a modified version of Horn's (1976) four stages of change in papers where Prochaska and DiClemente sought to demonstrate that stages and processes were related (DiClemente & Prochaska, 1982; Prochaska & DiClemente, 1983). In these papers, individuals were assigned to stages through a categorization algorithm. Papers providing "evidence" for the stages using the URICA scale were published thereafter (McConnaughy, DiClemente, Prochaska, & Velicer, 1989; McConnaughy et al., 1983). The categorization algorithm has undergone many revisions over the years (Farkas, Pierce, Gilpin, et al., 1996).

Later publications sought to integrate other constructs into the model. DiClemente et al. (1985) concluded that the self-efficacy construct is compatible with and important for the model. Prochaska and DiClemente (1984) further suggested that transtheoretical therapy problems are hierarchically organized across five different levels of change: (1) symptom/situational, (2) maladaptive cognitions, (3) current interpersonal conflicts, (4) family/systems conflicts, and (5) intrapersonal conflicts. Individuals are posited to attribute their problems to one of these levels. Norcross, Prochaska, Guadagnoli, and DiClemente (1984) proposed that these five levels could be measured using a Likert-like instrument. Later research expanded the number of levels to ten (Norcross, Prochaska, & Hambrecht, 1985). Levels of change dovetail nicely with different levels of intervention, but this aspect of the model has received the least attention. Most recently, it has been proposed that a decisional balance construct can be integrated with the model (Prochaska, Velicer, Rossi, et al., 1994).

## RESEARCH TO DATE

That the transtheoretical model has caught the interest of a significant number of researchers, clinicians, and educators is readily apparent from a survey of the literature. A comprehensive, though no doubt incomplete, search of the literature produced over 150 journal articles, book chapters, and monographs directly related to the transtheoretical model that were published between 1979 and 1995. As suggested in Figure 6.1, the model appears to have gained widespread acceptance at the beginning of the 1990s, as about two-thirds of publications were released in 1990 or later. Given that most of the publications related to developing and evaluating the model centered around substance use behaviors, it is not surprising to find that almost half (44%) of the publications are in the field of the addictions—primarily tobacco use and alcohol use (see Figure 6.2). It is interesting to note that although the model has its roots in the synthesis of common processes of different psychotherapies, psychotherapy-related publications only account for one-sixth (14%) of the publications. The model has also been applied to fields as diverse as exercise behavior, condom use, physician behavior, and even earthquake preparedness.

Research on the development of the transtheoretical model has been consistently produced over the years, and the model has grown incrementally to include a wider number of psychological constructs. However, the number of published articles related to the development or evaluation of the model is small in comparison to published studies that apply or describe the transtheoretical model.

Figure 6.3 categorizes publications according to the primary nature of the publication. Not all of the articles fit neatly into one category or another, but an overall pattern does emerge. Close to half (44%) of the publications took constructs from the transtheoretical model and applied them

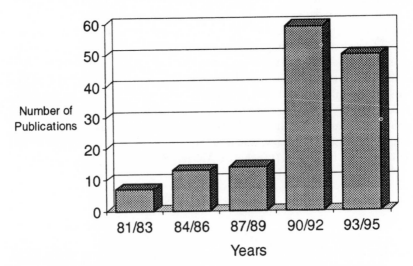

**FIGURE 6.1.** Number of publications on the transtheoretical model and stages of change during successive 3-year periods from 1981 to 1995.

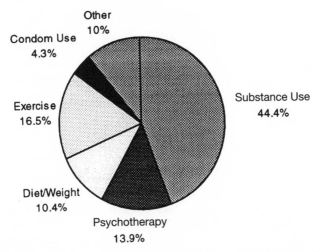

**FIGURE 6.2.** Publications on the transtheoretical model and stages of change categorized by the field of inquiry of each article.

without a critical analysis. These include (1) publications in which the authors claimed to be evaluating the model, but which in fact simply took constructs from the model and applied them to different fields of inquiry (Grimley et al., 1993), and (2) publications of studies in which construct characteristics (e.g., the number of stages) have been identified but not evaluated (Kirschenbaum et al., 1992). One-fourth (25%) of the publica-

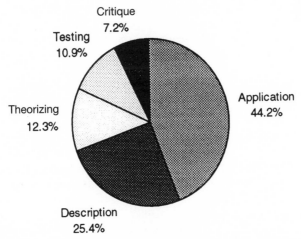

**FIGURE 6.3.** Publications on the transtheoretical model and stages of change categorized by the type of study or discussion.

tions simply described the model, and 12% theorized about potential applications or extensions of the model. Only 10 publications (7%) can be categorized as critiques or commentaries that delve into the strengths and weaknesses of the model. Most of these come from a 1992 issue of the *British Journal of Addiction*. A few such articles appeared in 1996 (Farkas, Pierce, Gilpin, et al., 1996; Farkas, Pierce, Zhu, et al., 1996; Sutton, 1996) and are referenced in this critique, but are not included in the summary of the research to date.

## EVALUATION

For purposes of this analysis, we view the transtheoretical model as one that integrates several theories.[1] Issues arising from an examination of the model have been grouped into two categories: conceptual and methodological. Conceptual issues addressed are (1) the validity of the underlying assumptions of the model, and (2) the degree to which the transtheoretical model meets expectations of a model of behavior change as defined by Prochaska and DiClemente. Methodological issues addressed are (1) the measurement and construct validity of the transtheoretical concepts, and (2) the quality of the empirical evidence to support the model to the exclusion of other models or theories.

Within this framework, we address popular criteria for the adequacy of a theory or a model; that is, is it internally consistent and free of contradictory derivations? Is it parsimonious? Does it fit it with prevailing theories in the field and, if not, is the conflict justifiable? Is there evidence for broad application or generalizability of the theory? Can the theory be tested? Does the theory have explanatory and predictive power? These are complex questions, some of which cross the boundary between conceptual and methodological issues. The reader is asked to keep these criteria in mind.

### Conceptual Issues

The transtheoretical model attempts to be a comprehensive model of behavior change. We begin with an evaluation of the model in terms of the issues that Prochaska and DiClemente outlined as being related to comprehensiveness, followed by comments on other issues that do not fall neatly under this umbrella.

Prochaska and DiClemente (1986) described characteristics for a comprehensive model of change with respect to addictive behaviors. A model should (1) account for the many ways people can change, (2) be applicable to an array of different behaviors, (3) address how change and failure to change occur, (4) be flexible enough to incorporate new developments, (5) help integrate the diverse population of available therapies, and (6) span the entire change process. The status of the transtheoretical model along each of these dimensions is evaluated next.

## Different Pathways to Change

In the transtheoretical model, an assumption is that behavior change processes are independent of the type of intervention (or even the receipt of an intervention). What is relevant is the impact each intervention has on the determinants of behavior change. Conclusive evidence for or against this assumption does not exist. Nevertheless, interventions studies conducted by Prochaska, DiClemente, Velicer, and Rossi (1993) suggest that the assumption is reasonable. The model appears to be encompassing enough to provide insight into the broad spectrum of ways in which people change their behavior, for example, through self-change, brief counseling, or intensive treatment. It appears that the processes of change can be broadly applied, thus supporting the generalizability of the model.

## Applicability to Different Behaviors

The model holds that behavior change processes generalize across different types of behavior, such as alcohol abuse, overeating, and smoking. Smoking cessation studies provided the initial empirical evidence for the transtheoretical model, but as indicated in the previous section, the model has now been applied across a diverse range of behaviors. The expanding use of the model in diverse domains is evidence for the widening appeal of the model, but to what extent can changes that have been made to assess stages and processes across behaviors be regarded as uncritical generalizations of the model? As we see in the next section, the bulk of the evidence for the stages of change is concentrated in a limited number of domains (smoking cessation, alcohol use). If the stages of change are applied to another behavior, such as condom use, but the number of stages is changed to three (see Bowen & Trotter, 1995), is this a legitimate extension of the model in another domain or an uncritical generalization of the model without empirical foundation?

## Explain Both Change and Failure to Change

Prochaska (1991) asserted that a large proportion of people fail to change their behavior (i.e., two-thirds of precontemplators were found to remain in precontemplation after 2 years of follow-up), but the model does not address this finding and instead focuses on how change occurs. The model's proponents have acknowledged the model's failure to contribute to knowledge about the nature, etiology, and development of addictive behavior (Prochaska, DiClemente, Velicer, & Rossi, 1992), but have justified this omission by claiming that too many theories of psychotherapy are theories about why people do not change rather than how people can change. As interesting as such a model may be, if a theory is to have explanatory and predictive power, as Kerlinger (1986) suggested, then the transtheoretical model should not be considered comprehensive if it fails to explain (1) why some people change and others do not, and (2) the circumstances under which change can be expected to occur.

The decisional balance measure appeared to have some predictive utility within the model (Prochaska, DiClemente, Velicer, Ginpil, & Norcross, 1985; Velicer, DiClemente, Prochaska, & Brandenburg, 1985). Incorporating into the model the expected costs or benefits of a behavior to identify who will change is consistent with many health behavior theories. However, this aspect of the model has not received as much attention as other aspects, and it does not address issues related to the timing of any change that occurs. This formulation also raises questions about how the decisional balance "pros and cons" shift over time, and how this relates to the predictive utility of the construct.

Thus, it seems that at this point the transtheoretical model should be considered a descriptive model. Some detractors go further and call the transtheoretical model a prescriptive model—a model of ideal change—rather than a descriptive model (Sutton, 1996).

## Flexibility to Integrate Developments

The transtheoretical model incorporates existing theoretical constructs including Bandura's (1977) work on the importance of self-efficacy in behavior change in therapy, Janis and Mann's (1977) model of decision making, and Horn's (1976) staging model of smoking behavior. The result is a multifaceted model of interacting constructs that appears to fit with existing theories. Viewed as a strength by its supporters, this integrating quality causes others to regard the model as unclear and without purposeful configuration (Davidson, 1992a). The architects of the model have argued that the days of searching for simple solutions to complex problems should be behind us (Prochaska & DiClemente, 1986). This argument notwithstanding, the challenge for any theory is to demonstrate parsimony. Is it the simplest model possible that will coherently describe and promote an understanding of the behavior change process? An integrative, complex model of behavior is acceptable if it accounts for an aspect of human psychology that certainly appears to be complex, but whether all theoretical constructs now encompassed by the model are optimal remains unclear.

Does the transtheoretical model have the ability to incorporate new conceptual and empirical developments in a coherent fashion? Not necessarily. The ability to incorporate new developments is largely dictated by their nature. Bandura (1995) has argued, without providing evidence, that the transtheoretical model has integrated various theories by ignoring the inherent contradictions in these theories. If this is true, the model necessarily lacks internal consistency and encompasses contradictory derivations.

What is clear is that the model has undergone numerous changes over the years, yet accounts of the changes, along with the reasons for them, are few. This poses difficulties for comparing early research on the model with research 10 years later, since changes have been made in, for example, the number of stages, the number of processes, and the items used to evaluate the stages and processes. The processes of change originally identified as underlying all psychotherapies are not the same as the processes of change now used in the relevant studies (Prochaska, 1988; Prochaska & DiClemente, 1984). Moreover, Farkas, Pierce, Gilpin, Zhu, et al. (1996) showed that the categorization algorithm often used to assign individuals to stages has undergone numerous changes across time and across studies. Specifically, the time frames for quit attempts and intentions have changed, and the primacy of the "intention" variable versus the "actual behavior" variable in the categorization algorithm has changed. Individuals who, prior to 1991, would have been assigned to the relapse category—which has never been "officially" designated as a stage, but has been treated as if it were one (see Prochaska & DiClemente, 1983)—are now divided among the other stages.

Thus, while the model draws from other theories and constructs, the nature of their incorporation has changed over time, making it difficult to assess their causal or predictive utility. Hence, the matter of whether the model can incorporate related developments is open to debate.

## Integrate Diverse Systems of Therapy

A key assumption in the development of the processes of change construct is that no system of therapy is superior to another (Prochaska et al., 1988). The impetus for this view is eclectic psychotherapy, which attempts to tailor methods of therapy to client characteristics by selecting intervention procedures from various psychotherapeutic approaches as needed, rather than prescribing a course of treatment based on adherence to one particular approach (Norcross, 1986). Eclecticism is appealing to the practicing psychotherapist or addictions counselor, who often encounters clients who are resistant to change using the methods prescribed in a particular type of therapy. Detractors of eclecticism (e.g., Arkowitz, 1995) have argued that there is as yet no convincing evidence for the causal role of common factors in psychotherapy outcome that would support such neglect of technical variations across therapies.

Held (1991) has asserted that the transtheoretical model, through its emphasis on the processes of change and its attempt to discard content, aspires to be a true process model. Process models often assume that it is not possible to know what causes different psychological problems and that such knowledge is irrelevant to knowing how to resolve these problems. Held further argued that while Prochaska and DiClemente would view the transtheoretical model as this type of process model, they ironically insinuate that research will reveal the formal content levels that cause different problems. They speak of a model that has the flexibility to choose the content level that appears actually to be causing a problem. However, in recent years, content constructs such as the levels of change have not received much attention, and this may be a reflection of the originators' deemphasis of content. Note that it can be argued that self-efficacy and decisional balance are content constructs and that their incorporation into the transtheoretical model simply involves exchange of one domain of content for another.

## Span the Entire Change Process

One of the most compelling contributions the model has made has been to expand the scope to address the broad continuum of behavior change. By successfully drawing attention to the fact that, at a given point in time, not every person with a maladaptive or risky behavior pattern is ready for change, the model suggests that interventions should be tailored or matched to the person's stage of change or level of motivation. Instead of treating behavior change as a dichotomous variable, for example, smoker to nonsmoker, the transtheoretical model more finely divides the change process into intervals or stages (Prochaska, 1991). Behavioral models that focus on action are directed at the minority of persons who are ready to change. The transtheoretical model broadens the focus to include the majority of individuals who are not yet thinking about change, are "stuck" in ambivalence, or have already changed but then relapsed (Prochaska & DiClemente, 1986). In the past, the therapist who encountered resistance in a client attributed the client's inaction to lack of motivation. The alternative working hypothesis of the transtheoretical model is that therapy should be tailored so that client and therapist are working at the same stage of change (Prochaska & DiClemente, 1986).

The model also spans the entire change process by stressing its iterative nature. This aspect of the model has ramifications for the time it takes to achieve permanent change. Relapse is often viewed as failure. The transtheoretical model views relapse as part of the process of cycling through the stages. Periodic relapse is common in many disorders, including addictive behaviors, and does not have to be construed as failure. In the journey toward permanent behavior change, the relapser is probably somewhere between a person who has not taken any action and a person who has maintained change. It may take some people more time than others to achieve stable change, as they relapse and then take action again, but stable change is within reach for many behaviors.

The implication of this alternative view of the behavior change process is that the success of an intervention should not be measured solely by the proportion of participants who achieve a goal of stable behavior change. Since the majority of smokers, for example, are in precontemplation and contemplation (Prochaska, 1991; Velicer, Hughes, Fava, Prochaska, & DiClemente, 1995), measuring the success of a program solely in terms of the proportion of smokers who quit misses the mark. A more sensitive evaluation would assess progress from one stage to the next as an outcome measure.

## Other Concerns

The preceding comments suggest that the transtheoretical model is comprehensive in some ways and not in others. What other observations can be made about the conceptualization of the model?

First, the transtheoretical model fails to acknowledge that individuals bring with them a personal history that can have a very powerful impact on the outcome of any professionally assisted or self-change program. Clients who have multiple addictions, or complex psychological problems (or comorbidity), present challenges to successful treatment that are not dealt with by the model. Substance abuse is known to be correlated with psychological and social problems, but the transtheoretical model fails to explain how this affects the behavior change process or modifies the probability of succeeding. Personal history may not completely predict success or failure in treatment in itself, but it is an important factor. A comprehensive model needs to take into account a person's life history and the current context. In this respect the transtheoretical model falls short.

Second, the transtheoretical model does not account for the impact of demographic factors, because they are assumed to offer little insight into predicting who will succeed in making permanent change. However, studies have shown that a socioeconomic status (SES) gradient exists for health behaviors such as cigarette smoking, physical inactivity, poor diet, and substance abuse (Adler et al., 1994). Prochaska and DiClemente (1984) have argued that how problems are acquired is often unrelated to how they are changed, suggesting that SES is not necessarily related to successful change. However, individuals with higher income and educational levels have been found to be more likely to try to quit again following a relapse (Wilcox, Prochaska, & Velicer, 1985). The study used a fairly homogeneous sample of middle-aged, middle-class adults from Rhode Island and Houston, Texas. If the sample been drawn from a population with greater variability in SES and ethnoracial background, then the utility of demographics in predicting change would likely have been even stronger. The fact that demographic characteristics are often static and not amenable to change does not justify ignoring the role they may play in health behavior change.

Finally, not enough thought has been given to how the social context affects an individual's potential to change behavior. The options for action that people have available to them are often limited by social and cultural forces and by their perceptions of control. If, as advocated by the transtheoretical model, the journey toward permanent change involves certain processes of change, then the fewer processes that are accessible to an individual, the more difficult or unlikely progress will be toward permanent change. Social context is more than the social-liberation process included in the model—it can expand or shrink the horizon of options for action. For example, in some cultures, cigarettes are viewed as a relaxant, whereas in others, cigarettes are viewed as a stimulant. A counterconditioning process item such as "I found other ways besides smoking to relax and deal with the tension and nervousness that would get me to smoke" (Di-Clemente & Prochaska, 1982) may have limited applicability in the latter context. Attempts to integrate the role of social support into the transtheoretical model have been made (Amick & Ockene, 1994). However, the focus has been on how social support activities relate to the processes of change, rather than how social context affects the basic assumptions of the model.

The levels of change, a concept introduced in the original versions of the model, addressed the social context of change, but this concept has been deemphasized in later versions. Because interpersonal and societal factors play a key role in change, we see the recent inattention that levels of change has received as unfortunate.

## Methodological Issues

The most significant methodological criterion for a good theory is its testability. The vast majority of studies related to the transtheoretical model, as discussed in the section on the research to date, have not tested the model but have simply applied it. Many published studies claim to provide evidence for the validity of the transtheoretical model, but most did not evaluate their results in light of alternative theories. In this section, we review evidence for the transtheoretical model, bearing in mind that good evidence supports the exclusion of other possibilities.

Although the processes of change was the first construct to be articulated, the stages of change construct now holds a more pivotal role in the transtheoretical model. Thus, much of the evidence we review centers around the stages of change. By adopting a stage-based model, Prochaska and DiClemente proposed a categorical structure that is distinguishable from other structural models, for example, hierarchical systems and dimensional systems (Skinner, 1981). In a hierarchical system, individuals are classified into subgroups, which are in turn classified into groups at higher levels in the hierarchy (i.e., an individual in a given group will necessarily have characteristics at all lower levels in the hierarchy). In dimensional systems, individuals are ordered along axes in a multidimensional space. The onus is on supporters of the transtheoretical model to provide empirical evidence to support the adoption of the categorical stage model over alternative models.

The simple staging model suggests that people move through ordered states that are qualitatively distinct. Passing from one state or stage to another occurs when a threshold (boundary) level is reached with respect to a particular stage. Important features of the transtheoretical model include the following:

1. There are five qualitatively distinct stages.
2. Movement occurs through the ordered stages over time, in a predicted pattern (not necessarily linear).
3. People at different stages have different behaviors, expectancies, and beliefs.
4. Variables influencing behavior at each stage can predict progress to other stages.

These features provide criteria against which evidence relevant to the transtheoretical model may be judged.

## Five Qualitatively Distinct Stages

Stage models have appeal because people find categories easier to use and understand. The transtheoretical model's emphasis on stages is no exception to this fundamental tendency toward organizing the world. However, the originators of the transtheoretical model have shifted back and forth on the number of stages. The authors claimed that, originally, five stages were identified, but in principal components analyses (McConnaughy et al., 1983, 1989), only four factors were found. The four factors were interpreted to mean that there were only four stages (note that evidence for distinct stages or categories is being adduced from a dimensional model and factor analysis). Seven years later, they realized that the cluster analyses (a categorical model) applied in the same studies had identified groups of individuals who were in the preparation stage. They felt their error was in placing too much value on the principal component analyses and too little on the cluster analyses, thereby ignoring evidence for the existence of the preparation stage (Prochaska, DiClemente, & Norcross, 1992).

Such flip-flopping about a central construct in the model is disconcerting. Also unsettling is the fact that while the principal empirical "evidence" for four qualitatively distinct stages of change (McConnaughy et al., 1983, 1989) has been published, the reanalyses of these studies that led Prochaska, DiClemente, and Norcross (1992) to argue for five stages have not been published to our knowledge. This is a noticeable gap in the evidence for the transtheoretical model.

Even if the reanalyses are made available, one must emphasize that factor analysis "imposes" a dimensional model on data, whereas cluster analysis "imposes" a categorical model (Skinner, 1981). Neither analysis by itself can be assumed to provide a more plausible fit to data. Skinner demonstrated that one can apply very different structural models (categorical vs. dimensional vs. hierarchical) to the same data with results that could support each model. These statistical techniques tend to impose a structure (and measure goodness of fit) rather than identify or confirm the "existence" of a structure. Since all measured variables have measurement error, it is difficult (and some would say impossible) for a given statistical analysis to provide a definitive test of a model.

If there is little published evidence for five distinct stages, is there at least evidence for a staging model of behavior change? While there is a wealth of literature on the application of the transtheoretical model in smoking studies using the popular categorical classifications (Hotz, 1995) and using other instruments such as the visual-analog scales (Rustin & Tate, 1993) and the contemplation ladder (Biener & Abrams, 1991), these instruments only demonstrate how to categorize individuals into distinct stages. They do not answer the fundamental question of whether behavior change follows well-defined stages. If behavior change is not adequately described by distinct stages, then there is little point in using categorical classifications to produce groups of participants.

In the original studies designed to provide evidence for the stages of change (McConnaughy et al., 1983, 1989), the investigators administered a 32-item Likert scale questionnaire (the URICA) to a sample of adult outpatients and conducted a cluster analysis on the scale. A cluster analysis seeks to arrange individuals into groups such that the individuals in each group resemble each other in values taken by variables more than they do individuals in different groups. If the stage model is correct, then

URICA-based subgroups (or profiles, as they are referred to) should relate to the hypothesized stages of change. Evidence in support of the stages would lie in the following:

1. A one-to-one correspondence between hypothesized stages of change and distinct sets of profiles.
2. A consistent set of profiles that are replicated across studies for a given behavior.
3. A consistent set of profiles obtained across behaviors.

*Correspondence between Stages and Profiles.* In the original published study that investigated the stages of change, McConnaughy et al. (1983) used a hierarchical clustering procedure to determine whether participants given the URICA questionnaire could be classified into a small number of cohesive groups. If the stages of change model adequately describes behavior change, then the number of distinct clusters should be very close to the number of stages in the model. The 18-cluster solution produced seven major and two minor profiles that were highly distinct but did not correspond exactly to the hypothesized stages of change. The authors stated that while several profiles were readily identifiable, other profiles needed more study. One cluster, a Noncontemplative Action profile, consisted of participants who endorsed both Precontemplation and Action but were below average on Contemplation and Maintenance (McConnaughy et al., 1983). This unexpected profile is clearly not consistent with a stages of change construct. Moreover, a profile that one might expect to find, the Action profile, was not forthcoming.

Other profile patterns indicated that it is possible for clients to be engaged in attitudes and behaviors described by more than one stage simultaneously. In a later replication study (McConnaughy et al., 1989), the authors claimed this straddling of stages showed that the progression from one stage to another involved a fluctuation in stage involvement at any given point in time. An equally compelling interpretation is that the results do not support a simple four- (or five-) stage model, but rather a continuous, dimensional model.

In another approach to evaluating the stages, Velicer et al. (1995) performed cluster analyses within stages as a critical test of the model. In their view, the model would be confirmed if a limited number of distinct clusters were found in each stage, at least one of which corresponded to the expected profile for that stage, and were interpretable within the context of the model. It can be argued that these criteria are weak given the fact that different clustering methods can provide very different results (since each imposes a method for finding clusters). There may be a need for a stronger measure of success such as one-to-one correspondence, as suggested earlier. The authors claimed that their analyses demonstrated the existence of subtypes within stages that were temporally ordered, yet they neither advocated replacing the 5-stage model with a 15- (or more) stage model, nor considered applying a continuous, multidimensional model.

Replicability across Studies. In the replication study, McConnaughy et al. (1989) stated that they hoped to cross-validate the stages of change using a new clinical sample. The same assessment instrument (URICA) and hierarchical clustering procedure were used as in the original study. The solution for eight clusters was judged to be the most clearly interpretable. One major cluster found in the original study, the Preparticipation profile, was not replicated, indicating some inconsistency across studies. As in the original study, a clear Action profile was not found. It may be argued that because of the brief nature of the Action stage, there were not enough clients at that stage in the sample to produce a distinct cluster. If this was the case, then a replication study with a much larger sample size, to support finding enough clients at each stage, should be conducted.

Replicability across Behaviors. In an attempt to demonstrate the cross-behavior nature of the stages of change, the URICA scale was given to new outpatients at an alcoholism treatment program (DiClemente & Hughes, 1990). A five-cluster solution was selected on the basis of the hierarchical tree and the clustering coefficients. One cluster, labeled the Ambivalent cluster, was described by the authors as "an anomalous profile with a high level of endorsement across the subscales." This profile was not found in the original McConnaughy et al. (1983) study and is not consistent with the stages of change model. This interpretation of this incongruous result is difficult. The findings may suggest that the stages of change are not entirely transferable across behaviors, or that the stages of change do not adequately describe behavior change.

Other relevant studies have used the SOCRATES, which was devised to provide a similar assessment to the URICA. Isenhart (1994) used a modified version of the SOCRATES to identify motivational subgroups as described by a stages of change model in an inpatient sample of substance abusers. Cluster analysis was performed using Ward's clustering method and squared Euclidean distance measures. Statistical methods that were not used in either the McConnaughy et al. (1983, 1989) or DiClemente and Hughes (1990) analyses provided estimates of the number of significant clusters. All of the cluster-analytic procedures were found to suggest the presence of three significant clusters or profiles, which were labeled Uninvolved, Ambivalent, and Active. Finding three profiles is consistent neither with the five stages of change, nor with the number of profiles found in the other studies. The fact that an Active profile was found is also inconsistent with the other studies.

Isenhart (1994) suggested the reason so many participants fit an Active profile is that the sample was drawn from inpatients who were participating in substance abuse treatment. However, the McConnaughy et al. and DiClemente and Hughes studies also used clinical samples, and no clear Active profile emerged from them. At issue, then, is whether the difference between the Isenhart study and the others is due to (1) the behavior studied (inpatients with mixed drugs of choice), (2) use of the SOCRATES versus URICA scale, (3) the statistical procedure used to determine the number of clusters, or some combination of these reasons. If it is the first, then the stages of change would not appear to apply across behaviors. If it is the second, it is unclear which scale is a better measure of readiness for change and thus which set of results is more compelling. If it is the third, then one can argue that the results are dependent on the specific clustering procedure used. This would be consistent with the assertion that the same data can produce different results depending on the method of defining clusters (Armitage & Berry, 1994; Skinner, 1981). If this is the case, then it is unclear which clustering method is the better one, if any, and thus which results are to be viewed as more credible.

Overall, these studies provide conflicting evidence for the stages of change and do not exclude the possibility of a continuous, multidimensional model, or possibly a hybrid, class-quantitative model. If a staging model of behavior change is "correct," strong evidence for the stages of change as advocated by the transtheoretical model is lacking. In any case, the URICA and SOCRATES have been used in a minority of studies. The vast majority of studies used categorical algorithms, and Sutton (1996) noted that the two methods have never been used together in a published study. Clearly, research is needed on how well these two measurement methods agree and, more generally, construct validation studies are needed using a multitrait–multimethod approach, where the different stages (traits) are assessed by two or more distinct methods. Then, evidence can be produced regarding the convergent and discriminant properties of methods that purport to assess the stages of change. In addition to self-report methods (whether the categorization algorithm or the URICA or SOCRATES), other distinct methods are needed (e.g., peer ratings, behavioral assessment) in order to evaluate a measurement model for the stages constructs.

## Movement Occurs through the Ordered Stages over Time in a Predicted Pattern

Evidence for the movement from stage to stage of participants, in the spiral pattern, would lend support to the staging of behavior change, as suggested by the transtheoretical model. A number of cross-sectional empirical studies reported a simplex pattern of higher correlation of adjacent "stages" with each other, than with other, more temporally distant stages (e.g., McConnaughy et al. 1989). This is what one would expect in a stage model, but cross-sectional studies cannot provide strong evidence for movement through the stages because individuals are not followed through time. More importantly, this sort of evidence does not exclude the possibility of a continuous, multidimensional model of behavior change. Also, it is impossible to evaluate the spiral pattern predicted by the transtheoretical model through cross-sectional studies, although the idea is intuitively appealing and the concept of relapse is well accepted (e.g., Marlatt & Gordon, 1985).

A handful of prospective studies allow comparison of the hypothesized and observed movement between stages. In one study, Prochaska and DiClemente (1992) reported a stage effect using smokers. Initial stage predicted cessation success at 12- and 18-month follow-ups. Participants in preparation were three to four times more likely than precontemplators to be abstinent, with participants in contemplation being midway between the two. In another paper, Prochaska et al. (1991) reported results from the longitudinal follow-up of participants over the 2-year interval. Examining those profiles with a sufficient sample size for interpretation, it appears that 85 of 494 participants (17%) showed a linear progression from one stage to a later stage over the 2 years of the study. Almost as large a group (67 of 494 participants, or 14%) moved back a stage or two, for example, from contemplation to precontemplation (these were not classified as recyclers). In another study of smoking cessation using young adults, Pallonen, Murray, Schmid, Pirie, and Luepker (1990) found that half of precontemplators moved to contemplation after 1 year and that three-fourths of contemplators moved to the action stage after 1 year. These results, while interesting, do not provide support for a staging model to the exclusion of a continuous, multidimensional model.

## People at Different Stages Show Different Behaviors, Beliefs, and Experiences

The rationale behind the stages of change is that individuals in different stages show unique patterns of behavior and hold unique beliefs in relation to their behavior. The instruments used to define the stages attempt to measure some of these beliefs and behaviors; other constructs such as the processes of change also may be able to differentiate individuals into different stages. While evidence of such differentiation cannot be interpreted to mean that a stage model is correct, it is fair to use it as supporting evidence in conjunction with the more direct evidence discussed in previous sections.

The earliest work aimed at demonstrating distinctions between individuals in different stages were studies that investigated the relation between the processes of change and the stages of change among smokers (DiClemente & Prochaska, 1982; Prochaska & DiClemente, 1983). It was suggested that certain processes are associated with earlier stages of change, and others are associated with later stages of change. Research published since these seminal articles provided support for the posited relation between the processes of change and the stages of change (Fava, Velicer, & Prochaska, 1995; Kristeller, Rossi, Ockene, Goldberg, & Prochaska, 1992). Individual processes were generally found to be associated with one of the stages or with two adjacent stages, and were not distributed widely across stages. However, it is difficult to assess the consistency of association between processes and stages because the comparison between studies is complicated by changes over the years in the number of stages included in the model and by modifications to the processes themselves. There does appear to be a general pattern in which the Contemplation stage is associated with cognitive processes such as consciousness raising and self-reevaluation; the Action stage is associated with processes such as self-liberation, reinforcement management, and stimulus control; and the Maintenance stage is associated with a decreased use of the processes of change (Prochaska & DiClemente, 1983; Prochaska, DiClemente, & Norcross, 1992). Perz et al. (1996) performed an analysis to show that two optimal patterns of process use were related to movement from two stages.

The relation between the processes and the stages of change has been found for other behaviors such as exercise (Marcus, Rossi, Selby, Niaura, & Abrams, 1992) and acquiring and maintaining a low-fat diet (Bowen, Meischke, & Tomoyasu, 1994). Prochaska and DiClemente (1985) found a similar relation between processes of change and stages of change across smoking cessation, weight control, and psychic distress. However, the frequency of use of particular processes varied across the different behaviors.

Other constructs within the transtheoretical model have been examined to determine whether a relationship with the stages of change exists. The self-efficacy construct, adapted from Bandura's (1977) research, is thought to relate to the stages of change in that low self-efficacy presumably is associated with earlier stages, and higher self-efficacy is associated with later stages (DiClemente et al., 1985). The decisional balance construct, which integrates motivational considerations into the transtheoretical model (Prochaska, Velicer, Rossi, et al., 1994), also is thought to relate to the stages. It is proposed that the ratings of the pros of changing a behavior increase with movement through the stages, while ratings of the cons of change for the same behavior decrease with movement (Prochaska, DiClemente, Velicer, Ginpil, et al., 1985; Rakowski, Fulton, & Feldman, 1993; Rakowski et al., 1992; Velicer et al., 1985). In summary, there are several lines of evidence to suggest that people at different stages use different processes and exhibit different characteristics.

## Factors Predicting Progress Differ According to Stage

Studies of factors that predict progress at each stage provide pertinent evidence. What supportive evidence is there that predictive factors, or values of predictive variables, differ by stage? In one of the first reported longitudinal studies (Prochaska, DiClemente, Velicer, et al., 1985), two processes of change (self-reevaluation and helping relationship), self-efficacy, and decisional balance were deemed to be the best predictor variables. Self-efficacy was useful in predicting movement into the action and maintenance stages, but was not relevant for earlier stage movement. Prediction of precontemplation and contemplation stage movement seemed to relate to decision making, as well as to cognitive processes of change.

The decisional balance measure appeared to be useful in predicting movement from precontemplation to contemplation and from contemplation to action. In the two groups that had already quit smoking, namely recent quitters and long-term quitters, decisional balance was not a useful predictor for movement. The authors suggested that perhaps once the decision to change has been made, other variables determine whether or not change is maintained (Velicer et al., 1985).

Results such as these are consistent with the notion that different factors predict progress at different stages of change. However, in another prospective study, the results are less supportive. Prochaska, Norcross, Fowler, Follick, and Abrams (1992) examined a behavioral intervention for weight control to identify predictors of percentage weight loss after treatment. The investigators concluded the stages and processes were good predictors of change (accounting for 18% and 26% of the variance in outcomes, respectively). Yet this was only true if processes were assessed midtreatment. When assessed prior to treatment, stages and processes accounted for only 2% and 6%, respectively, of the outcome variance. The transtheoretical model does not appear to be able to account for this unusual discrepancy. The best pretreatment predictor of outcome was social support from a friend (17% of the outcome variance). Pretreatment weight loss, age, and SES together accounted for 16% of the outcome variance. Thus, one could have alternatively concluded that the stages and processes are no better as predictor variables than appropriate combinations of other variables.

Farkas et al. (1996) evaluated the use of the stages of change construct as a predictor of smoking cessation at follow-ups conducted 1–2 years later by comparing it with a prediction equation based on quantity smoked and prior quit-attempt variables (addiction model). They concluded that the stages of change construct is not an independent predictor of smoking cessation and that an addiction model is a more appropriate theoretical basis for designing cessation interventions. In response, Prochaska and Velicer (1996) defended the transtheoretical model by noting that they have never been able to demonstrate the predictive effect of "addiction" variables, that the Farkas et al. analysis did not control for the potential confounder variable "length of follow-up," and that the failure of the stage effect may reflect the success of an intensive statewide antismoking campaign conducted during the period of the study.

This debate makes apparent the need for further studies on predictive factors. Ideally, these studies should employ a spectrum of designs. Most of the empirical studies on the transtheoretical model are cross-sectional in design, and only a handful are prospective. Also, since Prochaska and colleagues have focused primarily on self-changers, relevant randomized controlled clinical trials (RCTs) are rare. In one clinical trial, Prochaska et al. (1993) compared four different treatments (three of these were said to be for stage-matched groups), but there was no control group. The investigators argued that the best self-help program was used instead of a control group, because if new approaches could not outperform the best programs available, then there would be little reason to adopt the new programs (Prochaska & DiClemente, 1992). However, the criteria used to determine the "best" self-help program were not adequately described. Also, the groups in the study were not truly stage-matched, since individuals in each group not only received manuals for their specific stage of change, but for all subsequent stages as well (Prochaska et al., 1993). For example, if an individual in the action stage progressed to the maintenance stage, it was unclear whether the progression was due to the content of the action manual, the content of the maintenance manual, or both.

Ample opportunity exists for interesting and informative RCTs. The model suggests the processes of change used by individuals differ by stage and that it follows that interventions should be sensitive to the stage of an individual. A possible study design to test this hypothesis would be an RCT where an intervention specific to one stage was used across all stages in the intervention arm. If a significantly greater proportion of individuals progressed in the one stage of the intervention arm than in the same stage of the control arm, and if there were no difference between intervention and control arms for the other stages, one might consider this to be evidence for a stage model. An alternative RCT would use true stage-matched interventions and look for a significantly greater proportion of participants to progress through all stages of the intervention arm compared to the control arm. The assumption in these designs is that participants in an RCT use the same processes as self-changers and that these processes are amenable to facilitation through interventions.

In summary, there is some evidence that people at different stages exhibit different characteristics. However, claims regarding the predictive power of variables in the model (Prochaska, DiClemente, Velicer, et al., 1985) must be viewed in light of the preceding criticisms. Future efforts should be directed at expanding research beyond self-changers, since a central assumption in applications of the model is that interventions that promote the same processes used by self-changers can be effective.

## CONCLUSIONS

Prochaska and DiClemente have provided an intuitive and appealing framework for tailoring interventions to individuals' readiness for change. This review evaluated the model by considering both conceptual and methodological issues in the light of existing knowledge and the empirical evidence relevant to the model. Our decisional "balance sheet" for the transtheoretical model at this point in time is as follows:

*Pros of the transtheoretical model*
- Expands the scope and temporal perspective on the behavior change process to include preparatory and maintaining components that surround the act of changing behavior.
- Refines and expands the scope of interventions to include broader phases of the behavior change process.
- Emphasizes matching interventions to client readiness for change.
- Underscores that outcome measurement should not only include behavior change but also movement along the readiness for change continuum.
- Attempts to integrate influential concepts such as relapse, self-efficacy, and decisional balance.

*Cons of the transtheoretical model*
- Supporting evidence for distinct stages is weak and inconsistent.
- Evidence for the hypothesized relationship between processes and stages is mixed.
- Studies do not exclude the possibility of a continuous, multidimensional model.
- The model is descriptive rather than explanatory.
- The model does not consider individual characteristics and life

contexts surrounding behavior change (e.g., personal history, co-morbidities, SES, and social context).
- An expanded repertoire of study designs is needed to evaluate the model (e.g., construct validation studies, RCT designs for interventions).

These "cons" should be viewed as providing direction for further research and development of the transtheoretical model. For instance, more precise definitions are needed regarding inclusion–exclusion criteria for the various stages. What are the threshold values or boundaries between stages? Does a dimensional or even a hybrid model (e.g., class/quantitative) provide a more useful model, especially with certain populations (e.g., adolescents)?

Since both the categorical algorithm for staging and the URICA rely on a single method of measurement (self-report), a comprehensive multi-trait–multimethod analysis is needed to establish the convergent and discriminant validity properties. This would involve using more than one method of measurement, such as peer ratings and behavioral measures, as well as examining all five stages. This analysis could yield important information regarding the boundary issues among stages (discriminant validity), as well as whether a dimensional model may provide a more parsimonious representation of the data.

Further work is need to examine the extent to which stages or readiness for change are influenced by SES, demographic characteristics, and an individual's history. For example, how does chronicity or severity of a particular risk factor (e.g., alcohol abuse) figure into the model? An individual who is entering contemplation for the first time is likely to be quite different from someone who has a more long-term history of excessive drinking, has made numerous quit attempts, and is now in contemplation again.

Most research to date on the transtheoretical model has focused on a single behavior (e.g., cigarette smoking). How does stage or readiness for change with one risk behavior relate to an individual's readiness for change in another factor that is known to be correlated? For example, Skinner, Polzer, and Bercovitz (1997) found four distinct subgroups (factors) among 15 lifestyle areas in a sample of university students: Factor 1 (nutrition, physical activity, weight, sleep), Factor 2 (cigarettes, drugs, caffeine, alcohol), Factor 3 (social, emotional, work/leisure) and Factor 4 (driving habits, medical/dental care, sexual activities). Complex relationships probably exist within and across such domains of behavior, and it is possible that change in one behavior will be accompanied by change in others.

The transtheoretical model is innovative in many respects. It has stimulated a new era of research aimed at understanding and characterizing an individual's readiness for change and matching this with specific intervention approaches. Despite its considerable popularity, the transtheoretical model is in need of careful scrutiny, critical analysis, and empirical research. At this point, we need to redress the balance of efforts from simply applying the transtheoretical model to providing a more critical and constructive discourse.

## NOTE

1. Although the term "model" has many different uses and meanings (Earp & Ennet, 1991), Glanz et al. (1997) suggested that a model draws on a number of theories to help people understand a specific problem in a particular setting or context. Insofar as there is no single accepted definition of a theory, this definition of a model is somewhat vague. Nevertheless, Glanz et al. suggested that most definitions of a theory are consistent with a definition offered by Kerlinger (1986); that is, a theory is a set of interrelated concepts, definitions, and propositions that present a systematic view of events or situations by specifying relations among variables in order to explain and predict the events or situations.

The transtheoretical model, as the name suggests, is understood by many to be a model that integrates various theories to produce an understanding of the behavior change process. It is apparent, however, that Prochaska et al. view the model as a product of interrelated constructs. For example, with regard to the stages of change, Prochaska and colleagues have stated, "Stage is not a theory; it is a variable" (Prochaska, Redding, & Evers, 1997, p. 67), and "Stage is a variable; it is not a model" (Prochaska & Velicer, 1996, p. 1281). Although derived from theories of staging, Prochaska et al. thus consider stage to be a variable providing the operational definition of the stages of change construct within the transtheoretical model. The suggestion is that stage is a measure for a concept that is not a theory or model in itself, but becomes part of a model when it is related to what Prochaska et al. view as other constructs like the processes of change and decisional balance. Insofar as there is considerable variation in the definitions of theory and model, viewing stage as only a construct in a theory may be too limiting.

## REFERENCES

Adler, N. E., Boyce, T., Chesney, M. A., Cohen, S., Folkman, S., Kahn, R., & Syme, S. (1994). Socioeconomic status and health: The challenge of the gradient. *American Psychologist, 49,* 15–24.

Amick, T. L., & Ockene, J. K. (1994). The role of social support in the modification of risk factors for cardiovascular disease. In S. A. Shumaker & S. M. Czajkowski (Eds.), *Social support and cardiovascular disease* (pp. 259–278). New York: Plenum.

Arkowitz, H. (1995). Common factors or processes of change in psychotherapy? *Clinical Psychology Science and Practice, 2,* 94–100.

Armitage, P., & Berry, G. (1994). *Statistical methods in medical research*. Oxford, UK: Blackwell Scientific Publications.

Bandura, A. (1995, April). *Keynote address: Moving into forward gear in health promotion and disease prevention*. Presented at the meeting of the Society of Behavioral Medicine, St. Petersburg, FL.

Bandura, A. (1977). Self-efficacy: Toward a unifying theory of behavioral change. *Psychological Review, 84,* 191–215.

Biener, L., & Abrams, D. B. (1991). The contemplation ladder: Validation of a measure of readiness to consider smoking cessation. *Health Psychology, 10,* 360–365.

Bowen, A. M., & Trotter, R. (1995). HIV risk in intravenous drug users and crack cocaine smokers: Predicting stage of change for condom use. *Journal of Consulting and Clinical Psychology, 63,* 238–248.

Bowen, D. J., Meischke, H., & Tomoyasu, N. (1994). Preliminary evaluation of the processes of changing to a low-fat diet. *Health Education Research, 9,* 85–94.

Davidson, R. (1992a). Prochaska and DiClemente's model of change: A case study? *British Journal of Addiction, 87,* 821–822.

Davidson, R. (1992b). The Prochaska and DiClemente model: Reply to the debate. *British Journal of Addiction, 87,* 833–835.

DiClemente, C. C., & Hughes, S. O. (1990). Stages of change profiles in outpatient alcoholism treatment. *Journal of Substance Abuse, 2,* 217–235.

DiClemente, C. C., & Prochaska, J. O. (1982). Self change and therapy change of smoking behavior: A comparison of processes of change in cessation and maintenance. *Addictive Behaviors, 7,* 133–142.

DiClemente, C. C., Prochaska, J. O., & Gilbertini, M. (1985). Self-efficacy and the stages of self-change of smoking. *Cognitive Therapy and Research, 9,* 181–200.

Earp, J., & Ennet, S. T. (1991). Conceptual models for health education research and practice. *Health Education Research: Theory and Practice, 6,* 163–171.

Farkas, A. J., Pierce, J. P., Gilpin, E. A., Zhu, S., Rosbrook, B., Berry, C., & Kaplan, R. (1996). Is stage-of-change a useful measure of the likelihood of smoking cessation? *Annals of Behavioral Medicine, 18,* 79–86.

Farkas, A. J., Pierce, J. P., Zhu, S., Rosbrook, B., Gilpin, E., Berry, C., & Kaplan, R. (1996). Addiction versus stages of change models in predicting smoking cessation. *Addiction, 91,* 1271–1280.

Fava, J. L., Velicer, W. F., & Prochaska, J. O. (1995). Applying the transtheoretical model to a representative sample of smokers. *Addictive Behaviors, 20,* 189–203.

Glanz, K., Lewis, F. M., & Rimer, B. K. (Eds.). (1997). *Health behavior and health education: Theory, research, and practice* (2nd ed.). San Francisco: Jossey-Bass.

Grimley, D. M., Riley, G. E., Bellis, J. M., & Prochaska, J. O. (1993). Assessing the stages of change and decision making for contraceptive use for the prevention of pregnancy, sexually transmitted diseases, and acquired immunodeficiency syndrome. *Health Education Quarterly, 20,* 455–470.

Heather, N. (1992). Addictive disorders are essentially motivational problems. *British Journal of Addiction, 87,* 828–830.

Held, B. (1991). The process/content distinction in psychotherapy revisited. *Psychotherapy, 28,* 207–217.

Horn, D. (1976). A model for the study of personal choice health behavior. *International Journal of Health Education, 19,* 89–98.

Hotz, S. B. (1995). *Understanding and using the stages of change.* Ottawa: PTCC.

Isenhart, C. E. (1994). Motivational subtypes in an inpatient sample of substance abusers. *Addictive Behaviors, 19,* 463–475.

Janis, I. L., & Mann, L. (1977). *Decision making: A psychological analysis of conflict, choice and commitment.* New York: Free Press.

Kerlinger, F. N. (1986). *Foundations of behavioral research* (3rd ed.) Austin, TX: Holt, Rinehart & Winston.

Kirschenbaum, D. S., Fitzgibbon, M. L., Martino, S., Conviser, J. H., Rosendahl, D., & Laatsch, L. (1992). Stages of change in successful weight control: A clinically derived model. *Behavior Therapy, 23,* 623–635.

Kristeller, J. L., Rossi, J. S., Ockene, J. K., Goldberg, R., & Prochaska, J. (1992). Processes of change in smoking cessation: A cross-validation study in cardiac patients. *Journal of Substance Abuse, 4,* 263–276.

Luborsky, L., Singer, B., & Luborsky, L. (1975). Comparative studies of psychotherapies: Is it true that "Everyone has won and all must have prizes?" *Archives of General Psychiatry, 32,* 995–1008.

Marcus, B. H., Rossi, J. S., Selby, V. C., Niaura, R. S., & Abrams, D. (1992). The stages and processes of exercise adoption and maintenance in a worksite sample. *Health Psychology, 11,* 386–395.

Marlatt, G. A., & Gordon, J. (Eds.). (1985). *Relapse prevention: Maintenance strategies in the treatment of addictive behaviors.* New York: Guilford Press.

McConnaughy, E. A., DiClemente, C. C., Prochaska, J. O., & Velicer, W. F. (1989). Stages of change in psychotherapy: A follow-up report. *Psychotherapy, 26,* 494–503.

McConnaughy, E. A., Prochaska, J. O., & Velicer, W. F. (1983). Stages of change in psychotherapy: Measurement and sample profiles. *Psychotherapy: Theory, Research and Practice, 20,* 368–375.

Norcross, J. C. (1986). Eclectic psychotherapy: An introduction and overview. In J. C. Norcross (Ed.), *Handbook of eclectic psychotherapy* (pp. 3–18). New York: Brunner/Mazel.

Norcross, J. C., Prochaska, J. O., Guadagnoli, E., & DiClemente, C. C. (1984). Factor structure of the Levels of Attribution and Change (LAC) scale in samples of psychotherapists and smokers. *Journal of Clinical Psychology, 40,* 519–528.

Norcross, J. C., Prochaska, J. O., & Hambrecht, M. (1985). Levels of attribution and change (LAC) scale: Development and measurement. *Cognitive Therapy and Research, 9,* 631–649.

Pallonen, U. E., Murray, D. M., Schmid, L., Pirie, P., & Luepker, R. V. (1990). Patterns of self-initiated smoking cessation among young adults. *Health Psychology, 4,* 418–426.

Perz, C. A., DiClemente, C. C., & Carbonari, J. P. (1996). Doing the right thing at the right time? The interaction of stages and processes of change in successful smoking cessation. *Health Psychology, 15,* 462–468.

Piaget, J. (1926). *The language and thought of the child.* London: Routledge & Kegan Paul.

Prochaska, J. O. (1991). Assessing how people change. *Cancer, 67*(Suppl. 3), 805–807.

Prochaska, J. O. (1979). *Systems of psychotherapy: A transtheoretical analysis.* Homewood, IL: Dorsey Press.

Prochaska, J. O. (1984). *Systems of psychotherapy: A transtheoretical analysis* (2nd ed.). Homewood, IL: Dorsey Press.

Prochaska, J. O., & DiClemente, C. C. (1985). Common processes of change in smoking, weight control and psychological distress. In S. Shiffman & T. A. Wills (Eds.), *Coping and substance abuse* (pp. 345–363). New York: Academic Press.

Prochaska, J. O., & DiClemente, C. C. (1983). Stages and processes of self-change of smoking: Toward an integrative model of change. *Journal of Consulting and Clinical Psychology, 51,* 390–395.

Prochaska, J. O., & DiClemente, C. C. (1992). Stages of change in the modification of problem behaviors. In M. Hersen (Ed.), *Progress in behavior modification* (pp. 184–218). Sycamore, IL: Sycamore Publishing.

Prochaska, J. O., & DiClemente, C. C. (1984). *The transtheoretical approach: Crossing traditional boundaries of therapy.* Homewood, IL: Down Jones Irwin.

Prochaska, J. O., & DiClemente, C. C. (1986). Toward a comprehensive model of change. In W. R. Miller & N. Heather (Eds.), *Treating addictive behaviors: Processes of change* (pp. 3–27). New York: Plenum.

Prochaska, J. O., DiClemente, C. C., & Norcross, J. C. (1992). In search of how people change: Applications to addictive behaviors. *American Psychologist, 47,* 1102–1114.

Prochaska, J. O., DiClemente, C. C., Velicer, W. F., Ginpil, S., & Norcross, J. C. (1985). Predicting change in smoking status for self-changers. *Addictive Behavior, 10,* 395–406.

Prochaska, J. O., DiClemente, C. C., Velicer, W. F., & Rossi, J. S. (1992). Comments on Davidson's "Prochaska and DiClemente's model of change: A case study?" *British Journal of Addiction, 87,* 825–835.

Prochaska, J. O., DiClemente, C. C., Velicer, W. F., & Rossi, J. S. (1993). Standardized, individualized, interactive, and personalized self-help programs for smoking cessation. *Health Psychology, 12,* 399–405.

Prochaska, J. O., Norcross, J., Fowler, J., Follick, M., & Abrams, D. (1992). Attendance and outcome in a work site weight control program: Processes and stages of change as process and predictor variables. *Addictive Behaviors, 17,* 35–45.

Prochaska, J. O., Redding, C. A., & Evers, K. E. (1997). The transtheoretical model and stages of change. In K. Glanz, R. M. Lewis, & B. K. Rimer (Eds.), *Health behavior and health education* (pp. 60–84). San Francisco: Jossey-Bass.

Prochaska, J. O., & Velicer, W. F. (1996). Comments on Farkas et al.'s "Addiction versus stages of change models in predicting smoking cessation." *Addiction, 91,* 1281–82.

Prochaska, J. O., Velicer, W. F., DiClemente, C. C., & Fava, J. (1988). Measuring processes of change: Applications to the cessation of smoking. *Journal of Consulting and Clinical Psychology, 56,* 520–528.

Prochaska, J. O., Velicer, W. F., Guadagnoli, E., Rossi, J. S., & DiClemente, C. (1991). Patterns of change: Dynamic typology applied to smoking cessation. *Multivariate Behavioral Research, 26,* 83–107.

Prochaska, J. O., Velicier, W. F., Rossi, J. S., Goldstein, M., Marcus, B., Rakowski, W., Fiore, C., Harlow, L., Redding, C., Rosenbloom, D., & Rossi, S. (1994). Stages of change and decisional balance for 12 problem behaviors. *Health Psychology, 13,* 39–46.

Rakowski, W., Dube, C., Marcus, B., Prochaska, J., Velicer, W., & Abrams, D. (1992). Assessing elements of women's decisions about mammography. *Health Psychology, 11,* 111–118.

Rakowski, W., Fulton, J., & Feldman, J. (1993). Women's decision making about mammography: A replication of the relationship between stages of adoption and decisional balance. *Health Psychology, 12,* 209–214.

Rosenweig, S. (1936). Some implicit common factors in diverse methods of psychotherapy. *American Journal of Orthopsychiatry, 6,* 412–415.

Rustin, T., & Tate, J. (1993). Measuring the stages of change in cigarette smokers [Special Issue: Towards a broader view of recovery: Integrating nicotine addiction and chemical dependency treatments]. *Journal of Substance Abuse Treatment, 10,* 209–220.

Skinner, H., Polzer, J., & Bercovitz, K. (1997). *Readiness to change health behavior: A multidimensional perspective.* Unpublished manuscript, University of Toronto, Toronto, Canada.

Skinner, H. A. (1981). Toward the integration of classification theory and methods. *Journal of Abnormal Psychology, 90,* 68–87.

Stockwell, T. (1992). Models of change, heavenly bodies and weltanschauungs. *British Journal of Addiction, 87*(6), 830–832.

Sutton, S. (1996). Can "stage of change" provide guidance in the treatment of addictions? A critical examination of Prochaska and DiClemente's model. In G. Edwards & C. Dare (Eds.), *Psychotherapy, psychological treatments and the addictions.* New York: Cambridge University Press.

Velicer, W., DiClemente, C., Prochaska, J., & Brandenburg, N. (1985). A decisional balance measure for assessing and predicting smoking status. *Journal of Personality and Social Psychology, 48,* 1279–1289.

Velicer, W., Hughes, S., Fava, J., Prochaska, J., & DiClemente, C. (1995). An empirical typology of subjects within stage of change. *Addictive Behaviors, 20,* 299–320.

Wilcox, N., Prochaska, J., & Velicer, W. (1985). Subject characteristics as predictors of self-change in smoking cessation. *Addictive Behavior, 10,* 407–412.

# 7

## Behavioral Economics as a Framework for Organizing the Expanded Range of Substance Abuse Interventions

### RUDY E. VUCHINICH

This book articulates the necessity of expanding efforts to change addictive behaviors beyond individual-client clinical treatments to include multiple interventions at multiple levels. Achieving the pragmatic goals of this expansion will be partially determined by the degree to which it is guided by scientifically useful concepts and methods. This chapter argues that a behavioral economic analysis of substance abuse can contribute one such set of concepts and methods. The first section of the chapter briefly describes the development of behavioral economics and summarizes research that has applied these concepts to the study of substance abuse. A second section discusses some specific areas in which this research has practical utility. A final section argues that a cultural context more congenial to this expanded intervention agenda would be created by replacing the dominant disease and addiction metaphors for substance abuse with a more scientifically credible and pragmatically useful economic metaphor.

### DEVELOPMENT OF BEHAVIORAL ECONOMICS AND EXTENSIONS TO SUBSTANCE ABUSE RESEARCH

Behavioral economics originated in the basic science laboratory, where understanding the allocation of behavior (choice) among available activities is a crucial issue. A revolutionary change in studying choice was produced by the work of Premack (1965) and Herrnstein (1970). Premack showed that engaging in any activity depends on what other activities are also available and on their associated environmental constraints. Herrnstein showed that engaging in any given activity depends on its reinforcement relative to the reinforcement obtained from other activities. This work revealed the inadequacy of focusing on individual responses in accounts of choice, which had been the focus of prior work (e.g., Hull, 1943; Skinner, 1938), and demonstrated that behavioral allocation is critically affected by the more general context of environmental conditions that surrounds individual responses.

As the literature on choice developed (reviewed by Williams, 1988), it was soon recognized that the issue of understanding the behavioral allocation of animals in the laboratory was similar to the issues addressed by consumer demand theory in economics (e.g., Allison, 1979; Hursh, 1980; Rachlin, Green, Kagel, & Battalio, 1976; Staddon, 1980); that is, both animal subjects and human consumers allocate limited resources (time, behavior, money) to gain access to activities of varying value (eating, drinking, leisure) under conditions of variable environmental constraint. Recognizing this connection produced a merger of the behavioral analysis of choice and of microeconomic theory, which is now known as *behavioral economics* (e.g., Green & Kagel, 1987; Hursh, 1980; Kagel, Battalio, & Green, 1995; Staddon, 1980).

The potential contributions of behavioral economics for understanding substance abuse were recognized soon after its origin (Allison, 1979; Elsmore, Fletcher, Conrad, & Sodetz, 1980; Vuchinich, 1982), and research applications to substance abuse have flourished (e.g., Bickel, De-Grandpre, & Higgins, 1993; Green & Kagel, 1996; Vuchinich, 1997). From the behavioral economic perspective, patterns of substance abuse emerge, develop, and change over time within temporally extended environmental contexts that are characterized by stability and change in access to substance use and activity opportunities unrelated to substance use. This is a *molar* level of analysis, in which the concepts and empirical relations represent contextually embedded behavior patterns. This is in contrast to a *molecular* level of analysis, in which the concepts and empirical relations represent events inside the individual that immediately precede substance use episodes (Vuchinich, 1995; Vuchinich & Tucker, 1996a). This molar view directs attention to two broad classes of variables as critical influences on substance abuse (cf. Vuchinich & Tucker, 1988): (1) environmental constraints on access to the abused substance (e.g., availability and price), and (2) the availability of and constraints on access to alternative, non-substance-related activities (e.g., intimate, family, or social relations; vocational or academic success). Research findings from each of these domains are summarized next.

## Constraints on Access to the Abused Substance

Although it has been known for some time that consumption of abused substances varies inversely with their cost (e.g., Griffiths, Bigelow, & Henningfield, 1980; Ornstein, 1980), behavioral economic research can coherently organize these relations under the rubric of demand curve analysis. Demand is the primary dependent variable in microeconomics and refers to the amount of a commodity that is purchased (and presumably consumed). Given that the primary concern in substance abuse is excessive consumption, the focus of behavioral economics on demand renders the framework especially applicable to substance abuse research (Hursh, 1993). The basic demand curve plots consumption of a commodity as a function of its price, and the general economic Law of Demand states that there is an inverse relation between consumption and price. A central concept in demand curve analysis is *own-price elasticity* of demand, which is defined as the ratio of proportional changes in consumption to proportional changes in price (cf. Hursh, 1993); it thus provides a quantitative measure of how consumption changes as a function of price. Commodities can be distinguished along the continuum of demand elasticities. *Inelastic demand* refers to little or no changes in consumption as price changes, and *elastic demand* refers to substantial changes in consumption as price changes. Typically, commodities show mixed elasticity along the range of price changes, with demand being more inelastic at low prices and more elastic at high prices.

Two central empirical issues for an application of behavioral economics to substance abuse are (1) whether abused substances obey the Law of Demand, and (2) whether the quantitative properties of the demand curve (e.g., own-price elasticity) aid in the description and analysis of substance consumption. Research on this issue has yielded a positive answer on both counts. In human and animal laboratory preparations designed to study these relations, participants typically must emit a specified number of responses in order to receive a specified dose of the substance. Thus, the number of responses is the empirical interpretation of price.

Bickel, DeGrandpre, Higgins, and Hughes (1990), Bickel et al. (1993), and DeGrandpre, Bickel, Hughes, Layng, and Badger (1993) reanalyzed data from numerous, earlier drug self-administration experiments (including cocaine, codeine, *d*-amphetamine, ethanol, ketamine, methohexital, morphine, pentobarbital, phencyclidine, and procaine) that did not employ a demand curve analysis when first reported but did manipulate relevant variables (including multiple drug doses and the response requirement to receive each dose). The important generalization that emerged from these reanalyses was that the demand curves all showed the typical mixed elasticity, with demand being inelastic at lower prices and elastic at higher prices. Similar results were obtained in a reanalysis of 17 studies of human cigarette smoking (DeGrandpre, Bickel, Hughes, & Higgins, 1992) and in an experiment with human cigarette smokers that explicitly employed a demand curve analysis (Bickel, DeGrandpre, Hughes, & Higgins, 1991). This same inverse relation between substance consumption and (monetary) price has also been observed in the natural environment for alcoholic beverages (e.g., Leung & Phelps, 1993) as well as illicit drugs (e.g., Chaloupka, Grossman, & Tauras, in press; Saffer & Chaloupka, in press).

Research on this first variable class has repeatedly demonstrated a quantifiable inverse relation between substance use and abuse and direct constraints on access to the substance (Bickel et al., 1993; DeGrandpre & Bickel, 1996). This relationship has generality across species, substances of abuse, normal and clinical populations, and laboratory and natural environments. Importantly, these behavioral economic analyses of demand for abused substances as a function of direct constraints indicate that consumption of them can be accurately described with the same analytic tools that apply to all commodities. This suggests that the demand for abused substances is but one instance of a "ubiquitous behavioral process" (Bickel et al., 1993, p. 181) and that drugs are not a special class of commodities that requires unique concepts for analysis.

## Reinforcement Context and Demand for Abused Substances

The research just discussed studied demand for abused substances in situations devoid of opportunities for engaging in other activities. Although some important regularities have emerged from this work, the laboratory settings used lack a potentially critical feature of the contexts in which substance abuse typically develops; that is, strong preferences for abused substances arise in natural environments that contain opportunities to engage in a variety of other activities. Understanding the conditions under which substance consumption emerges as a highly preferred activity from among an array of qualitatively different activities is a basic problem for substance abuse research (Vuchinich & Tucker, 1988). Moreover, the latter class of contextual variables may be more important for understanding substance abuse patterns in natural environments, because substance availability typically is minimally constrained and constant in most natural environments relative to the considerable variability that exists in access to valued alternative activities.

In general, the behavioral economic perspective suggests that demand for abused substances should vary inversely with the availability of alternative activities and directly with constraints on access to those alternatives. Numerous laboratory experiments have demonstrated these relationships. With animals, for example, the consumption of cocaine (Nader & Woolverton, 1991), phencyclidine (Carroll, Carmona, & May, 1991), and ethanol (Samson & Lindberg, 1984) varied inversely with the availability of food, saccharin, and sucrose, respectively. Similar relations have been found with humans. For example, Bickel, DeGrandpre, Higgins, Hughes, and Badger (1995) found that smokers demanded fewer cigarette puffs in a condition in which an alternative response produced either money or access to video games than in a condition in which only smoking was available. Other studies have found that cocaine (Hatsukami, Thompson, Pentel, Flygare, & Carroll, 1994) and alcohol consumption (Chutuape, Mitchell, & de Wit, 1994; Vuchinich & Tucker, 1983) varied inversely with the amount of money participants could earn during experimental sessions.

This research clearly demonstrates that there are important qualitative relations between demand for drugs and the availability of alternative reinforcers. However, behavioral economic concepts also can precisely quantify how drug demand interacts with the availability of and demand for other reinforcers. These concepts concern *substitutability relations* between commodities (e.g., Green & Freed, 1993), which categorize and quantify how consumption of one commodity changes as a function of price-induced changes in the consumption of another commodity. Demand for *substitutable commodities* varies inversely (e.g., coffee and tea), and demand for *complementary commodities* varies directly (e.g., flour and baking powder). For example, if commodities $A$ and $B$ are available for consumption, demand for $A$ would be reduced if its own price were increased. If demand for $B$ increased when demand for $A$ decreased, even though the price of $B$ was unchanged, $B$ would be a substitute for $A$. If, under the same circumstances, demand for $B$ decreased when demand for $A$ decreased, $B$ would be a complement of $A$. *Cross-price elasticity of demand* quantifies these relations across commodities and is defined as the ratio of proportional changes in consumption of one commodity to proportional changes in the price of another commodity (cf. Hursh, 1993).

In order to demonstrate the utility of this concept, Bickel, DeGrandpre, and Higgins (1995) conducted a reanalysis of 16 drug self-administration studies that permitted an evaluation of substitutability relations between drug consumption (including caffeine, nicotine, cocaine, etonitazene, ethanol, heroin, methadone, morphine, pentobarbital, and phencyclidine, or PCP) and alternative drug and nondrug reinforcers (e.g., food, sucrose, water). This reanalysis showed that these drugs enter into relations with other reinforcers at all points along the substitutability continuum. For example, in separate studies, substitutable relations were found between sucrose and ethanol, etonitazene and water, and PCP and ethanol, whereas complementary relations were found between heroin and cigarettes, alcohol and cigarettes, heroin and food, and ethanol and water. Thus, these behavioral economic concepts are useful for understanding how drug consumption interacts with demand for other commodities.

These laboratory studies involving choice between drug and nondrug reinforcers have yielded consistent findings. However, because the abused substance and the alternative activity typically are both available at the same time, they also lacked a contextual element that may be important for understanding substance abuse in the natural environment. In the natural environment, the abused substance and the activities with which it competes typically are available at different times; that is, individuals choose between substance use, which typically is readily available with little delay, and engaging in behavior that will produce access to more valuable activities (e.g., vocational or academic success, satisfying intimate and social relations) that usually are available only after delays that sometimes may be considerable. Thus, it is critical to incorporate theory and research on *intertemporal choice,* that is, choice between smaller sooner rewards (SSR) and larger later rewards (LLR) (e.g., Ainslie, 1992; Rachlin, 1974), into a behavioral economic analysis of substance abuse.

As an illustration, Figure 7.1A depicts a simple intertemporal choice between an SSR of Amount 3 available at Time 6 and an LLR of Amount 6 available at Time 12. The SSR and LLR are viewed as analogous, respectively, to substance use and more valuable but delayed activities that do not involve substance use (e.g., vocational success, personal relations) (Vuchinich & Tucker, 1988). The curves to the left of the rewards represent their value during the times before they are available; the reward with the highest value curve at the time of choice will be preferred. It is important to note that the value of the rewards varies inversely with their delay. Thus, the value of a delayed reward today is less than what its value will be when it is received in the future (i.e., its present value is discounted). The curves in the figure are drawn according to a *hyperbolic temporal discounting function,* which has extensive empirical support (e.g., Ainslie, 1992). A key choice dynamic produced by hyperbolic discounting is that preference between the LLR and SSR will reverse simply with the passage of time. This is indicated by the crossing of the reward value curves between Time 4 and Time 5 in Figure 7.1A. Thus, the LLR would be preferred before that time and the SSR would be preferred after that time.

The choice dynamics depicted in Figure 7.1A are consistent with two important aspects of substance abuse patterns. First, given a constant reward structure in the environment, individuals will display ambivalence in that their preference for substance use will vary over time depending on

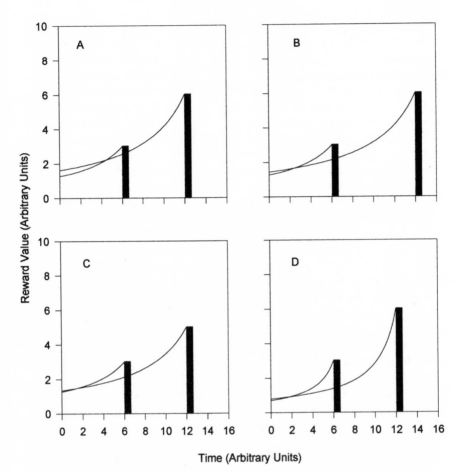

**FIGURE 7.1.** An illustration of intertemporal choice between smaller sooner rewards (SSR) and larger later rewards (LLR), which are analogous, respectively, to substance use and more valuable activities that do not involve substance use. Rewards are vertical bars; height represents value, and abscissa location represents time of availability. The curves represent reward value during times before availability and are drawn according to a hyperbolic discount function. The reward with the highest value curve at the time of choice will be preferred. The SSR in each panel is of Amount 3 and is available at Time 6. *Panel A:* Choice between the SSR and an LLR of Amount 6 that is available at Time 12. Hyperbolic temporal discounting results in preference reversal with the passage of time. *Panel B:* Choice between the SSR and an LLR of Amount 6 that is available at Time 14. The longer delay to LLR availability results in a stronger preference for substance use in panel B than in panel A. *Panel C:* Choice between the SSR and an LLR of Amount 5 that is available at Time 12. The smaller LLR results in a stronger preference for substance use in panel C than in panel A. *Panel D:* Rewards are the same as in panel A, but with a higher degree of delayed reward discounting than in panel A. This results in a stronger preference for substance use in panel D than in panel A.

the temporal distance to the availability of the substance and the alternative activity. The LLRs will be preferred before the point where the reward value curves cross, and substance use will be preferred after that point. But, once the person exits the situation involving substance availability, preference will revert back to the LLRs, and the individual may regret the substance use episode. Second, the LLRs that enter into these intertemporal choice dynamics with substance use will likely differ across individuals and across time for the same individual (Vuchinich & Tucker, 1996b). Such variability is consistent with the diversity of life–health problems associated with substance abuse in populations of alcohol and drug abusers (e.g., Maisto & McCollum, 1980).

The other three panels in Figure 7.1 illustrate variables that have been shown to influence the consumption of abused substances. One such variable is the delay until receipt of the LLR, as seen by comparing panel B with panel A. In panel A, an LLR of Amount 6 is available at Time 12, but in panel B, the same-amount LLR is not available until Time 14. This produces an earlier preference shift toward the SSR in panel B compared to panel A, which should lead to more consumption of the abused substance. Such a relation was found by Vuchinich and Tucker (1983) and by Vuchinich, Tucker, and Rudd (1987), who gave human participants the choice between consuming alcohol and earning money, and manipulated the delay with which any money earned would be received.

Another relevant choice dynamic that influences the consumption of abused substances is shown in panels C and A, which depict different amounts of the LLR. In panel A, an LLR of Amount 6 is available at Time 12, but in panel C, an LLR of Amount 5 is available at Time 12. Again, this produces an earlier preference shift toward the SSR in panel C compared to panel A, which should lead to more consumption of the abused substance. Such relationships were found in the laboratory studies mentioned earlier (Bickel et al., 1995; Carroll et al., 1991; Chutuape et al., 1994; Hatsukami et al., 1994; Nader & Woolverton, 1991; Samson & Lindberg, 1984; Vuchinich & Tucker, 1983)

The choice dynamics illustrated by comparing panels B and C with A are relevant to understanding relapse and recovery processes. Panels B and C both represent situations in which access to the LLR is more constrained than in panel A. The reward value curves cross much earlier in panel B and C than in A, which yields a stronger preference for substance use (the SSR), even when access to the abused substance remains constant. Thus, the risk of relapse would increase when the reward structure in an individual's environment goes through a transition from the situation depicted in panel A to that depicted in panels B or C; that is, preference for substance use should increase if valued alternatives unrelated to substance use become more constrained. Such relationships were found in a prospective study of life events and drinking episodes in problem drinkers during a 6-month interval after treatment (Vuchinich & Tucker, 1996b). Moreover, drinking episodes preceded by events that signaled increased constraints on valued nondrinking alternatives were found to be more severe than drinking episodes that were not associated with events and presumably did not involve a change in the overall reward structure. This suggests an environmental basis for distinguishing the controlling variables of lapses and relapses. O'Connell and Martin (1987) found similar relationships with respect to smoking cessation attempts.

Decreasing substance abuse and maintaining the change (i.e., recovery) can be conceptualized as involving the reverse process wherein the reward structure transitions from the situation depicted in panels B or C to that depicted in panel A. If initial abstinence or reduced substance use increases access to valuable alternatives unrelated to substance use, then preference for substance use should decrease and remain low except in situations where drug availability is imminent. As reduced substance use or abstinence is maintained and as access to valued non-substance-related activities is forthcoming, then the LLR reward value curve should supersede the value curve for substance use at almost all points in time. Such relationships between the maintenance of recovery and increased access to valued nondrinking rewards were found in both treated and untreated problem drinkers who had abstained continuously for several years (Tucker, Vuchinich, & Gladsjo, 1994; Tucker, Vuchinich, & Pukish, 1995).

Another relevant variable concerns the degree to which the value of delayed rewards are discounted during the times before they are available. Greater degrees of temporal discounting produce a stronger preference for the SSR, which leads to more substance use. This relationship is shown by comparing panels D and A in Figure 7.1. The amounts and delays of the rewards are the same in both panels, but the rewards are discounted to a greater degree in D than in A. The greater discounting in panel D produces lower reward value curves, which result in an earlier preference shift toward the SSR in panel D compared to panel A. This suggests that substance use should be positively correlated with the degree of temporal discounting. Individuals with a relatively low degree of discounting, as in panel A, would spend more time behaving in ways that produce access to the nondrug rewards and less time preferring substance use. Individuals with a relatively high degree of discounting, as in panel D, would spend less time behaving in ways that produce access to the rewards unrelated to substance use and more time preferring substance use.

Preliminary support has been found for a such a positive relation between temporal discounting and substance use. Vuchinich and Simpson (1998) compared heavy social and problem drinkers with light social drinkers on the degree to which they discounted the value of delayed amounts of money. The light drinkers discounted the value of delayed money significantly less than the heavy or problem drinkers. The same relationship was found in a similar study that compared the delayed monetary discounting of opioid-dependent and control participants (Madden, Petry, Badger, & Bickel, 1997). Also, in a prospective follow-up of problem drinkers who were attempting to resolve their problem without treatment (Tucker & Vuchinich, 1997), successful maintenance for a year or more was predicted by a monetary index of the extent to which individuals organized a portion of their behavior around delayed outcomes when they were drinking heavily. Individuals who remained resolved had saved about 10 times as much money during the year prior to the initiation of abstinence or nonproblem, moderate drinking compared to those who resumed problem drinking, even though the two outcome groups were similar in their total preresolution income and expenditures, and in their preresolution drinking practices. This discounting–substance abuse relation suggests that individuals who more heavily discount the value of delayed outcomes may be more susceptible to developing substance abuse and, once a problem exists, they may be less likely to resolve it.

## Summary

Research derived from the behavioral economic perspective has produced a broad array of theoretically coherent empirical relations on various aspects of substance abuse that have considerable generality. This research indicates that the two classes of variables highlighted by a behavioral economic analysis have important effects on substance use and abuse. Thus, for purposes of encouraging reduced substance use, this perspective emphasizes increasing constraints on access to abused substances, increasing access to valued activities other than substance use, or both. However, because of pragmatic limitations on constraining access to abused substances, increasing access to valued activities other than substance use may be preferable. Moreover, such increased access would increase individuals' motivation to change substance abuse behavior patterns and would aid in the prevention or minimization of relapse. The applied implications of a behavioral economic analysis of substance abuse, which are discussed next, are derived from these themes.

## APPLIED IMPLICATIONS FOR BROADENING THE BASE OF SUBSTANCE ABUSE INTERVENTIONS

An attractive feature of the behavioral economic framework for guiding applications is that its concepts can be applied consistently across the range of relevant situations; that is, behavioral allocation, in general, and substance use, in particular, by animals and humans in laboratory preparations, and by humans in the natural environment, can be described with the same theoretical terms, although their empirical interpretations differ across the different situations. The generality of relations found in one situation therefore can be evaluated by extending the same theoretical terms, with appropriate empirical interpretations, to other situations. Thus, the merger of the behavioral analysis of choice and of microeconomic theory that formed behavioral economics has been extended to encompass under one umbrella behavioral economic and econometric analyses of substance use and abuse (Chaloupka, Bickel, Grossman, & Saffer, in press). The applicability of the same theoretical terms in situations that range from animals in the laboratory to humans in the natural environment greatly enhances the generality of discovered empirical relations. The applied implications summarized in this section demonstrate the utility of behavioral economic concepts for broadening the base of substance abuse interventions.

## Assessing Abuse Liability of Drugs and Developing Pharmacological Interventions

The quantitative properties of drug demand curves in laboratory preparations may provide valuable information in assessing abuse liability and in developing pharmacological interventions. For example, the quantification of own-price elasticity of demand for different drugs, or of the same drug under different conditions, provides a common metric for evaluating the ease with which drugs may come to be used in an abusive manner (Hursh, 1993). Bickel et al. (1993) reanalyzed some of the data from a study by Goldberg, Hoffeister, Shlichting, and Wuttke (1971) and showed that demand for pentobarbital was over 12 times more responsive to price increases than was demand for cocaine. Thus, demand for pentobarbital was much more elastic than demand for cocaine, which implies that pentobarbital has less abuse potential compared to cocaine, a finding that matches casual observation regarding the abuse potential of the two drugs. Thus, elasticity coefficients derived from demand curve analyses in the laboratory may provide a useful metric to compare and contrast the motivational properties of different drugs.

Own-price elasticity of drugs also may be useful in the development and use of pharmacotherapies for drug abuse. Such treatments typically employ agonists or antagonists of the abused substance (Bickel et al., 1993). Agonists mimic and antagonists block drug effects (e.g., methadone is an agonist and naltrexone is an antagonist of heroin). As a demonstration of the potential utility of behavioral economics in this area, Bickel et al. (1993) showed that, at low prices of heroin, methadone did not change demand for heroin, but naltrexone increased demand for heroin. At higher heroin prices, both drugs made demand for heroin more elastic. Such findings imply that if the street-price of heroin is low, methadone may have minimal effects on heroin demand and naltrexone may actually increase heroin demand (a countertherapeutic effect). At higher heroin prices, the presence of either methadone or naltrexone would facilitate decreases in the demand for heroin, which would be a therapeutic effect. This suggests that the use of these common pharmacotherapies for heroin dependence should be sensitive to the price and availability of street-procured heroin.

In addition, studying relations between substance use and alternative reinforcers in controlled laboratory situations also may reveal important pharmacotherapeutic implications. The quantification of commodity substitutability relations through cross-price elasticity of demand coefficients, as discussed earlier, may be a metric useful in the identification of the neurochemical substrates of reinforcement and incentive systems, including drugs (e.g., Green & Rachlin, 1991; Hursh, 1991). This, in turn, may be critical information in the development of new pharmacotherapies for drug abuse (e.g., George & Ritz, 1993).

## Psychological Assessment and Individual Client Interventions

A simple yet potentially powerful implication of the behavioral economic perspective is that in characterizing the determinants of substance abuse and in developing psychological interventions to reduce it, more attention should be paid to the *molar context of substance use* (Vuchinich & Tucker, 1996a). This context is defined by the availability of valuable activities other than substance use and by the extent to which access to these activities is contingent upon abstinence or reduced substance use.

The research summarized earlier clearly shows that the variety and availability of valuable activities other than substance use can have a critical influence on substance consumption. These relations have relevance for clinical assessment procedures. Given that reductions in access to valued activities (e.g., intimate and family relationships) are correlated with resumption of problem drinking after alcohol treatment (Vuchinich & Tucker, 1996b), and given that increases in access to such activities are correlated with treatment-assisted and natural recovery from alcohol problems (Tucker et al., 1995), it is important to assess these relations explicitly in clinical populations for purposes of treatment planning (Vuchinich & Tucker, 1996a; Vuchinich, Tucker, & Harllee, 1988).

The inverse relation between substance use and valued activities unrelated to it also has important implications for interventions delivered at the level of the individual client. Such treatments should move rapidly to improve clients' access to alternative activities that would reduce demand for substance use, rather than focusing nearly exclusively on reducing or eliminating drug use, as is common practice. Cox and Klinger (1988, p. 176) stated the importance of this general intervention principle: "Any treatment technique will be doomed to failure if it enables alcoholics to stop drinking but does not provide them with alternative sources of . . . satisfaction." The conceptually compatible and highly effective Community Reinforcement Approach, which increases clients' access to nondrug reinforcers in the natural environment (e.g., Higgins et al., 1991; see Chapter 12, this volume), illustrates this principle and may include increasing access to employment, drug-free housing, and drug-free social interactions.

It is not always possible, of course, for a clinician to modify directly activities other than substance use that are available to clients in their natural environments, or the constraints that exist on access to them. Also, some clients have sufficiently rich life circumstances but fail to engage them in a positive fashion. Thus, in many cases, motivating and enabling the client to exploit better the alternative activities that are available are the more appropriate goal of treatment. Motivating and enabling contact with available nondrug activities may be an important contribution to the effectiveness of brief interventions (e.g., Heather, 1989), especially those based on motivational interviewing (e.g., Miller, 1996). In such interventions, the clinician is empathic and nonjudgmental, and attempts to generate client interest in, and motivation for, behavior change by emphasizing discrepancies between current substance use patterns and longer term goals (among other techniques). Such verbal manipulations may modify clients' perceptions of their choice options or may reduce the degree to which longer term positive outcomes are discounted (see Figure 7.1D). Although highly speculative, this interpretation is suggested by the behavioral economic perspective and may shed some light on the processes through which motivational interviewing exerts its positive effects, which are poorly understood (Miller, 1996). In any case, the emphasis of these interventions on valuable activities other than substance abuse is consistent with the behavioral economic perspective.

## Prevention, Community, and Public Policy Interventions

Epidemiological studies indicate that the vast majority of substance users and abusers establish patterns of consumption during a several-year period in adolescence (Kandel & Logan, 1984). This developmental period therefore is the primary target of prevention efforts. From the present perspective, the development of substance abuse in adolescence should be influenced by variables that (1) modify constraints on access to abused substances, or (2) modify constraints on access to valuable alternative activities. Hawkins, Catalano, and Miller's (1992) review of risk factors in adolescent substance abuse reported many variables that fall into these categories, broadly conceived. Regarding the first category, they found that lower prices of abused substances, greater substance availability in the community, and substance use by family members and peers—all of which lower direct constraints on substance use—were risk factors for the development of substance abuse. Regarding the second category, they found that economic deprivation, low bonding in the family, academic failure, and peer rejection—all of which increase constraints on access to valuable alternative activities—also were risk factors for adolescent substance abuse.

The finding that such variables are risk factors for the development of substance use and abuse strongly suggests that explicit manipulation of them could prevent substance abuse in some individuals. Indeed, substance abuse prevention programs that have shown positive results (e.g., Botvin, Baker, & Dusenbury, 1990; Perry, Williams, & Forster, 1993) include a combination of intervention components that change these two classes of variables in ways that shift preferences away from abused substances and toward more constructive alternative activities. A particularly impressive community-level program of this sort is the Midnight Basketball project that was implemented in several urban localities in the early 1990s (United States Department of Housing and Urban Development, 1994; United States Government Printing Office, 1992). Program participants received immediate access to valuable activities unrelated to substance use (e.g., membership in a basketball league) if they refrained from substance use and involvement in criminal activities. Participants also were required to engage in employment skills training and other educational programs that would increase their ability to engage effectively in constructive activities that did not involve substance use. Such interventions have had impressive success in promoting program retention and long-term positive outcomes in a population that is at extremely high risk for substance abuse and criminal involvement (United States Government Printing Office, 1992). The success of programs of this sort contrasts with more typical prevention programs that focus on education regarding abused substances, such as the DARE program, which has been found to be ineffective (e.g., Ennett, Tobler, & Ringwalt, 1994).

Public policy interventions to reduce substance use and abuse typically have focused on increasing constraints on access to substances. The U.S. War on Drugs clearly is an attempt to minimize the availability of illicit drugs and to maximize their cost. Similar examples of such efforts against licit drugs include raising taxes on alcoholic beverages and tobacco products (e.g., Leung & Phelps, 1993), raising the legal age for alcohol consumption (e.g., Wagenaar, 1993), and increasing penalties for inappropriate alcohol use (e.g., Hingson, Heeren, & Winter, 1994). Such programs somewhat reduce drug consumption and associated problems, but their effectiveness would almost certainly be enhanced if they incorporated procedures that increased access to valuable activities other than drug use. The behavioral economic literature is clear that substantially reducing substance use and abuse depends critically on increasing access to valued activities other than drug use (Carroll, 1996; Vuchinich & Tucker, 1988). Simply increasing the constraints on access to substances usually will not significantly reduce or eliminate use, especially under natural conditions when the price of substances is relatively low. Indeed, constraining access to substances or increasing their price without also providing alternative activities intensifies drug-seeking behavior, which creates its own set of problems, including increased criminal activity (Bickel & DeGrandpre, 1996; Hursh, 1991).

The effects of various prevention, community-level, and public policy interventions can be readily interpreted in light of behavioral economic concepts. Even though those concepts did not generate the initial design of these programs, their explicit consideration may lead to the design of more effective programs. As noted by Higgins (1997, p. 426):

> Policy makers, behavioral scientists, and clinicians invested in resolving the public health problems of [substance] abuse should think seriously and creatively about how the presence and absence of alternative, nondrug reinforcers is involved in the genesis and maintenance of this disorder and what kinds of creative interventions might be devised to curtail it. The extant scientific evidence suggests that an open and creative approach to these concepts and principles could result in some important gains.

## Developing New Services

As detailed throughout this book, the heterogeneity of substance abuse problems and the limited absolute effectiveness of clinical treatments have made an expansion of services a high priority (e.g., Institute of Medicine, 1990). As discussed by Marlatt, Tucker, Donovan, and Vuchinich (1997), a primary goal of these expanded services is to attract more substance abusing individuals into helping environments, especially the underserved majority with less severe problems. In other words, in the terms of behavioral economics, the expanded care system must increase demand for services. Help-seeking research (Marlatt et al., 1997) has repeatedly shown that the abstinence-oriented, U.S. service delivery system has not created sufficient demand for services, in that only about 20% of persons with substance-related problems seek any kind of help.

Several factors probably contribute to this low demand for current services, including the stigma associated with substance abuse and its treatment, the general lack of effective intervention alternatives, and the typical requirement that clients abstain if they are to receive help (see Chapters 1 and 3, this volume, for more extended discussion of these issues). The accessibility and cost of treatment do not appear to be important factors, and most substance abusers seek help for problems caused by and related to their substance use, rather than because of excessive substance use itself (Marlatt et al., 1997). From the behavioral economic perspective, one way to increase demand for services would be to relax the traditional abstinence requirement under some circumstances. The choice dynamics discussed earlier and shown in Figure 7.1 indicate that by requiring abstinence for entry into an intervention, the substance abuser must forgo consumption of a readily available, valued commodity (i.e., substance use) in order to gain access to more valuable but delayed and probabilistic outcomes (i.e., benefits of treatment or abstinence). The fact that a small minority of substance abusers seek services strongly suggests that the discounted value of the delayed and probabilistic treatment effects usually do not outweigh the value of the more immediate and certain substance use (compare Figure 7.1D with 7.1A). This suggests that the abstinence requirement could be relaxed until the client's access to valued activities other than substance use is increased, unless that access is dependent upon abstinence, or if there are imminent health reasons for abstaining. This provides a functional basis for initial goal selection and is responsive to the forces that often promote help-seeking (addressing problems related to the substance use).

Another implication of the behavioral economic perspective is that service providers for substance abusing persons should attend more to the needs and preferences of the consumers of those services, including those who are not interested in stopping substance use but who wish to reduce the harm associated with it. This follows directly from an economic perspective, in which demand for a commodity (i.e., substance abuse services) can be increased by minimizing constraints on access to the commodity and by maximizing its attractiveness. This theme is shared by harm reduction (e.g., Marlatt & Tapert, 1993) and motivational (e.g., Miller, 1996) interventions that emphasize "meeting clients where they are." Thus, the behavioral economic and harm reduction perspectives converge in promoting the development of services that are more accessible, make greater use of social and community resources, and facilitate the natural forces that promote behavior change (Marlatt et al., 1997).

## Summary

Behavioral economic concepts and research have potentially important implications for substance abuse applications that range from specific recommendations for altering current practices to the design of new services and new interventions. The implementation of these recommendations across this range has the potential for guiding the development of more effective and humane policies for dealing with substance abuse problems. As discussed in the next section, however, there are nonscientific, cultural impediments to the realization of these positive changes.

# CREATING A SOCIAL CONTEXT FOR BROADENING THE BASE OF SUBSTANCE ABUSE INTERVENTIONS

Implementing the "broadening-the-base" agenda discussed throughout this book will require the cooperation of many individuals and groups. In addition to the scientists who study substance abuse and the clinicians who treat it, the effort will depend on policy analysts and other experts, as well as on the executives, administrators, and elected officials, who will decide on the allocation of financial and other necessary resources. Successfully coordinating these complex activities and interactions would be greatly facilitated if all parties shared a common set of concepts and beliefs regarding the nature of substance abuse that could direct attention toward key variables to change in the service of achieving pragmatic goals.

If our culture has anything approaching such a core set of beliefs, it is derived from concepts such as disease and addiction (e.g., Peele, 1990). Such beliefs, unfortunately, are serious impediments to realizing the full potential of the behavioral economic analysis of substance abuse. For example, Bickel and DeGrandpre (1995) recommended some specific policy initiatives to reduce substance use and abuse, including programs to develop activities other than substance use for current and potential substance abusers. As discussed earlier, such a recommendation derives naturally and obviously from the behavioral economic perspective, and there are plenty of data to support its effectiveness. Bickel and DeGrandpre also noted, however, that

> while such a programme may have appeal, adoption and application of this principle may prove difficult. . . . [P]roviding alternative reinforcers as an intervention to decrease drug use is not intuitively obvious to politicians or constituents because it does not directly focus on drugs

or their use. . . . [P]oliticians may view efforts to improve the availability of competing nondrug reinforcers as "coddling the drug addict" or as "pork." (p. 103)

They were quite correct in their assessment of how such initiatives would be viewed, as evidenced by the "midnight basketball" programs being "reviled as pork and denied federal funding" (Anonymous, 1996, p. 32) during the budget debate in the U.S. Congress in 1996.

Such programs are not "intuitively obvious," because the relevant intuitions are derived from currently dominant disease and addiction metaphors for substance abuse, which have led to conceptions of the critical variables that control substance abuse as residing *inside* the individual as either corporeal or psychological mechanisms. Any suggestion for dealing with substance abuse that does not address such internal causes therefore will not be intuitively appealing. These intuitions remain intact even though the disease concept of substance abuse has long since outlived its scientific credibility and practical utility (e.g., Pattison, Sobell, & Sobell, 1977; Peele, 1989), and even though convincing evidence now exists that substance use and abuse are a function of variables best characterized as residing *outside* the individual in environmental contexts and in the individuals' interactions with those contexts (e.g., Green & Kagel, 1996; Moos, Finney, & Cronkite, 1990; Tucker, Vuchinich, & Gladsjo, 1990/1991). This indicates the need for an alternative metaphor for substance abuse that can readily incorporate the relevant environmental contextual factors and that can replace the disease and addiction metaphors. A metaphor based on economic choice—resource allocation under conditions of environmental constraint—can fill this need.

## Disease and Addiction Metaphors for Substance Abuse

Metaphor is "the use of a term for one thing to describe another because of some kind of similarity between them" (Jaynes, 1976, p. 48). The crucial role of metaphor in language, lay and scientific concepts, and behavior has only recently begun to be fully recognized:

> Metaphor is for most people a device of the poetic imagination and the rhetorical flourish—a matter of extraordinary rather than ordinary language. . . . For this reason, most people think they can get along perfectly well without metaphor. We have found, on the contrary, that metaphor is pervasive in everyday life, not just in language but in thought and action. Our ordinary conceptual system, in terms of which we both think and act, is fundamentally metaphorical in nature.

The concepts that govern our thoughts . . . also govern our everyday functioning, down to the most mundane details. Our concepts structure what we perceive, how we get around in the world, and how we relate to other people. Our conceptual system thus plays a central role in defining our everyday realities. If we are right in suggesting that our conceptual system is largely metaphorical, then the way we think, what we experience, and what we do every day is very much a matter of metaphor. (Lakoff & Johnson, 1980, p. 3)

Metaphor is as central to scientific activity as it is to normal language and behavior, which is as true of physics (Holton, 1988) as it is of psychology (Jaynes, 1976; Sarbin, 1968).

The disease and addiction metaphors for substance abuse were originated by British clergy in the early 17th century in reference to excessive alcohol consumption (Warner, 1994). These "preachers and moralists had long been in the habit of labeling excessive drinkers as 'addicted' . . . and had additionally described habitual drunkenness as a 'disease' in its own right" (Warner, 1994, p. 689). The familiar term for one thing, an actual disease that damages health and constructive behavior, was used to describe another thing, excessive drinking, which also damages health and behavior. The metaphorical character of the term "disease" in this context is obvious, because 350 years ago, biomedical science had not discovered any corporeal mechanism that produced excessive drinking (some have argued that this remains as true today as it was then, e.g., Peele, 1989). Thus, the preachers were not arguing that certain persons drank to excess *because* they had a disease. They were instead saying that these persons were drinking *as if* they had a disease. The disease metaphor of excessive drinking immediately forces a look inside individuals for the variables that control drinking, because that is where "real" diseases are.

The disease metaphor has been a powerful concept for organizing information about substance abuse and for guiding efforts to deal with it over the last 300 years and, by the mid-1800s, it was the prevailing view among professionals and laypersons alike (Levine, 1978; Warner, 1994). Leaders in the medical community merged with the Temperance movement to work toward a social policy rather than a clinical intervention solution, which culminated in Prohibition in the early 20th century. The failure of Prohibition left a large gap, but by then, medicine was organized well enough to exercise the intervention implications of its disease metaphor. However, the inadequacies of a medical approach to substance abuse have been convincingly argued by numerous authors (e.g., Pattison et al., 1977; Peele, 1989). Fundamentally, substance abuse disorders are not actual diseases, and medicine's conceptual structure and technological delivery system therefore are ill equipped to deal with them.

The addiction metaphor for substance abuse has been more popular than the disease metaphor in the social and behavioral sciences. Although the addiction metaphor was not necessarily internalized like the disease metaphor, it has followed the same course. MacAndrew (1988) and Gori (1996) noted that the term "addiction" has not always denoted a "thing" that someone "has" that is "bad." Initially, the term denoted an obligation, such as a bank loan or military service, which clearly includes a feature of an environmental context in the description and explanation of the relevant action; that is, one repays a loan or enters the military *because* one is addicted (i.e., obligated) to do so. The term then became a metaphor for describing an individual's strong preferences for a given activity by noting that he or she behaves "as if addicted" (i.e., obligated) to the activity. Thus, the familiar term for one thing, an obligation that requires considerable time and behavior, was used to describe another thing, substance abuse, which also involves considerable time and behavior. This use of the term obviously does not mean that persons engage in the activity *because* they are addicted to it, only that they are behaving *as if* they are addicted to it.

Unlike the disease metaphor, the addiction metaphor does not entail a locus of the causes of the behavior. Nevertheless, there is a strong tendency for metaphors of this sort to be reified, internalized, and attributed causal significance (Sarbin, 1968). This clearly has occurred with the term addiction, which has gone from being a metaphorical description of devotion to a particular activity, to being an internal entity whose existence is revealed by that devotion, and, finally, to being the internalized cause of that devotion. Psychological analyses typically stop short of explaining the excessive behavior by the corporeal instantiation of addiction. There has been, nevertheless, a similar trend towards internalization of the addiction metaphor in terms of psychological mechanisms (Vuchinich, 1995; Vuchinich & Tucker, 1996a). Contemporary usage of the term addiction clearly implies that the excessive substance consumption occurs *because* of some internal entity or process to which the individual is "obligated," not simply *as if* they had such an obligation.

## An Economic Metaphor for Substance Abuse

The core idea of an economic metaphor for substance abuse is that individuals maximize utility under given conditions of resources and environmental constraints. From this perspective, the observation of excessive consumption would not produce a search for internal corporeal or psychological causes of the excessive consumption, as in the disease and addiction metaphors. Instead, an economic metaphor would produce a search for causes among those resources and environmental constraints. Thus, excessive consumption is seen as resulting from a particular vortex of contextual forces rather than from internal compulsion. Interventions at all levels, from the clinic to the public policy level, that are aimed at reducing or preventing excessive consumption would proceed by modifying those environmental constraints so that behavior is allocated away from excessive consumption toward more constructive alternatives, and by providing individuals with the resources necessary to exploit those alternatives.

The historical development of behavioral economics raises an important point that distinguishes an economic metaphor for substance abuse from the disease and addiction metaphors. The latter metaphors gained ascendance in the U.S. culture without the benefit of any scientific foundation whatsoever; in fact, they proliferated long before science was widely applied to human affairs. It therefore is not surprising that the extensive research on substance abuse during the 20th century has revealed them as inadequate characterizations of the problem (e.g., Peele, 1990). The dominance of the disease and addiction metaphors has resulted in an inadequate cultural response to substance use disorders, which has resulted in the broadening-the-base agenda of this book. An economic metaphor for substance abuse follows the opposite path, in that it provides a framework for understanding substance abuse only after having garnered considerable scientific support. The behavioral economics of substance abuse is nested within a much more general theoretical and empirical literature on behavioral allocation, intertemporal choice, and economics (e.g., Ainslie, 1992; Kagel et al., 1995; Loewenstein & Elster, 1992). As applied to substance abuse, this scientific foundation has produced the evidence summarized earlier, as well as formal behavioral economic theories of excessive consumption (Becker & Murphy, 1988; Herrnstein & Prelec, 1992; Rachlin, 1997). This scientific activity will continue to evolve and reveal new facts, and an economic metaphor for substance abuse, which followed rather than preceded a scientific database, is much less vulnerable to outstripping its scientific validity, as occurred with the disease and addiction metaphors.

The tenacity of the disease and addiction metaphors in the face of overwhelming contrary evidence is probably due in part to the absence of a compelling alternative metaphor that can organize the scientific evidence, capture the imagination of the professional and lay communities, and guide the implementation of practical solutions to substance abuse problems. The core ideas of the behavioral economic perspective have the potential to provide such a metaphor; that is, the potential exists to replace our culture's dominant yet ineffective metaphors for substance abuse— disease and addiction—with a more conceptually cohesive, scientifically credible, and practically useful metaphor based on economic choice— resource allocation under conditions of environmental constraint. An economic metaphor would lead to a conception of excessive consumption in terms of contextually determined behavioral allocation (choice) rather than in terms of internally driven compulsion (disease or addiction), which in turn would make sensible the specific practical implications of the behavioral economic perspective. For people who understand substance abuse in terms of an economic metaphor, regardless of whether they be scientist, clinician, or politician, programs such as those recommended by Bickel and DeGrandpre (1995) and in this chapter would be intuitively obvious.

## SUMMARY AND CONCLUSIONS

Despite its recency, research guided by behavioral economic concepts has revealed a number of empirical regularities regarding substance use and abuse that can guide the development and coordination of interventions at multiple levels, ranging from the individual in treatment to the community and health services system to public policy. There are two general ways in which these positive contributions can be viewed. First, one could acknowledge the effect of these variables on substance use and abuse, add them to the already long list of variables known to influence drug taking, and agree with provisional implementation of some of the specific recommendations. Such an incremental, eclectic stance could be adopted regardless of one's own theory of the nature of substance abuse—disease, addiction, or whatever—while continuing to maintain that theory. A second view would go further and recognize that behavioral economics provides a significant step forward in the evolution of scientific concepts and empirical evidence regarding excessive consumption that demand a fundamental revision in our culture's conceptions of the nature of substance use and abuse. The former view may bolster the armamentarium of procedures to address substance abuse problems, but it would not facilitate the coherence of the broadening-the-base agenda. The latter view would do both, and therein lies the general practical implications of the behavioral economics of substance abuse.

### REFERENCES

Ainslie, G. (1992). *Picoeconomics: The strategic interaction of successive motivational states within the person.* Cambridge, UK: Cambridge University Press.
Allison, J. (1979). Demand economics and experimental psychology. *Behavioral Science, 24,* 403–415.
Anonymous. (1996). 'Round midnight. *Sports Illustrated, 85*(8), 32.

Becker, G. S., & Murphy, K. M. (1988). A theory of rational addiction. *Journal of Political Economy, 96,* 675–700.

Bickel, W. K., & DeGrandpre, R. J. (1995). Price and alternatives: Suggestions for drug policy from psychology. *International Journal of Drug Policy, 6,* 93–105.

Bickel, W. K., & DeGrandpre, R. J. (1996). Modeling drug abuse policy in the behavioral economics laboratory. In L. Green & J. H. Kagel (Eds.), *Advances in behavioral economics: Vol. 3. Substance use and abuse* (pp. 69–95). Norwood, NJ: Ablex.

Bickel, W. K., DeGrandpre, R. J., & Higgins, S. T. (1993). Behavioral economics: A novel experimental approach to the study of drug dependence. *Drug and Alcohol Dependence, 33,* 173–192.

Bickel, W. K., DeGrandpre, R. J., & Higgins, S. T. (1995). The behavioral economics of concurrent drug reinforcers: A review and reanalysis of drug self-administration research. *Psychopharmacology, 118,* 250–259.

Bickel, W. K., DeGrandpre, R. J., Higgins, S. T., & Hughes, J. R. (1990). Behavioral economics of drug self-administration: I. Functional equivalence of response requirement and drug dose. *Life Sciences, 47,* 1501–1510.

Bickel, W. K., DeGrandpre, R. J., Higgins, S. T., Hughes, J. R., & Badger, G. J. (1995). Effects of simulated employment and recreation on human drug taking: A behavioral economic analysis. *Experimental and Clinical Psychopharmacology, 3,* 467–476.

Bickel, W. K., DeGrandpre, R. J., Hughes, J. R., & Higgins, S. T. (1991). Behavioral economics of drug self-administration: II. A unit-price analysis of cigarette smoking. *Journal of the Experimental Analysis of Behavior, 55,* 145–154.

Botvin, G. J., Baker, E., & Dusenbury, L. (1990). Preventing adolescent drug abuse through a multimodal cognitive-behavioral approach: Results of a 3-year study. *Journal of Consulting and Clinical Psychology, 58,* 437–446.

Carroll, M. E. (1996). Reducing drug abuse by enriching the environment with alternative nondrug reinforcers. In L. Green & J. Kagel (Eds.), *Advances in behavioral economics: Vol. 3. Substance use and abuse* (pp. 37–68). Norwood, NJ: Ablex.

Carroll, M. E., Carmona, G. G., & May, S. A. (1991). Modifying drug-reinforced behavior by altering the economic conditions of the drug and the non-drug reinforcer. *Journal of the Experimental Analysis of Behavior, 56,* 361–376.

Chaloupka, F. J., Bickel, W. K., Grossman, M., & Saffer, H. (Eds.). (in press). *The economic analysis of substance use and abuse: An integration of econometric and behavioral economic perspectives.* Chicago: University of Chicago Press.

Chaloupka, F. J., Grossman, M., & Tauras, J. A. (in press). The demand for cocaine and marijuana by youth. In F. J. Chaloupka, W. K. Bickel, M. Grossman, & H. Saffer (Eds.), *The economic analysis of substance use and abuse: An integration of econometric and behavioral economic perspectives.* Chicago: University of Chicago Press.

Chutuape, M. A. D., Mitchell, S. H., & deWit, H. (1994). Ethanol preloads increase ethanol preference under concurrent random-ration schedules in social drinkers. *Experimental and Clinical Psychopharmacology, 2,* 310–318.

Cox, M., & Klinger, E. (1988). A motivational model of alcohol use. *Journal of Abnormal Psychology, 97,* 168–180.

DeGrandpre, R. J., & Bickel, W. K. (1996). Drug dependence as consumer demand. In L. Green & J. H. Kagel (Eds.), *Advances in behavioral economics: Vol. 3. Substance use and abuse* (pp. 1–36). Norwood, NJ: Ablex.

DeGrandpre, R. J., Bickel, W. K., Hughes, J. R., & Higgins, S. T. (1992). Behavioral economics of drug self-administration: III. A reanalysis of the nicotine regulation hypothesis. *Psychopharmacology, 108,* 1–10.

DeGrandpre, R. J., Bickel, W. K., Hughes, J. R., Layng, M. P., & Badger, G. (1993). Unit price as a useful metric in analyzing effects of reinforcer magnitude. *Journal of the Experimental Analysis of Behavior, 60,* 641–666.

Elsmore, T. F., Fletcher, D. V., Conrad, D. G., & Sodetz, F. J. (1980). Reduction in heroin intake in baboons by an economic constraint. *Pharmacology Biochemistry and Behavior, 13,* 729–731.

Ennett, S. T., Tobler, N. S., & Ringwalt, C. L. (1994). How effective is drug abuse resistance education? A meta-analysis of Project DARE outcome evaluations. *American Journal of Public Health, 84,* 1394–1401.

George, F. R., & Ritz, M. C. (1993). A psychopharmacology of motivation and reward related to substance abuse treatment. *Experimental and Clinical Psychopharmacology, 1,* 7–26.

Goldberg, S. R., Hoffeister, F., Shlichting, U. U., & Wuttke, W. (1971). A comparison of pentobarbital and cocaine self-administration in rhesus monkeys: Effect of dose and fixed-ratio parameter. *Journal of Pharmacology and Experimental Therapeutics, 179,* 277–283.

Gori, G. B. (1996). Failings of the disease model of alcoholism. *Human Psychopharmacology, 11,* S33–S38.

Green, L., & Freed, D. E. (1993). The substitutability of reinforcers. *Journal of the Experimental Analysis of Behavior, 60,* 141–158.

Green, L., & Kagel, J. H. (Eds.). (1987). *Advances in behavioral economics: Vol. 1.* Norwood, NJ: Ablex.

Green, L., & Kagel, J. H. (Eds.). (1996). *Advances in behavioral economics. Vol. 3: Substance use and abuse.* Norwood, NJ: Ablex.

Green, L., & Rachlin, H. (1991). Economic substitutability of electrical brain stimulation, food, and water. *Journal of the Experimental Analysis of Behavior, 55,* 133–143.

Griffiths, R. R., Bigelow, G. E., & Henningfield, J. E. (1980). Similarities in human and animal drug-taking behavior. In N. K. Mello (Ed.), *Advances in substance abuse: Behavioral and biological research* (Vol. 1, pp. 1–90). Greenwich, CT: JAI Press.

Hatsukami, D. K., Thompson, T. N., Pentel, P. R., Flygare, B. K., & Carroll, M. E. (1994). Self-administration of smoked cocaine. *Experimental and Clinical Psychopharmacology, 2,* 115–125.

Hawkins, J. D., Catalano, R. F., & Miller, J. Y. (1992). Risk and protective factors for alcohol and other drug problems in adolescence and early adulthood: Implications for substance abuse prevention. *Psychological Bulletin, 112,* 64–105.

Heather, N. (1989). Brief intervention strategies. In R. K. Hester & W. R. Miller (Eds.), *Handbook of alcoholism treatment approaches: Effective alternatives* (pp. 93–116). New York: Pergamon.

Herrnstein, R. J. (1970). On the law of effect. *Journal of the Experimental Analysis of Behavior, 13,* 243–266.

Herrnstein, R. J., & Prelec, D. (1992). A theory of addiction. In G. Loewenstein & J. Elster (Eds.), *Choice over time* (pp. 331–360). New York: Russell Sage Foundation.

Higgins, S. T. (1997). The influence of alternative reinforcers on cocaine use and abuse: A brief review. *Pharmacology Biochemistry and Behavior, 57,* 419–427.

Higgins, S. T., Delaney, D. D., Budney, A. J., Bickel, W. K., Hughes, J. R., Foerg, F., &

Fenwick., J. W. (1991). A behavioral approach to achieving initial cocaine abstinence. *American Journal of Psychiatry, 148,* 1218–1224.

Hingson, R., Heeren, T., & Winter, M. (1994). Lower legal blood alcohol limits for young drivers. *Public Health Reports, 109,* 738–744.

Holton, G. (1988). *Thematic origins of scientific thought: Kepler to Einstein.* Cambridge, MA: Harvard University Press.

Hull, C. L. (1943). *Principles of behavior.* New York: Appleton-Century.

Hursh, S. R. (1980). Economic concepts for the analysis of behavior. *Journal of the Experimental Analysis of Behavior, 34,* 219–238.

Hursh, S. R. (1991). Behavioral economics of drug self-administration and drug abuse policy. *Journal of the Experimental Analysis of Behavior, 56,* 377–393.

Hursh, S. R. (1993). Behavioral economics of drug self-administration: An introduction. *Drug and Alcohol Dependence, 33,* 165–172.

Institute of Medicine. (1990). *Broadening the base of treatment for alcohol problems.* Washington, DC: National Academy Press.

Jaynes, J. (1976). *The origin of consciousness in the breakdown of the bicameral mind.* Boston: Houghton Mifflin.

Kagel, J. H., Battalio, R. C., & Green, L. (1995). *Economic choice theory: An experimental analysis of animal behavior.* New York: Cambridge University Press.

Kandel, D. B., & Logan, J. A. (1984). Patterns of drug use from adolescence to young adulthood: Periods of risk for initiation, continued use, and discontinuation. *American Journal of Public Health, 74,* 660–666.

Lakoff, G., & Johnson, M. (1980). *Metaphors we live by.* Chicago: University of Chicago Press.

Leung, S. -F., & Phelps, C. E. (1993). "My kingdom for a drink . . . ?" A review of the estimates of the price sensitivity of demand for alcoholic beverages. In M. E. Hilton & G. Bloss (Eds.), *Economics and the prevention of alcohol-related problems* (pp. 1–31) (NIAAA Research Monograph No. 25, NIH Pub. No. 93-3513). Rockville, MD: U.S. Department of Health and Human Services.

Levine, H. G. (1978). The discovery of addiction: Changing conceptions of habitual drunkenness in America. *Journal of Studies on Alcohol, 39,* 143–174.

Loewenstein, G., & Elster, J. (Eds.). (1992). *Choice over time.* New York: Russell Sage Foundation.

MacAndrew, C. (1988). On the possibility of an addiction-free mode of being. In S. Peele (Ed.), *Visions of addiction: Major contemporary perspectives on addiction and alcoholism* (pp. 163–182). Lexington, MA: Lexington Books.

Madden, G. J., Petry, N. M., Badger, G. J., & Bickel, W. K. (1997). Impulsive and self-control choices in opioid-dependent patients and non-drug-using-control participants. *Experimental and Clinical Psychopharmacology, 5,* 256–263.

Maisto, S. A., & McCollum, J. B. (1980). The use of multiple measures of life health to assess alcohol treatment outcome: A review and critique. In L. C. Sobell, M. B. Sobell, & E. Ward (Eds.), *Evaluating alcohol and drug abuse treatment effectiveness* (pp. 15–76). New York: Pergamon.

Marlatt, G. A., & Tapert, S. R. (1993). Harm reduction: Reducing the risks of addictive behaviors. In J. S. Baer, G. A. Marlatt, & R. McMahon (Eds.), *Addictive behaviors across the lifespan* (pp. 243–273). Newbury Park, CA: Sage.

Marlatt, G. A., Tucker, J. A., Donovan, D. M., & Vuchinich, R. E. (1997). Help-seeking by substance abusers: The role of harm reduction and behavioral economic approaches to facilitate treatment entry and retention. In L. S. Onken, J. D. Blaine, & J. J. Boren (Eds.), *Beyond the therapeutic alliance: Keeping the drug dependent individual in treatment* (NIDA Research Monograph No. 165, pp. 44–84). Rockville, MD: National Institute on Drug Abuse.

Miller, W. R. (1996). Motivational interviewing: Research, practice, puzzles. *Addictive Behaviors, 21,* 835–842.

Moos, R. H., Finney, J. W., & Cronkite, R. C. (1990). *Alcoholism treatment: Context, process, and outcome.* New York: Oxford University Press.

Nader, M. A., & Woolverton, W. L. (1991). Effects of increasing the magnitude of an alternative reinforcer on drug choice in a discrete-trials choice procedure. *Psychopharmacology, 105,* 169–174.

O'Connell, K. A., & Martin, E. J. (1987). Highly tempting situations associated with abstinence, temporary lapse, and relapse among participants in smoking cessation programs. *Journal of Consulting and Clinical Psychology, 55,* 367–371.

Ornstein, S. I. (1980). Control of alcohol consumption through price increases. *Journal of Studies on Alcohol, 41,* 807–818.

Pattison, E. M., Sobell, M. B., & Sobell, L. C. (1977). *Emerging concepts of alcohol dependence.* New York: Springer.

Peele, S. (1989). *Diseasing of America: Addiction treatment out of control.* San Francisco: Jossey-Bass.

Peele, S. (1990). Addiction as a cultural concept. *Annals of the New York Academy of Sciences, 602,* 205–220.

Perry, C. L., Williams, C. L., & Forster, J. L. (1993). Background, conceptualization, and design of a community-wide research program on adolescent alcohol abuse: Project Northland. *Health Education Research: Theory and Practice, 8,* 125–136.

Premack, D. (1965). Reinforcement theory. In D. Levine (Ed.), *Nebraska Symposium on Motivation* (pp. 123–180). Lincoln: University of Nebraska Press.

Rachlin, H. (1974). Self-control. *Behaviorism, 2,* 94–107.

Rachlin, H. (1997). Four teleological theories of addiction. *Psychonomic Bulletin and Review, 4,* 462–473.

Rachlin, H., Green, L., Kagel, J., & Battalio, R. (1976). Economic demand theory and psychological studies of choice. In G. Bower (Ed.), *The psychology of learning and motivation* (Vol. 10, pp. 129–154). New York: Academic Press.

Saffer, H., & Chaloupka, F. J. (in press). Demographic differentials in the demand for alcohol and illicit drugs. In F. J. Chaloupka, W. K. Bickel, M. Grossman, & H. Saffer (Eds.), *The economic analysis of substance use and abuse: An integration of econometric and behavioral economic perspectives.* Chicago: University of Chicago Press.

Samson, H. H., & Lindberg, K. (1984). Comparison of sucrose–sucrose to sucrose–ethanol concurrent responding in the rat: Reinforcement schedule and fluid concentration effects. *Pharmacology Biochemistry and Behavior, 20,* 973–977.

Sarbin, T. R. (1968). Ontology recapitulates philology: The mythic nature of anxiety. *American Psychologist, 23,* 411–418.

Skinner, B. F. (1938). *The behavior of organisms: An experimental analysis.* Englewood Cliffs, NJ: Prentice-Hall.

Staddon, J. E. R. (Ed.). (1980). *Limits to action: The allocation of individual behavior.* New York: Academic Press.

Tucker, J. A., & Vuchinich, R. E. (1997). [Unpublished data.] Auburn University, AL.

Tucker, J. A., Vuchinich, R. E., & Gladsjo, J. A. (1990/1991). Environmental influences on relapse in substance abuse disorders. *International Journal of the Addictions*, 25, 1017–1050.

Tucker, J. A., Vuchinich, R. E., & Gladsjo, J. A. (1994). Environmental events surrounding natural recovery from alcohol-related problems. *Journal of Studies on Alcohol*, 55, 401–411.

Tucker, J. A., Vuchinich, R. E., & Pukish, M. A. (1995). Molar environmental contexts surrounding recovery from alcohol problems by treated and untreated problem drinkers. *Experimental and Clinical Psychopharmacology*, 3, 195–204.

United States Department of Housing and Urban Development. (1994). *Midnight basketball: How to give young people a chance*. Washington, DC: Author.

United States Government Printing Office. (1992). *The risky business of adolescence: How to help teens stay safe, part II*. Hearing before the Select Committee on Children, Youth, and Families. House of Representatives, 102nd Congress, First Session (pp. 65–82).

Vuchinich, R. E. (1982). Have behavioral theories of alcohol abuse focused too much on alcohol consumption? *Bulletin of the Society of Psychologists in Substance Abuse*, 1, 151–154.

Vuchinich, R. E. (1995). Alcohol abuse as molar choice: An update of a 1982 proposal. *Psychology of Addictive Behaviors*, 9, 223–235.

Vuchinich, R. E. (1997). Behavioral economics of drug consumption. In B. A. Johnson & J. D. Roache (Eds.), *Drug addiction and its treatment: Nexus of neuroscience and behavior* (pp. 73–90). Philadelphia: Lippincott–Raven.

Vuchinich, R. E., & Simpson, C. A. (1998). Hyperbolic temporal discounting in social drinkers and problem drinkers. *Experimental and Clinical Psychopharmacology*, 6, 292–305.

Vuchinich, R. E., & Tucker, J. A. (1983). Behavioral theories of choice as a framework for studying drinking behavior. *Journal of Abnormal Psychology*, 92, 408–416.

Vuchinich, R. E., & Tucker, J. A. (1988). Contributions from behavioral theories of choice to an analysis of alcohol abuse. *Journal of Abnormal Psychology*, 97, 181–195.

Vuchinich, R. E., & Tucker, J. A. (1996a). The molar context of alcohol abuse. In L. Green & J. Kagel (Eds.), *Advances in behavioral economics: Vol. 3. Substance use and abuse* (pp. 133–162). Norwood, NJ: Ablex.

Vuchinich, R. E., & Tucker, J. A. (1996b). Alcoholic relapse, life events, and behavioral theories of choice: A prospective analysis. *Experimental and Clinical Psychopharmacology*, 4, 19–28.

Vuchinich, R. E., Tucker, J. A., & Harllee, L. (1988). Behavioral assessment (of alcohol dependence). In D. Donovan & G. A. Marlatt (Eds.), *Assessment of addictive behaviors* (pp. 51–93). New York: Plenum.

Vuchinich, R. E., Tucker, J. A., & Rudd, E. J. (1987). Preference for alcohol consumption as a function of amount and delay of alternative reward. *Journal of Abnormal Psychology*, 96, 259–263.

Wagennar, A. C. (1993). Minimum drinking age and alcohol availability to youth: Issues and research needs. In M. E. Hilton & G. Bloss (Eds.), *Economics and the prevention of alcohol-related problems* (NIAAA Research Monograph No. 25, NIH Publication No. 93-3513, pp. 175–200). Rockville, MD: National Institute on Alcohol Abuse and Alcoholism.

Warner, J. (1994). "Resolv'd to drink no more" : Addiction as a preindustrial construct. *Journal of Studies on Alcohol, 55,* 685–691.

Williams, B. A. (1988). Reinforcement, choice, and response strength. In R. C. Atkinson, R. J. Herrnstein, G. Lindzey, & R. D. Luce (Eds.), *S. S. Stevens' handbook of experimental psychology* (Vol. 2, pp. 167–244). New York: Wiley.

# II

## EXPANDING THE RANGE OF BEHAVIOR CHANGE INITIATIVES

# 8

## Public Health Perspective on Addictive Behavior Change Interventions: Conceptual Frameworks and Guiding Principles

SUSAN J. CURRY
ELEANOR L. KIM

Public health approaches to addictive behavior change encompass a wide range of interventions. Building from the classic agent–host–environment triad, a basic tenet of the public health perspective is that reduction in premature morbidity and mortality associated with addictive behaviors will result from population-based implementation of interventions that address interactions among the addictive substance (agent), individual characteristics (host), and the physical and social context (environment) (Winett, King, & Altman, 1989). Discussions of public health approaches to health behavior often distinguish among different levels of intervention (Abrams, Emmons, Niaura, Goldstein, & Sherman, 1991; Winett et al., 1989). For example, Winett and colleagues describe a continuum of four levels: individual, interpersonal, organizational, and societal, with corresponding intervention approaches that could include self-help programs, worksite wellness programs and policies, mass media programs, and legislation. Typically, it is interventions at the organizational and societal levels that are thought of as "public health."

A basic premise of this chapter is that the public health perspective is important not only for developing mass media, policy, and legislative approaches to addictive behaviors, but is also important to consider in developing more individually focused intervention programs. The emerging view of addictive behaviors as a continuum of involvement with substance use is a key impetus for considering the public health perspective in developing addictive behavior change programs (Institute of Medicine, 1990). As illustrated in Figure 8.1, addictive behaviors can be defined along a spectrum of consumption that ranges from none to substantial and heavy levels of use that define substance abuse and addiction. Although most severe problems occur among highly dependent individuals at the apex of this continuum, moderate to substantial health, social, and economic problems occur even among nondependent moderate substance users. Indeed, the combined public health impact of the spectrum of addictive behaviors is considerable. Addictive behaviors, including alcohol, drug, and tobacco use, are the single largest cause of premature morbidity and mortality in the United States, accounting for more than 25% of deaths each year (Institute for Health Policy, 1993). The estimated combined economic costs of substance abuse are well over $200 billion per year (Institute for Health Policy, 1993). These include not only medical and treatment costs, but also costs associated with loss of productivity, crime, and destruction of property.

Moving from dichotomous definitions of addiction and substance abuse to defining levels of use and associated medical, social, and psychological consequences along a continuum has important implications for

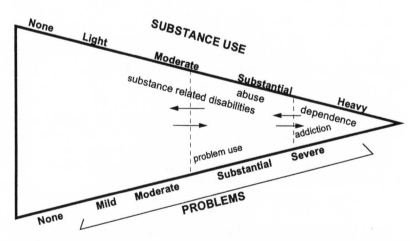

**FIGURE 8.1.** Continuum of substance use and problems. Reprinted with permission from Institute of Medicine (1990). Copyright 1990 by the National Academy of Sciences. Courtesy of the National Academy Press, Washington, DC.

reducing the individual and social costs of addictive behaviors. As high-lighted in the Institute of Medicine (IOM) report on broadening the base of treatment for alcohol problems, the availability of a range of intervention approaches that are appropriate for different points along this continuum is critical. Recent estimates are that fewer than 25% of individuals who need treatment for addictive behaviors receive it (Institute for Health Policy, 1993). One of the reasons for our failure to meet these treatment needs may be an overreliance on an intensive, clinical model of treatment as distinct from taking a public health perspective. A comparison of the clinical and public health perspectives is summarized in Table 8.1, which was adapted from Lichtenstein and Glasgow (1992).

Essentially, a clinical perspective focuses primarily on individual factors and lifestyle issues in addictive behavior change. The target population for interventions includes those individuals who self-refer or who respond to recruitments for interventions. The treatment setting is medical or psychotherapeutic, and treatments are provided by professionals with special training in addictive behaviors. The interventions are intensive, usually involving multiple sessions. Treatment outcome studies are usually comparative "horse race" studies in which alternative treatments are compared. These types of interventions often produce relatively high rates of change among the select sample of participants; however, their cost-effectiveness for producing population-based reductions in addictive behaviors is relatively low because of their low penetration into the population.

In a public health perspective, the target population is neither self-

**TABLE 8.1. Clinical and Public Health Perspectives on Addictive Behavior Change**

| Characteristic | Clinical perspective | Public health perspective |
| --- | --- | --- |
| Problem definition | Individual, lifestyle | Community, environment |
| Target population | Self-referred or recruited | Populations or high-risk groups |
| Setting | Specialty, clinical | Natural environments |
| Provider | Trained professional | Lay, automated |
| Intervention | Intensive, multisession | Brief, low cost |
| Research design | Component analysis, comparative studies | "Best shot" or special intervention versus usual care |
| Outcome | Higher rates of change | Lower rates of change |
| Cost effectiveness | Lower | Higher |

*Note.* Adapted from Lichtenstein and Glasgow (1992). Copyright 1992 by the *Journal of Consulting and Clinical Psychology*. Adapted by permission.

referred nor recruited, but includes all individuals with addictive behavior problems, regardless of their motivation to change their behavior. Interventions are delivered in natural settings, and the providers of interventions will not necessarily be specialists in the treatment of addictive behaviors. Treatment outcome studies typically compare a new intervention to usual care. In a public health context, interventions can be brief and low cost in order to reach the largest potential proportion of the target population. Consequently, rates of change in these programs are often much lower than in intensive clinical programs.

It is important to note that the public health perspective is not competitive with, or antithetical to, the clinical approach. Indeed, the primary purpose of this chapter is to facilitate better integration of these perspectives by describing crosscutting conceptual models and principles. As noted earlier, there are multiple levels of intervention that one can consider from a public health perspective. In Figure 8.2, we illustrate the levels that will be considered in this chapter: individual, provider/practitioner, and organizational.

Organizational-level interventions comprise policies (e.g., worksite drug testing policies, smoking bans, health care benefits packages for treatment of addictive behaviors), resource allocation for the development of treatment innovations, and community outreach or involvement in community initiatives outside of the organization. Provider-level interventions may focus on training of nonspecialists to identify and intervene with addictive behavior problems, develop and implement practice guidelines, and automate office-based systems for population-based tracking of individuals with addictive behavior problems. And, there are the more familiar individual-level interventions that include the array of minimal to in-

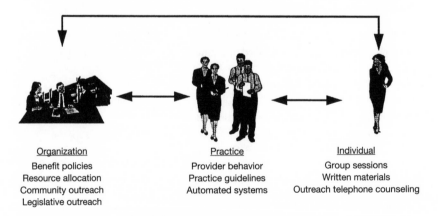

| Organization | Practice | Individual |
|---|---|---|
| Benefit policies | Provider behavior | Group sessions |
| Resource allocation | Practice guidelines | Written materials |
| Community outreach | Automated systems | Outreach telephone counseling |
| Legislative outreach | | |

**FIGURE 8.2.** Levels of intervention.

tensive treatment programs available to help people make and maintain behavior changes. These include individual and group interventions, self-help interventions, outreach telephone counseling, and computer-based programs. A viable public health approach to addictive behavior change interventions will include a great deal of interaction among these levels. Each of these levels is necessary, but none alone is sufficient to provide a broad base of treatment at the population level.

There are many challenges at each of these levels for developing and sustaining addictive behavior change interventions. Among the important challenges at the individual level are understanding factors associated with motivation for behavior change, particularly among the majority of substance users/abusers who do not self-refer for treatment (see Chapters 4–5, this volume). Furthermore, it is important to know how to translate this knowledge into intervention protocols that can be delivered on a wide scale. Practice-level challenges include ways to train nonspecialist providers both to screen for individuals at risk for or with current addictive behavior problems and to implement practice-based stepped-care treatment models that offer interventions of graded levels of intensity that consider the current needs and past experiences of patients. Organizational level challenges include ways of building commitment for providing resources to evaluate programs and enacting policies to institutionalize those interventions that are proven effective.

Our strategy for demonstrating the integration of the clinical and public health approaches is to move from this overview of the traditional clinical and public health perspectives to a summary of the various theoretical models that target multiple levels—spanning from individuals to large populations. In our review of some of the major conceptual frameworks, it is important to note that although we have presented the models separately, there is overlap in many of their components. We use the natural convergence of these conceptual models to delineate guidelines for working toward a more integrated model in which principles of both the clinical and public health perspective can be applied to intervene with addictive behaviors. We also provide a case example to demonstrate more specifically how these guidelines were utilized to develop a tobacco addiction treatment program in a health maintenance organization.

## CONCEPTUAL FRAMEWORKS

Conceptual models in the behavioral sciences can help guide practical and effective solutions to the aforementioned challenges. A common misconception regarding the public health approach is that, unlike clinical approaches, it is not theory driven. In this section, we review several major conceptual models that are often applied in public health intervention models. Clearly, because of the complexity of factors involved, no single theory is likely to underlie a comprehensive public health approach to addictive behaviors (cf. Winett, 1995; Abrams, Emmons, & Linnan, 1995). Rather, theoretical models are best incorporated as part of more integrative conceptual frameworks that can guide the development, implementation, and evaluation of public health intervention strategies (Curry & Emmons, 1994). There are a number of comprehensive models for planning and integrating public health approaches to health behavior change that the interested reader can refer to, including work by Green and Kreuter (1991), Winett et al. (1989), and Walsh and McPhee (1992). In this section, we provide brief descriptions of several major theoretical paradigms that are often incorporated into these general conceptual frameworks. The purpose of these descriptions is to familiarize the reader with the core concepts in these models. More detailed presentations of these and other models can be found in an excellent book, *Health Behavior and Health Education: Theory, Research and Practice* (Glanz, Lewis, & Rimer, 1995). The models reviewed here include value–expectancy theories, social cognitive theory, social marketing theory, communication theory, and diffusion theory.

## Value-Expectancy Theories

Value–expectancy theories (Fishbein & Ajzen, 1975; Hochbaum, 1958; Rosenstock, 1960, 1966, 1974), with their emphasis on the decision-making process, can help us understand factors associated with motivation for behavior change, particularly among substance users/abusers who do not self-refer for treatment. From the value–expectancy perspective, an individual's motivation to engage in behavior change is the result of his or her subjective *value* of an outcome and of the subjective probability or *expectation* that a particular action will attain the outcome. The two most prominent value–expectancy theories are the health belief model (HBM) and the theory of reasoned action (TRA).

Since it was first developed in the 1950s by social psychologists in the U.S. Public Health Service (Hochbaum, 1958; Rosenstock, 1960, 1966, 1974), the HBM has evolved into a psychosocial model that proposes three main components in an individual's motivation for making health-related actions: (1) perceived *susceptibility* to a disease, or the subjective risks of contracting a serious illness; (2) perceived *severity* of an illness, both in terms of medical and lifestyle consequences; and (3) belief that specific behaviors will reduce the perceived threat and that the associated benefits of those behaviors will outweigh the perceived costs or barriers. The degree of perceived susceptibility and severity is based largely on an individual's concern about health or the value placed on health, as well as on knowledge of a disease and its potential outcome (Rosenstock, 1974).

Within a health belief framework, addictive behaviors can be viewed as risk factors for serious illness (e.g., cigarette smoking as a risk factor for cancer and cardiovascular disease) or as the illness themselves (e.g., alcoholism as a disease or a maladaptive behavior pattern). From the former perspective, for example, there is evidence that the likelihood of smoking cessation among patients with smoking-related illnesses such as myocardial infarction is related to their perceived susceptibility to future ill health (Marshall, 1990). This study also found a significant difference between the ex-smokers and continued smokers on a benefits versus barriers to change measure, with ex-smokers perceiving greater benefits of quitting smoking compared to continued smokers.

The HBM also recognizes the potential importance of "cues to action." While perceived susceptibility and severity provide the force for action, and the perceived benefits and barriers indicate a preferred course of action, cues to action can start the process of behavior change (Rosenstock, 1974). These cues to action may be internal (e.g., feeling less energetic or motivated to complete activities after drinking) or external (e.g., a recommendation from a doctor to stop smoking). Determining the required intensity of the cue depends on the level of susceptibility and severity perceived by the individual. For instance, Bardsley and Beckman (1988) assessed "cues to action" in problem drinkers who had and had not entered treatment by asking whether they had seen an advertisement for alcoholism treatment in the last month, experienced social pressure to enter treatment, or experienced unusual events (e.g., new physical symptoms, a car accident while drunk). Compared to participants who were not in treatment, those who were in treatment had experienced relatively more "unusual events" in the previous month and tended to view their problem as being more serious. These results suggest that individuals may have been moved to take action to enter treatment because of these events and perceptions of problem severity (see Chapters 3 and 4, this volume, on barriers to, and incentives for, help-seeking).

The concept of self-efficacy from Bandura's social cognitive theory was added to HBM in 1984 (Janz & Becker, 1984). Perceived self-efficacy refers to "beliefs in one's capabilities to organize and execute the courses of action required to produce given attainments" (Bandura, 1995, p. 3). This concept was added to acknowledge the importance of not only believing that an action can benefit one's health at an acceptable cost, but also the belief that one has the skills and ability to implement that change.

The Theory of Reasoned Action (TRA) is another value–expectancy theory that provides a framework for assessing the factors that an individual may consider in deciding whether to pursue a specific behavior or action. This theory, originally proposed by Fishbein and Azjen (1975), provides a mathematical description of the relationship among beliefs, attitudes, intention, and behavior.

According to the model, the best single predictor of behavior is the behavioral intention regarding that specific behavior; other factors that may influence behavior are mediated through intentions. More specifically, the TRA posits that the strength of an individual's behavioral intention is a function of two subcomponents: (1) the person's *attitude* toward the behavior (i.e., whether the person has positive or negative feelings about engaging in the behavior), and (2) *subjective norms* regarding the behavior (i.e., the person's perception of the social pressures to perform or not perform the behavior and his or her motivation to comply with these normative referents). The beliefs and attitudes components of the TRA parallel the constructs of perceived benefits and severity that are postulated in the HBM. Both models require knowledge of the salient primary beliefs on which an attitude is based to create behavior change. Despite the similar emphasis on beliefs in the two models, the TRA goes beyond the exclusive focus of the HBM on the individual's assessment of risk also to include assessment of the social normative context. The TRA postulates that changing the beliefs underlying attitudes or norms leads to changes in behavioral intentions, which ultimately produce a change in behavior.

In recent years, Ajzen (1985; Ajzen & Madden, 1986) revised the original Fishbein and Ajzen (1975) theory to incorporate the self-efficacy concept. Renamed the theory of planned behavior (TPB), the revision emphasizes that it is not only important to know an individual's intention to perform a given behavior, but also the belief that he or she can actually perform the behavior (self-efficacy) is an additional factor that contributes to the practice of preventive health behaviors. This factor was added to account for behaviors over which individuals had limited personal control.

Overall, theories such as the HBM, TRA, and TPB can enhance our understanding of motivation for changing addictive behaviors, but it is important to acknowledge their potential limitations. First, these models assume a rational decision-making process, which is not always the case. Second, they focus primarily on health concerns as motivators, whereas addictive behavior change is often motivated more by negative psychosocial consequences and a desire for self-control than by health problems, particularly among younger individuals who are not physically dependent. Third, the emphasis of these models on cognitive factors needs to be augmented by models that take into account behavioral (e.g., skills) and environmental (e.g., situational determinants of substance use) components of the behavior change process. With this in mind, we turn to a brief description of social cognitive theory.

## Social Cognitive Theory

The cognitive-behavioral intervention model that is the cornerstone of most state-of-the-art intervention programs has its conceptual roots in social cognitive theory (SCT) (Bandura, 1986). Called social learning theory (SLT) until 1986, when Bandura renamed it SCT (Perry, Baranowski, & Parcel, 1990), SCT goes beyond the primarily cognitive, intraindividual focus of the value expectancy theories and incorporates both behavioral and environmental components as equally important determinants of behavior. Although the terms SLT and SCT have been used interchangeably in the literature, the change in terminology reflects the growing acknowledgment of the important role that both cognitive and social factors play in determining behavior. SCT has a rich history that includes many significant contributors such as Miller and Dollard (1941) in their work on the imitation of behavior, as well as Hull (1943), who studied motivation and the role of reinforcement in the learning process. Some of the theory's main ideas and key concepts are reviewed here to provide a sample of how it has been applied to the health domain.

From a social cognitive perspective, there are three factors that predict an individual's behavior: behavioral, cognitive, and environmental. Behavioral factors comprise individuals' experiences with the target behavior (e.g., history of substance use, prior attempts to stop or modify use) as well as their general repertoire of behavioral skills (e.g., assertiveness, coping strategies, interpersonal skills, etc.). Cognitive factors include knowledge, attitudes, and beliefs, as outlined in the value–expectancy models along with more specific cognitive representations of situational factors (e.g., the perceived effect of alcohol as a social enhancer). Environmental factors relate to influences that are external to the person, such as the actions of family members, physicians and peer groups, plus more global environmental influences including advertising/media, availability of substances, and regulations/restrictions on the use and availability of substances.

Bandura (1978) also introduced the crucial concept of reciprocal determinism to describe the way in which the environment, person, and behavior are continually interacting. Reciprocal determinism highlights the importance of considering these components to be part of an open system in which each is mutually affected. Each component can be changed as a result of the transactions that occur among them.

The concept of self-efficacy, described earlier in the discussion of value–expectancy models, emerged out of social cognitive theory to describe the way in which an individual self-regulates or exercises behavioral control over his or her behavior. Bandura (1995) posited that self-efficacy affects three basic phases of change, starting with the initiation of the be-havior, moving to the mobilization toward successful behavior change, and attaining the maintenance of the habits an individual has already changed. Marlatt, Baer, and Quigley (1995) reviewed the way self-efficacy theory is specifically relevant to addictive behavior change by expanding a taxonomy originally proposed by DiClemente and colleagues (Di-Clemente, Fairhurst, & Piotrowski, in press). They described five cate-gories of self-efficacy: (1) resistance self-efficacy refers to individuals' per-ceived ability to resist pressure to drink or use drugs; (2) harm reduction self-efficacy refers to individuals' perceived ability to reduce risks associat-ed with use of alcohol or other drugs; (3) action self-efficacy refers to indi-viduals' belief in their ability to achieve the desired goal of abstinence or controlled use; (4) coping self-efficacy refers to individuals' belief in their ability to cope with high-risk situations that might lead to relapse; and (5) recovery self-efficacy refers to individuals' belief in their ability to cope with lapses or slips as they continue to work toward their behavioral goals. Presumably, once individuals are equipped with the behavioral skills and cognitive self-efficacy in these various areas, they will be able to make be-havior changes in the direction of their behavioral goals.

Although SCT has been most commonly used as an interpersonal model, Bandura recently extended the concept of self-efficacy to groups through his conceptualization of collective efficacy and its potential im-pact on policymaking. Bandura posited that communities with a sense of collective efficacy will be able to mobilize their efforts and resources to cope with external obstacles to the changes they seek (Bandura, 1995).

Thus far, we have described theories that focus primarily on individ-ual-level factors. Although limited in scope in this respect, these models make important contributions to the development of outreach strategies to identify individuals at risk for, or with, current addictive behavior problems and for intervention programs designed to enhance motivation and skills for changing addictive behaviors. We now turn to three frameworks that ad-dress behavior change in communities and populations. Although discussed separately, these multilevel models are not mutually exclusive. The commu-nity-level models focus on larger populations, but the principles described by SCT and value–expectancy theories fill the gaps regarding how these approaches ultimately affect individual behavior. Similarly, although the in-dividual-level change strategies may rely heavily on individual-level change principles, such individualized strategies often rely on community-level dis-semination to increase their reach to a greater number of participants.

## Social Marketing

Social marketing theory emerged in the late 1960s when researchers be-gan to envision new avenues for the application of marketing strategies

(Frederiksen, Solomon, & Brehony, 1984). Kotler (1984) defined "social marketing" as the application of commercial marketing principles to the advancement of social causes, ideas, and behaviors. Because professional marketers have demonstrated success in shaping consumer behavior, these principles have been applied to behavior change in the field of public health. The social marketing framework has been used in the area of health behavior change for developing, implementing, and improving programs based on consumer need, perception, preference, and satisfaction.

There are two primary areas in public health that are advanced by the application of social marketing. The first area is the design of programs and services that are desired by consumers and fit with their needs. For example, the development of a primary-care-based prevention program for people who are at risk for developing alcohol problems may incorporate principles of social marketing to assess consumers' tastes and needs. Once the product is developed, the second major area to consider is selling the product to appropriate intermediaries that can implement the procedures or product effectively. Possible intermediaries include health professionals (e.g., counselors or health care providers) who work with patient populations, as well as administrative personnel in health care and other organizational settings, who make decisions about what types of addictive behavior change programs to disseminate.

In general, the marketing framework emphasizes the importance of *market research*, which refers to a clearly developed plan of objectives and strategies. It also relies on *market segmentation* for identifying consumers, investigates *consumer benefits* or rewards for engaging in a particular behavior, and builds a product personality that can be recognized across presentation styles (Brehony, Frederiksen, & Solomon, 1984).

The marketing mix of tools for developing a product personality is remembered by the mnemonic, the four "P's" (Brehony et al., 1984). The first P is the *product*, which might be in the form of a program, service, or other focus of transaction between the marketer and the target audience. Reading materials, physician waiting-room computerized assessment and feedback technology, and worksite skills training programs are all examples of interventions that have been developed into "products" to be marketed to consumers. As the products become more specific, the market size becomes more narrow. The price refers to the amount of money, time, and effort, as well as the psychological and social costs, associated with adopting a product. For example, people may not join a smoking cessation group because of the time and distance involved. However, they may be more likely to join such a group and ultimately quit smoking if they could receive assistance with minimal cost (e.g., visit with their health provider or get assistance via telephone). The *place* refers to how the product is made available to consumers. For example, community-based smoking cessation programs may target a wide variety of public places such as grocery stores, bars, or churches, to deliver a particular health message. The fourth P is *promotion*, which refers to the means of informing people about the product and persuading them to adopt it. This includes more formal methods of advertising, publicity, and availability of incentives, as well as informal methods such as personal communications. Winett (1995) added two other "P's" that also are important to consider. *Positioning* refers to creating a unique niche for the product, and *politics* refers to the social and economic climate that can affect the success of the marketing process.

The marketing process itself involves several stages. The process begins with *analyzing the market* at the economic, consumer, and institutional levels. Defining the market involves a study of the market's size, geographical scope, and available resources. The consumer-level analysis, in particular, involves an assessment of the demographic, geographic, and psychosocial characteristics of consumers, such as lifestyle behaviors, readiness to change a particular behavior, and user status. The institutional analysis involves gathering data regarding whether the health organization has the resources and organizational commitment to implement an intervention package. The marketing process then moves to the second *planning* stage, which requires the planning group to figure out the structure of the program and determine who will undertake the marketing efforts. The third stage is comprised of *product development*, testing product components (e.g., package designs, pricing, etc.), and *program refinement*. Program refinement involves the evaluation of the product prototype with a small sample in order to get a sense of what the market reaction would be if the product were distributed in a real-world setting. Larger scale testing would normally follow and might involve distributing the prototype to a test market community, such as a town or city. Marketers then can distribute the product regionally (e.g., at the county or state level) to test how it might be received before full-scale national distribution. The fourth and final stage involves the *implementation* of the action plan or execution of the full program, which is accompanied by careful monitoring of the *in-market effectiveness*. Although the areas for assessing effectiveness would depend on the unique goals of a product, the effectiveness is typically assessed using measures of consumer reaction and response, retailer response, health professional response, communication penetration and impact, and financial impact. The marketing process is circular, so the final stage incorporates the feedback to the first stage, where the cycle begins again.

The social marketing approach can be applied to persuade consumers to adopt an idea or behavior, not just to purchase tangible products. The marketing strategies demand that we learn more about the consumer rather than making assumptions about what is best for the communities to be served. The approach also does not assume that "one size fits all" and provides a technique and rationale for tailoring specific messages to particular segments of the target population in order to create a better match between product and consumer. This conceptualization forces consideration of demographic and cultural differences in the design, development, and distribution of a product, whether it be a tangible commodity or a behavior change program that focuses on smoking cessation, needle exchange, methadone maintenance, or alcohol use reduction.

## Communication Theory

Communication theory is a major framework used in the area of health promotion. Human communication contexts range from the intrapersonal and interpersonal to the public and mass communication levels. Communication theory has been used to understand and guide interactions that span diverse communication contexts, including the patient–provider relationship in the health care setting (Northouse & Northouse, 1985), as well as in educating and mobilizing larger communities to respond to widespread problems such as substance abuse (Backer, Rogers, & Sopory, 1992) and HIV infection (Ratzan, 1993).

A classic model of the communication process is Hovland's information-processing model of attitude and behavior change (Hovland, Janis, & Kelley, 1953; Hovland, Lumsdaine, & Sheffield, 1949). McGuire (1968, 1972, 1978) elaborated on Hovland's original model and developed the "persuasion matrix" as a way of conceptualizing the relationship between the inputs and outcomes of persuasive communication. According to this model, *inputs* refer to the components of the communication process, such as the characteristics of the message source. For example, the social psychological and communications research literatures indicate that a persuasive message has the most impact on attitude change if it is delivered by multiple sources of high credibility and similarity to the receiver. Research has also identified effective characteristics of other input factors, which include message, channel, receiver, and destination factors. The research literature suggests that the message content be repeated often and consistently, and that the delivery or channeling of the message utilize multiple media at times and locations that are accessible to receivers. The receivers are more likely to be receptive to the message if it is personally relevant or consistent with their value structures. Beyond these individual input characteristics, McGuire also described the importance of factors that incorporate interactions between the components of the communication process. For example, high fear arousal in a message is more effective for low anxiety receivers (McGuire, 1969). A review of the literature (Flay, DiTecco, & Schlegel, 1980) on the effectiveness of media campaigns revealed additional components that are conducive to belief or attitude change. These included arousing participation in the issue and motivating receivers to change, presenting the message in a novel way to maintain receiver interest, targeting specific issues, providing alternatives, and producing high-quality materials to promote attention.

The outcomes in McGuire's persuasion matrix refer to changes in knowledge, attitudes, or behavior in the receivers. McGuire outlined six steps in the process of persuasion through communication strategies, including (1) exposure to a persuasive message, (2) attending to or being aware of a message, (3) gaining knowledge by comprehending the message content, (4) forming beliefs and attitudes by yielding to the appeal of the message, (5) maintaining new attitude changes, and (6) demonstrating behavior change. McGuire further assumed that the pathways between each of these six steps are automatic (i.e., that changes in beliefs automatically lead to changes in attitudes, intentions, and behavior), but this assumption has been criticized by Flay et al. (1980), who also reconceptualized the model to incorporate intermediate processes that must occur before receivers can attain awareness, knowledge, or beliefs, and explicitly acknowledged that the paths leading to changes in attitudes, intentions, and behaviors are tentative.

The application of communication theory principles to the area of health promotion has led to the development of health communication. This area is specifically concerned with how individuals in society seek to maintain and deal with health-related issues (Northouse & Northouse, 1985). The mass media, in particular, have been embraced by public health approaches because of their ability to touch upon communication at all levels, from the interpersonal to large-scale social institutions and systems. Mass media channels define how a message is delivered to a receiver through visual, auditory, or written texts (e.g., television, newspapers, radio, pamphlets, or on the Internet). Four primary objectives of mass media campaigns from a public health approach have been outlined in the literature (Flora & Cassady, 1990). One objective is to employ media campaigns as the *primary change agent*. For example, an advertising campaign describing the harmful effects of smoking may have the goal of encouraging individuals to stop smoking. Media presentation has also been used as a *complement to other interventions*. For example, media campaigns such as posters and videos may have been used in conjunction with school-based skills aimed at delaying or reducing adolescent experimentation with drugs and alcohol. Media campaigns have also been used to *recruit and promote services and programs*. For example, smoking cessation programs available through Employee Assistance Programs may be advertised through public service announcements, internal electronic mail notices, or newsletters. Media messages are also applied to provide *support for lifestyle changes*. For example, media messages could reinforce a person for making and maintaining behavior change by publicizing personal testimonials of the challenges and rewards experienced by individuals who have or are in the process of cutting down on their alcohol consumption.

In summary, social marketing utilizes mass media communication as a conduit for the dissemination and promotion of programs and services. Similarly, mass media communication uses social marketing techniques to direct the development of a product, to determine the target audience, and to create avenues of communication. Together, these theories can guide diffusion of innovative intervention approaches at the individual, practice, and organizational levels. These are only some of the strategies that can facilitate the progression from intervention development and evaluation to incorporating and institutionalizing the interventions at the organizational and community levels. These issues are central to the study of diffusion of innovations, which is discussed in the following section.

## Diffusion of Innovations

Diffusion of innovations models focus on factors that characterize the successful implementation of innovations in real-world settings (Orlandi, Landers, Weston, & Haley, 1990). Diffusion theory emphasizes a broad contextual framework that utilizes organizational, economic, and environmental strategies in addition to individualized skills training, in order to achieve program adoption and behavior change (Portnoy, Anderson, & Eriksen, 1989). Diffusion theory is at the core of the public health approach because, like the public health perspective in general, it targets multiple levels across many different settings, and it uses multiple change strategies. The theory relies on aspects of social marketing and mass media to accomplish its goals.

An innovation is an "idea, practice or object that is perceived as new by an individual or other unit of adoption" (Rogers, 1983, p. 11). Diffusion is "the process by which an innovation is communicated through certain channels over time among the members of a social system" (p. 5). A combination of both formal and informal communication channels and the implementation of strategies through a variety of settings and systems are critical for the diffusion to be effective (Oldenberg, Hardcastle, & Kok, 1997).

Early work in the area of diffusion theory focused on the characteristics of both the adopter and the innovation itself as predictors of diffusion patterns. Rogers (1983) identified five adopter categories (i.e., innovators, early adopters, early majority adopters, late majority adopters, and laggards) to direct the design and implementation of intervention strategies to particular groups of individuals. The attributes of the innovation that have been predictive of successful diffusion include the innovation's relative advantage compared to other products, compatibility with the intended adopter, complexity, trialability, and observability. Characteristics of the innovation, such as the risk and uncertainty, the investment of time required, and the capacity for its modification, have been identified as possible barriers to its diffusion (Zaltman & Duncan, 1977). In addition to understanding the aspects of the innovation and adopter, Orlandi et al. (1990) described the importance of having a linking agent, which is a person or group bridging the gap between the promoters of a program and the potential users of the program. Incorporating users into the decision-making process not only improves the development of the innovation, but it also builds a sense of ownership and commitment on the part of the adopter.

Recently, four stages of diffusion have been proposed based on the literature on diffusion theory (Oldenberg et al., 1997). The *dissemination* stage encompasses the transfer of the innovation from the resource system to the user system. This stage requires the identification of the available communication systems. For example, local public service announcements or billboards may be targeted as possible channels. The *adoption* stage refers to the identification of potential adopters and the acceptance of the programs by these individuals. The *implementation* stage refers to the initial use of the innovation. It emphasizes the importance of improving the self-efficacy and skills of adopters. The *maintenance* stage encourages sustained program use. *Institutionalization* is the last stage, which entails the formalization of innovations into policies.

## Summary

We have provided an overview of various conceptual models that contribute to the theoretical base used to understand health behavior change, to translate that understanding into behavior change interventions, and to facilitate widescale dissemination of the interventions to appropriate target populations. As is evident in the array of factors highlighted by the different models, a comprehensive, public health perspective on addictive behavior change interventions is complex and cannot be informed by a single model. As noted earlier, there is overlap in many of the models, and they often use different terms for the same constructs. For example, the terms "consumer" (from social marketing), "receiver" (from communication theory), and "adopter" (from diffusion theory) all refer to the individual or group who is being targeted for a particular product, message, or innovation, which could be an intervention program (at the individual level) or a training program (at the provider level). Our intent in presenting these models is not to encourage professionals involved in the development and dissemination of addictive behavior interventions to select and uncritically apply one theory. Rather, the maximal utility of these conceptual frameworks occurs when their components converge to provide consistent guidelines for directing the development of addictive behavior interventions from a public health perspective. We turn to this application in the next section.

## GUIDING PRINCIPLES FOR DEVELOPING INTERVENTIONS WITH A PUBLIC HEALTH PERSPECTIVE

Key concepts from the frameworks outlined in the previous section, combined with practical experience, can be distilled into several common principles for addressing practical issues and challenges for addictive behavior interventions at the individual, practice, and organizational levels. In this section, we outline those principles that have emerged from our experience in developing and implementing conceptually based addictive behavior interventions within a public health perspective.

### Individual-Level Principles

From a public health perspective, the *impact* of an intervention is a product of its reach into the target population and the effectiveness of interventions offered (Abrams et al., 1995). To illustrate, a smoking cessation intervention that reaches 30% of smokers and has a 30% quit rate would have an impact of 9% ($0.3 \times 0.3$). In comparison, an intervention that reaches only 5% of the population but has a 60% quit rate would have an impact of 3%. Thus, our goal is not only to have programs that have high success rates, but also to have ways of providing those programs to as high a percentage of the target population as possible. Consequently, maximizing reach through population-based screening and having effective interventions that can be disseminated on a broad scale are two important challenges at the individual level. Our conceptual frameworks suggest applying the following principles to meet these challenges in developing interventions that are delivered directly to individuals.

1. *Use nonthreatening screening methods that involve minimal time and effort.* Population-based identification of individuals who are appropriate for addictive behavior interventions typically include some form of "risk assessment." Social marketing theory highlights not only the importance of the amount of time and effort that are required to complete such assessments, but also that of minimizing the psychological and social costs involved. Whether individuals complete paper-and-pencil assessments or use innov-

ative touch-screen computer technologies, it is important to keep assessment time to a minimum and to ensure that there is sufficient privacy for
their confidential completion. It is often helpful to distinguish among the
levels of information needed to (a) ascertain whether an individual en-
gages in an addictive behavior; (b) understand how motivated he or she is
to modify the behavior; (c) understand the level of impairment in order to
recommend a treatment strategy (e.g., minimal vs. more intensive); and (d)
conduct a detailed intake assessment for intensive treatment. Disaggregat-
ing these levels of assessment can make population-based screening brief
as well as avoid giving individuals messages about the target behavior that
may be inappropriate for their level of use (e.g., individuals who are at risk
for future drinking problems but who are not alcohol dependent may be
put off by lengthy assessments that assume very high levels of alcohol consumption).

2. *Address different levels of motivation to change.* If population-based
screening efforts are successful, a large proportion of individuals who are
identified as candidates for addictive behavior interventions will be unmotivated for treatment. Using terminology and data from Prochaska and
DiClemente's stages of change model (e.g. Prochaska & DiClemente,
1983; Prochaska, Redding & Evers, 1995; see Chapter 6, this volume),
only about 20% of individuals are ready to actively attempt to change
their behavior at a given point in time. The remaining 80% are fairly
evenly split between those who have no interest or motivation to change
their behavior (i.e., are precontemplative) and those who are seriously considering changing, but not in the near future (i.e., are contemplative). Such
individuals are unlikely to accept interventions that assume relatively high
levels of motivation and intentions to change. In dissemination theory
terms, they would be viewed as "laggards." Thus, a full complement of interventions will include components aimed at enhancing motivation to
change in addition to traditional action-oriented programs.

3. *Emphasize positive results and avoid high-threat communications.* Value–
expectancy theories underscore the importance of believing that recommended actions will have positive results. However, trying to motivate people to take those actions through fear and anxiety can backfire. There are
a number of intervention approaches that provide alternatives to high-
threat communications. For example, the FRAMES paradigm in motivational interviewing proposes that motivation and commitment to change
is triggered by (a) providing feedback, (b) enhancing personal responsibility, (c) giving advice with a menu of options, (d) being empathic, and (e)
supporting self-efficacy by using the success of others as encouragement
(Miller & Rollnick, 1991).

4. *Provide specific behavioral skills.* State-of-the-art intervention pro-

grams must include relevant skills training components. Even minimal intervention programs, such as self-help manuals (e.g., Curry, 1993), can include such skills training components as self-monitoring, goal setting and contracting, planning for high-risk situations, problem-solving approaches to identify strategies for coping with high-risk situations, methods of enlisting social support, and relaxation exercises (Marlatt & Gordon, 1985).

5. *Provide meaningful supports.* Facilitative environmental factors such as positive social norms and encouragement and support from significant others are emphasized by both value–expectancy and social cognitive theories. Nonspecialist practitioners such as primary health care providers can give meaningful support by praising patients' efforts to change and by including consistent and repeated follow-up as part of routine care. At the macro-level, mass media can play an important role in reinforcing social norms that support addictive behavior change (e.g., reinforce nonsmoking norms or norms against drinking and driving).

6. *Provide opportunities for individual tailoring.* The social marketing approach tells us that "one size does not fit all." Credible, effective minimal intervention strategies must offer individuals the opportunity to tailor program components. Tailoring can occur with regard to selection of treatment goals (e.g., abstinence, controlled use, harm reduction), treatment format (e.g., written materials with supportive telephone counseling, participation in group sessions, interactive video), and specific treatment components (e.g., individuals concentrate on different parts of a written intervention program, such as motivational exercises, assertiveness training components, and stress management strategies, based upon a self-assessment).

## Practice-Level Principles

Public health interventions are often delivered in natural settings by providers who are not necessarily specialists in the treatment of addictive behaviors. The most common setting in which these interventions are incorporated is a primary health care delivery system. Recognition of the potential public health impact of primary-care-based screening and intervention for addictive behavior change is evident in the dissemination of guidelines for providers, such as the recently released *Smoking Cessation Clinical Practice Guideline* (Fiore, Bailey, Cohen, et al., 1996) and the *Physician's Guide to Helping Patients with Alcohol Problems* (National Institute on Alcohol Abuse and Alcoholism, 1995). Among the core features of these guidelines are recommendations to screen patients (Ask), give advice to change (Advise), offer help to motivated patients (Assist), and monitor progress (Arrange follow-up). Thus, in this section, we discuss principles related to implementation of a primary-care-based addictive behavior change approach that involves population-based screening and dissemination of intervention materials to patients who screen positive for the target behavior. The conceptual frameworks variously suggest applying the following principles to ensure implementation at the practice level.

1. *Define roles for all practice team members.* Practice team members include not only the primary health care providers (e.g., physicians, nurses, medical assistants, health educators/counselors) but also key support staff such as receptionists and administrative assistants. All of the components of a public health intervention need not be implemented by the primary provider. For example, in a primary care medical setting, a receptionist can be assigned the role of giving patients screening instruments as they register for their appointments, the medical assistant can quickly scan and tally the screening instrument as patients are placed in the examining room, and the primary care provider can deliver a motivational message and advice to change behaviors to those patients with positive screening scores and can give patients written self-help materials to take home. The practice nurse can provide postvisit follow-up, either in person or by telephone, to assess progress with the self-help program. In addition to roles related to patient interactions, it is important to assign specific responsibilities to each team member to maintain key components of the intervention (e.g., ensuring a handy supply of written materials, entering patient information into computerized systems).

2. *Provide role-relevant training for service providers.* The content of training for service providers can be informed by many of the same concepts on which individual-level interventions are based. For example, consistent with value–expectancy models, primary care providers will be more likely to screen for addictive behaviors and to provide advice and intervention materials to patients if they believe that such behaviors pose serious health risks (this is particularly true for screening and intervention with individuals who are on the less severe portion of the continuum of substance use and problems), and if they believe that the intervention materials (e.g., self-help booklets, videotapes) are effective. From a social cognitive perspective, it is important to provide role-playing opportunities during training sessions in order to enhance self-efficacy and to give providers the opportunity to learn from observing others.

3. *Provide information and tracking systems.* Implementing public health interventions in natural settings to which individuals return over time provides an opportunity for consistent and repeated follow-up. However, in settings such as general medical practices, follow-up is unlikely to occur in

the absence of information and tracking systems that cue providers to monitor progress. Such systems need not be elaborate. There are some excellent models in the smoking cessation area that include components such as chart stickers and vital sign stamps that cue physicians to assess smoking status at each visit (Fiore et al., 1996).

4. *Have state-of-the-art supportive materials available.* From a communication theory perspective, health care providers can provide a highly credible, personalized, persuasive message to change behavior. While these messages can change individuals' attitudes toward the target behavior and raise intentions to make changes, many patients need more specific guidance in making changes, and providers may be reluctant to raise the need for change because they neither feel competent nor have the time to provide sufficient guidance for implementing change. Fortunately, there are numerous minimal intervention protocols and supportive materials that can provide such guidance to patients (e.g., Glynn, Boyd, & Gruman, 1991; Sanchez-Craig, 1993; National Institute on Alcohol Abuse and Alcoholism, 1996). Making such materials and referral sources readily accessible to providers and their patients is crucial.

## Organizational-Level Principles

Organizational-level factors are of primary importance for the last two stages of diffusion—*maintenance*, or sustained program implementation, and *institutionalization*, wherein intervention programs are incorporated into the organization through formalized policies. The social marketing approach suggests several principles for successful institutionalization of addictive behavior change interventions at the organizational level.

1. *Assess and build organizational commitment.* Innovative interventions are often introduced to organizations through funded treatment outcome evaluations. Researchers and program advocates are often dismayed to find that when the grant funding goes away, even highly successful programs are not maintained by the organization. Thus, it is important to assess and build organizational commitment for interventions, starting with the research and development phase. A first step in this process is to identify divisions and people in the organization whose support is critical for maintaining the program. Questions to consider during this phase are: (a) What division(s) in the organization would have responsibility for maintaining the program (e.g., in a work site, it could be the occupational health program; in a managed care system, it could be a center for health promotion or a specialized drug treatment program)? (b) Who controls resources that would have to be allocated for program implementation? (c)

Is there a marketing division that would have an interest in this program as a potential marketing tool? (d) Who would be on the front lines delivering the program? (e) Are there committees in the organization whose endorsement is critical for institutionalizing the program? Building organizational commitment can begin with including discussion of the program on regular meeting agendas in order to identify people interested in developing institutional policies to maintain it.

2. *Coordinate and share resources.* As implied in the preceding principle, addictive behavior interventions are likely to crosscut organizational and budgetary divisions. For example, in a health care organization, tertiary care for alcoholics may be provided by a specialty service with its own budget, whereas primary and secondary prevention efforts may occur through primary care or centralized health promotion services, each with separate budget allocations. All of these divisions could appropriately contribute to costs associated with provider training, population-based screening, and computerized tracking of individuals who are appropriate for treatment. Achieving coordination and sharing of resources for these efforts invokes Winett's (1995) additional social marketing "P's" of positioning and politics. All members of relevant units need to believe that the proposed intervention components enhance their existing efforts to offer services and that sharing resources will not detract from their other priority areas.

3. *Evaluate the impact of organizational interventions at the individual and practice levels.* If an organization is going to commit resources to a program, it will want assurances that the investment was worthwhile. Defining important outcomes is one way conceptual models can make a major contribution to organizations. Demonstrating changes in the target behavior is clearly important, and there are other outcomes that may be important to assess. At the individual level, evaluation can focus on whether there are changes in factors such as knowledge, attitudes, beliefs, and skills that mediate addictive behavior change. Other relevant outcomes include patient satisfaction, utilization of other services, and psychosocial functioning (e.g., employment, family relations). Feedback of positive, individual-level outcomes to providers can motivate continued program implementation. Relevant outcomes at the provider level also include changes in knowledge, attitudes, beliefs, and skills relevant to intervention delivery, as well as provider satisfaction, productivity, and retention. Organizational-level outcomes could include changes in costs associated with addictive behaviors (e.g., decreases in employee absenteeism following worksite implementation of screening and intervention programs). An important principle to keep in mind regarding evaluation is that it does not have to be expensive or elaborate. Often, meaningful data can be obtained simply by including systematic recordkeeping as part of program implementation.

## CASE EXAMPLE: TREATMENT OF TOBACCO ADDICTION IN A HEALTH MAINTENANCE ORGANIZATION

Group Health Cooperative of Puget Sound (GHC) is a consumer-governed, staff-model health maintenance organization with over 490,000 members and over 1,000 physicians. GHC's initiatives for treatment of tobacco addiction over the past decade provide several concrete examples of the application of the individual-, practice-, and organizational-level principles outlined in the previous section.

GHC's initiatives in smoking cessation began in the mid-1980s with participation as the clinical site for a randomized evaluation of a self-help smoking cessation program, Free and Clear (Orleans et al., 1991). The project was funded by the National Cancer Institute (NCI) and involved a comparative study of a self-help booklet alone, a self-help booklet along with special social support materials for another person, a self-help booklet along with four outreach telephone counseling calls, and a minimal treatment condition that received referrals to community programs and a brief bibliotherapy guide. The telephone counseling was delivered by lay personnel with special training. The study participants were volunteers who were recruited through advertisements in a bimonthly publication, *View* magazine, that was sent to all GHC enrollees. The trial results showed significantly higher quit rates for the group who received the self-help booklet plus telephone counseling compared to all of the other treatment conditions. The long-term abstinence rate in this group was 18% at a 16-month follow-up (Orleans et al., 1991).

Comparisons of the smokers who volunteered for the Free and Clear intervention with the characteristics of smokers in the general GHC population (Wagner et al., 1990) indicated that the volunteers represented approximately 4% of the smokers enrolled in GHC, and that the volunteers were older, sicker, and heavier smokers than the population of smokers as a whole. Thus, by the late 1980s, GHC had a minimal intervention that was proven effective in a select sample of smokers and that had the potential to be disseminated on a broad scale. The challenges remaining from a public health perspective included (1) increasing the reach of the program through population-based screening and referral of smokers for treatment; (2) developing practice guidelines, training, and information systems at the practice level; (3) building organizational commitment to provide resources to sustain the program beyond the initial funding period and to institute benefit policies that provided incentives for smokers to participate in the program; and (4) assessing individual-, practice-, and organizational-level outcomes such as patient satisfaction, changes in health care utilization associated with smoking cessation, and the cost-effectiveness of providing coverage for smoking cessation services.

By the mid-1990s, significant progress has been made on all of these fronts. A comprehensive practice guideline for addressing tobacco use during primary care visits was developed as part of the work of GHC's Committee on Prevention (COP) (Thompson, Taplin, McAfee, Mandelson, & Smith, 1995). The practice guideline customized the "4-A model" (Ask, Advise, Assist, Arrange) disseminated by the NCI as a result of several randomized trials of physician interventions for smoking cessation (Glynn & Manley, 1990). The guideline recommends screening for tobacco use at all primary care visits by including tobacco use as a vital sign. In addition, the guideline applies all of the practice-level principles outlined in the previous section, including defining roles for all practice team members, providing training, having information, tracking systems (e.g., chart stickers), and state-of-the-art supportive materials available. Supportive materials at GHC include prescriptions (referral forms) for the Free and Clear program for smokers who are motivated to participate in treatment and clinic-based copies of NCI's *Clearing the Air* pamphlet, which was reprinted and customized for GHC enrollees. Staff from the Center for Health Promotion, which houses the Free and Clear program, have provided in-clinic training sessions on the guideline for all providers.

Organizational commitment has been continued through a Tobacco Use Steering Committee that meets quarterly and includes representatives from clinics, pharmacies, administration, and research. The committee assists in establishing protocols for tracking compliance with the guideline and providing feedback to providers (e.g., quarterly chart reviews to assess the percentage of patient charts with smoking status noted and whether visit notes indicate that smoking cessation was addressed with patients identified as smokers). Other activities include adding to the regular patient-satisfaction surveys an assessment of smoking status, provider advice to quit smoking, and satisfaction with smoking cessation services offered at GHC. Based on the work of the COP and subsequent Tobacco Use Steering Committee, GHC's Cooperative Benefit's Committee approved coverage of smoking cessation services beginning in 1993. The benefit provides 50% coverage for the cost of the Free and Clear program (enrollees pay a $42.50 copayment). In addition, smokers who enroll in Free and Clear have full coverage of nicotine replacement therapy.

Several innovative research projects have been implemented along with these treatment initiatives, and we highlight a few of them here. First, a randomized trial evaluated the impact of the self-help materials and outreach telephone counseling on nonvolunteer smokers who were identified through health surveys with a random sample of nearly 6,000 GHC enrollees (Curry, McBride, Grothaus, Louie, & Wagner, 1995). This study found promising effects of self-help materials along with outreach telephone counseling, particularly among less motivated smokers. The outreach telephone counseling significantly improved 3-month cessation rates among all smokers and long-term cessation rates among smokers who indicated at the baseline survey that they were not seriously considering quitting smoking in the next 6 months (Curry et al., 1995).

A second study (Wagner, Curry, Grothaus, Saunders, & McBride, 1995) examined the impact of smoking and quitting on health care use by using automated data on utilization of health services and smoking cessation data from participants in two randomized trials of smoking cessation interventions that were conducted at GHC. These analyses indicate that successful smoking cessation stops the progressive increase in use of health services associated with continued smoking within a 4-year period.

Finally, a recently completed study (Curry, Grothaus, McAfee, & Pabiniak, 1998) compared rates of utilization and cost-effectiveness of the standard coverage of smoking cessation services to three alternative coverage structures that varied copayments on behavioral and pharmacological treatments. This study found that adding a copayment for nicotine replacement therapy (NRT) reduced use of the cessation services and that fewer service users filled NRT prescriptions. Removing all copayments (i.e., no copayments for the behavioral program or NRT) had the highest impact on the overall population of smokers. In this group, rates of program utilization more than doubled (approximately 5% with standard coverage compared to approximately 12% in the full-coverage group), while quit rates did go down (6-month abstinence rates were approximately 38% with standard coverage and 28% with full coverage). The lower quit rate in the group with full coverage resulted in higher costs per quit to GHC ($795 standard vs. $1,162 full coverage). However, the utilization and cessation percentages translated into population-level impacts of 2% ($0.05 \times 0.38$) versus 3% ($0.12 \times 0.28$), which is a 50% increase in impact for the full-coverage structure. Thus, the nearly 50% increase in costs to the organization are offset by a comparable 50% in overall impact.

Applying a public health perspective to the development, evaluation, and implementation of addictive behavior interventions does not require that all organizations conduct all of the research summarized in this section. Nevertheless, our hope is that results from carefully controlled research in an organization such as GHC can be used to justify comparable approaches in other settings.

## CONCLUSIONS

Because of the multiple levels of intervention and the many factors that can be important to address within and across levels, the public health perspective can seem quite complicated. In this chapter, we have attempted to simplify the conceptual and practical considerations from a public health perspective by providing an overview of conceptual models and guiding principles, as well as examples of their application to tobacco addiction interventions in a health maintenance organization. The underlying theme of this chapter has been that applying these conceptual models and guiding principles to program development and implementation may help to broaden the base and reach of current and future intervention approaches. Innovation in services for addictive behaviors is likely to occur when the clinical and public health perspectives are merged. The following chapters describe a number of intervention approaches that illustrate this merger.

## ACKNOWLEDGMENTS

Preparation of this chapter was supported in part by the National Institute on Alcohol Abuse and Alcoholism, Grant No. AA09175, and the National Heart, Lung, and Blood Institute, Grant No. HL48121 to Susan J. Curry.

## REFERENCES

Abrams, D. B., Emmons, K. M., & Linnan, L. A. (1995). Health behavior and health education: The past, present and future. In K. Glanz, F. M. Lewis, & B. K. Rimer (Eds.), *Health behavior and health education: Theory, research and practice* (pp. 453–478). San Francisco: Jossey-Bass.

Abrams, D. B., Emmons, K. M., Niaura, R., Goldstein, M. G., & Sherman, C. B. (1991). Tobacco dependence: An integration of individual and public health perspectives. In B. McCrady (Ed.), *Annual review of addictions research and treatment* (pp. 391–436). New York: Pergamon.

Ajzen, I. (1985). From intentions to actions: A theory of planned action. In J. Kuhl & J. Beckman (Eds.), *Action control: From cognition to behavior* (pp. 11–39). New York: Springer-Verlag.

Ajzen, I., & Madden, T. J. (1986). Prediction of goal-directed behavior: Attitudes, intentions, and perceived behavioral control. *Journal of Experimental Social Psychology, 22,* 453–474.

Backer, T. E., Rogers, E. M., & Sopory, P. (1992). *Designing health communication campaigns: What works?* Newbury Park, CA: Sage.

Bandura, A. (1978). The self system in reciprocal determinism. *American Psychologist, 33,* 344–358.

Bandura, A. (1986). *Social foundations of thought and action.* Englewood Cliffs, NJ: Prentice-Hall.

Bandura, A. (1995). Exercise of personal and collective efficacy in changing societies. In A. Bandura (Ed.), *Self-efficacy in changing societies* (pp. 1–45). New York: Cambridge University Press.

Bardsley, P. E., & Beckman, L. J. (1988). The health belief model and entry into alcoholism treatment. *International Journal of the Addictions, 23*(1), 19–28.

Brehony, K. A., Frederiksen, L. W., & Solomon, L. J. (1984). Marketing principles and behavioral medicine: An overview. In L. W. Frederiksen, L. J. Solomon, & K. A. Brehony (Eds.), *Marketing health behavior: Principles, techniques, and applications* (pp. 3–22). New York: Plenum.

Curry, S. J. (1993) Self-help interventions for smoking cessation. *Journal of Consulting and Clinical Psychology, 61*(5), 790–803.

Curry, S. J., & Emmons, K. M. (1994). Theoretical models for predicting and improving compliance with breast cancer screening. *Annals of Behavioral Medicine, 16*(4), 302–316.

Curry, S. J., Grothaus, L. C., McAfee, T., & Pabiniak, C. (1998). Utilization and cost effectiveness of smoking cessation services under four insurance coverage structures in a health maintenance organization. *New England Journal of Medicine, 339*(10), 673–679.

Curry, S. J., McBride, C. M., Grothaus, L. C., Louie, D., & Wagner, E. H. (1995). A randomized trial of self-help materials, personalized feedback and telephone counseling with nonvolunteer smokers. *Journal of Consulting and Clinical Psychology, 63*(6), 1005–1014.

DiClemente, C. C., Fairhurst, S. K., & Piotrowski, N. A. (1995). The role of self-efficacy in the addictive behaviors. In J. Maddux (Ed.), *Self efficacy, adaptation, and adjustment: Theory, research, and application* (pp. 109–142). New York: Plenum.

Finnegan, J. R., & Viswanath, K. (1995). Communication theory and health behavior change: The media studies framework. In K. Glanz, F. M. Lewis, & B. K. Rimer (Eds.), *Health behavior and health education: Theory, research, and practice* (2nd ed., pp. 313–341). San Francisco: Jossey-Bass.

Fiore, M. C., Bailey, W. C., Cohen, S. J., Dorfman, S. F., Goldstein, M. G., Gritz, E. R., Heyman, R. B., Holbrook, J., Jaen, C. R., Kottke, T. E., Lando, H. A., Mecklenburg, R., Mullen, P. D., Nett, L. M., Robinson, L., Stitzer, M., Tommasello, A. C., Villejo, L., & Wewers, M. E. (1996). *Smoking cessation* (Clinical Practice Guideline No. 18, AHCPR Publication No. 96-0692). Rockville, MD: U.S. Department of Health and Human Services, Public Health Service, Agency for Health Care Policy and Research.

Fishbein, M., & Ajzen, I. (1975). *Belief, attitude, intention and behavior: An introduction to theory and research.* Reading, MA: Addison-Wesley.

Flay, B. R., DiTecco, D., & Schlegel, R. P. (1980). Mass media in health promotion: An analysis using an extended information-processing model. *Health Education Quarterly, 7*(2), 127–147.

Flora, J. A., & Cassady, D. (1990). Roles of media in community-based health promotion. In N. Bracht (Ed.), *Health promotion at the community level* (pp. 143–157). Newbury Park, CA: Sage.

Frederiksen, L. W., Solomon, L. J., & Brehony, K. A. (1984). *Marketing health behavior: Principles, techniques, and applications.* New York: Plenum.

Glanz, K., Lewis, F. M., & Rimer, B. K. (1995). *Health behavior and health education: Theory, research and practice* (2nd ed.). San Francisco: Jossey-Bass.

Glynn, T. J., Boyd, G. M., & Gruman, J. C. (1991). *Self-guided strategies for smoking cessation: A program planners guide* (NIH Publication No. 91-3104, National Cancer Institute, Smoking and Tobacco Control Program). Washington, DC: U.S. Department of Health and Human Services.

Glynn, T. J., & Manley, M. W. (1990). *How to help your patients stop smoking: A national cancer institute manual for physicians* (National Cancer Institute, NIH Publication No. 90-3064). Bethesda, MD: U.S. Department of Health and Human Services, Public Health Service, National Institutes of Health.

Green, L. W., & Kreuter, M. W. (1991). *Health promotion planning: An educational and environmental approach* (2nd ed.). Mountain View, CA: Mayfield.

Hochbaum, G. M. (1958). *Public participation in medical screening programs: A sociopsychological study* (Public Health Service Publication No. 572). Washington, DC: U.S. Government Printing Office.

Hovland, C. I., Janis, I. L., & Kelley, H. H. (1953). *Communication and persuasion.* New Haven, CT: Yale University Press.

Hovland, C. I., Lumsdaine, A. A., & Sheffield, F. D. (1949). *Experiments on mass communication.* Princeton, NJ: Princeton University Press.

Hull, C. L. (1943). *Principles of behavior.* East Norwalk, CT: Appleton & Lange.

Institute for Health Policy, Brandeis University. (1993). *Substance abuse: The nation's number one health problem: Key indicators for policy.* Princeton, NJ: Robert Wood Johnson Foundation.

Institute of Medicine. (1990). *Broadening the base of treatment for alcohol problems: A report of a study by a committee of the Institute of Medicine, Division of Mental Health and Behavioral Medicine.* Washington, DC: National Academy Press.

Janz, N. K., & Becker, M. H. (1984). The health belief model: A decade later. *Health Education Quarterly, 11,* 1–47.

Kotler, P. (1984). Social marketing of health behavior. In L. W. Frederiksen, L. J. Solomon, & K. A. Brehony (Eds.), *Marketing health behavior: Principles, techniques, and applications* (pp. 23–38). New York: Plenum.

Lichtenstein, E., & Glasgow, R. E. (1992). Smoking cessation: What have we learned over the past decade. *Journal of Consulting and Clinical Psychology, 60,* 518–527.

Marlatt, G. A., Baer, J. S., & Quigley, L. A. (1995). Self-efficacy and addictive behavior. In A. Bandura (Ed.), *Self-efficacy in changing societies* (pp. 289–315). New York: Cambridge University Press.

Marlatt, G. A., & Gordon, J. R. (1985). *Relapse prevention.* New York: Guilford Press.

Marshall, P. (1990). "Just one more . . . !" A study into the smoking attitudes and behaviour of patients following first myocardial infarction. *International Journal of Nursing Studies, 27*(4), 375–387.

McGuire, W. J. (1968). Personality and susceptibility to social influence. In E. F. Borgatta & W. W. Lambert (Eds.), *Handbook of personality theory and research* (pp. 1130–1187). Chicago: Rand McNally.

McGuire, W. J. (1969). The nature of attitudes and attitude change. In G. Lindzey & E. Aronson (Eds.), *The handbook of social psychology* (2nd ed., Vol. 3, pp. 136–314). Reading, MA: Addison-Wesley.

McGuire, W. J. (1972). Attitude change: The information processing paradigm. In C. G. McClintock (Ed.), *Experimental social psychology.* New York: Holt, Rinehart & Winston.

McGuire, W. J. (1978). An information-processing model of advertising effectiveness. In H. L. Davis & A. J. Silk (Eds.), *Behavioral and management science in marketing* (pp. 1130–1187). New York: Wiley.

Miller, N. E., & Dollard, J. (1941). *Social learning and imitation.* New Haven, CT: Yale University Press.

Miller, W. R., & Rollnick, S. (1991). *Motivational interviewing: Preparing people to change addictive behaviors.* New York: Guilford Press.

National Institute on Alcohol Abuse and Alcoholism. (1995). *The physician's guide to helping patients with alcohol problems* (NIAAA Publication No. 95-3769). Bethesda, MD: U.S. Department of Health and Human Services, Public Health Service, National Institutes of Health, National Institute on Alcohol Abuse and Alcoholism.

National Institute on Alcohol Abuse and Alcoholism. (1996). *How to cut down on your drinking* (NIH Publication No. 3770). Bethesda, MD: Author.

Northouse, P. G., & Northouse, L. L. (1985). *Health communication: A handbook for health professionals.* Englewood Cliffs, NJ: Prentice-Hall.

Oldenberg, B., Hardcastle, D., & Kok, G. (1997). Diffusion of health promotion and education programs. In K. Glanz, F. M. Lewis, & B. K. Rimer (Eds.), *Health behavior and health education: Theory, research, and practice* (2nd ed., pp. 270–286). San Francisco: Jossey-Bass.

Orlandi, M. A., Landers, C., Weston, R., & Haley, N. (1990). Diffusion of health promotion innovations. In K. Glanz, F. M. Lewis, & B. K. Rimer (Eds.), *Health behavior and health education: Theory, research, and practice* (pp. 288–313). San Francisco: Jossey-Bass.

Orleans, C. T., Schoenbach, V. J., Wagner, E. H., Quade, D., Salmon, M. A., Pearson, D. C., Fiedler, J., Porter, C. Q., & Kaplan, B. H. (1991). Self-help quit smoking interventions: Effects of self-help materials, social support instructions and telephone counseling. *Journal of Consulting and Clinical Psychology, 59,* 439–448.

Perry, C. L., Baranowski, T., & Parcel, G. S. (1990). How individuals, environments, and health behavior interact: Social learning theory. In K. Glanz, F. M. Lewis, & B. K. Rimer (Eds.), *Health behavior and health education: Theory, research, and practice* (pp. 161–186). San Francisco: Jossey-Bass.

Portnoy, B., Anderson, D. M., & Eriksen, M. P. (1989). Application of diffusion theory to health promotion research. *Family and Community Health, 12*(3), 63–71.

Prochaska, J. O., & DiClemente, C. C. (1983). Stages and processes of self-change of smoking: Toward an integrative model. *Journal of Consulting and Clinical Psychology, 51,* 390–395.

Prochaska, J. O., Redding, C. A., & Evers, K. E. (1995). The transtheoretical model and stages of change. In K. Glanz, F. M. Lewis, & B. K. Rimer (Eds.), *Health behavior and health education: Theory, research, and practice* (2nd ed., pp. 60–84). San Francisco: Jossey-Bass.

Ratzan, S. C. (1993). *AIDS: Effective health communication for the 90s.* Washington, DC: Taylor & Francis.

Rogers, E. (1983). *Diffusion of innovations.* New York: Free Press.

Rosenstock, I. M. (1960). What research in motivation suggests for public health. *American Journal of Public Health, 50,* 295–301.

Rosenstock, I. M. (1966). Why people use health services. *Milbank Memorial Fund Quarterly, 44,* 94–124.

Rosenstock, I. M. (1974). Historical origins of the health belief model. *Health Education Monographs, 2*(4), 328–335.

Sanchez-Craig, M. (1993). *Saying when: How to quit drinking or cut down* (2nd ed., rev.). Toronto: Addiction Research Foundation.

Thompson, R. S., Taplin, S. H., McAfee, T. A., Mandelson, M. T., & Smith, A. E. (1995). Primary and secondary prevention services in clinical practice: Twenty years' experience in development, implementation and evaluation. *Journal of the American Medical Association, 273*(14), 1130–1135.

Wagner, E. H., Curry, S. J., Grothaus, L., Saunders, K. W., & McBride, C. M. (1995). The impact of smoking and quitting on health care use. *Archives of Internal Medicine, 155*, 1789–1795.

Wagner, E. H., Schoenbach, V. J., Orleans, C. T., Grothaus, L. C., Saunders, K. W., Curry, S. J., & Pearson, D. C. (1990). Participation in a smoking cessation program: A population-based perspective. *American Journal of Preventive Medicine, 6,* 258–266.

Walsh, J. M., & McPhee, S. J. (1992). A systems model of clinical preventive care: An analysis of factors influencing patient and physician. *Health Education Quarterly, 19*(2), 157–175.

Winett, R. A., King, A. C., & Altman, D. G. (1989). *Health psychology and public health.* New York: Pergamon.

Winett, R. A. (1995). A framework for health promotion and disease prevention programs. *American Psychologist, 50*(5), 341–350.

Zaltman, G., & Duncan, R. (1977). *Strategies for planned change.* New York: Wiley.

# 9

# Brief Interventions for Alcohol and Drug Problems

## ALLEN ZWEBEN
## MICHAEL F. FLEMING

## BROADENING THE BOUNDARIES
## OF SUBSTANCE ABUSE SERVICES

Recognition is growing that individuals with substance use problems are a diverse population with differing levels of severity of alcohol- or drug-related problems and varying capabilities and resources to cope with them (Institute of Medicine, 1990). Within this vulnerable population, a sizable proportion occasionally drink or use drugs in a manner that could cause serious harm to themselves and to others but as yet have only experienced mild to moderate negative consequences. Such problems may entail missing a few days of work each month, marital and other interpersonal problems, and guilt or anxiety about substance use. Other individuals who use alcohol or drugs experience more serious problems such as medical complications, psychiatric disorders (e.g., depression), physiological difficulties (e.g., tolerance and withdrawal symptoms), and legal difficulties (Institute of Medicine, 1990; Heather, 1995a; Skinner & Allen, 1982). Persons with mild to moderate difficulties comprise the majority of persons with substance-related problems, but they have not been the target of conventional intensive treatments. The potential for averting future serious problems and associated costs with this group is enormous, and they are the main target of brief interventions.

As the definition of alcohol and drug abuse has expanded, so have the boundaries of alcohol and drug treatment services. More persons with substance-related problems are being identified at earlier stages and are receiving services in a variety of settings (Rose, Zweben, & Stoffel, in press). For example, screenings for substance abuse have been incorporated into the intake assessments of many managed care organizations (MCOs), into the medical history forms used in hospital emergency departments, as part of referrals to employee assistance programs (EAPs), and as part of evaluating the needs of welfare recipients. Individuals with alcohol and drug problems of varying severity are receiving services in an expanded range of settings, including emergency departments of general hospitals, public schools, child protection agencies, legal services, and EAPs (Zweben & Rose, in press). Many of these programs are aimed at identifying and treating alcohol and drug problems *before* they become more serious. Public health policies have similarly expanded to include a focus on individuals with mild to moderate substance use problems, along with those having more serious problems (Higgins-Biddle & Babor, 1996; Institute of Medicine, 1990).

The diverse needs and capacities of individuals with alcohol and drug problems necessitate a continuum of services that are responsive to their varying levels of problem severity, coping capacities, and social resources, along with the preferences of clients (Institute of Medicine, 1990). Rather than focus exclusively on eliminating drinking or drug use, as in traditional treatments, newer services are often geared to reducing the harmful consequences of the abuse (e.g., prevention of spousal violence, HIV transmission, and motor vehicle accidents) (Marlatt, Larimer, Baer, & Quigley, 1993; Zweben & Cisler, 1996). Within this approach, it is deemed appropriate for some individuals to cut down on their substance use and for others to abstain entirely.

In the United States, practitioners have often resisted these recommendations and have continued to rely on conventional, abstinence-oriented treatments. This contrasts with the scope of services offered in many European countries, Canada, and Australia, which have expanded to serve better the diversity of clients' needs. Conventional treatments often are not highly successful or cost-effective, particularly with individuals who have less severe alcohol or drug problems (e.g., Miller et al., 1995). Such individuals often have not had serious enough substance-related problems to motivate them to accept or undertake the changes required in conventional treatments (Sobell & Sobell, 1993). Required changes typically involve acceptance of the "alcoholic" or "addict" label, a commitment to lifelong abstinence, regular attendance of Alcoholics Anonymous or Narcotics Anonymous meetings, and participation in intensive treatment that consists of education on chemical dependency and individual or group therapy. As a result, many individuals with less severe problems refuse to enter or to remain in intensive treatments that are designed to serve alcohol or drug-dependent clients (Cooney, Zweben, & Fleming, 1995; Zweben & Barrett, 1997).

It is within this context that brief interventions for substance abuse have been devised and utilized. The approach was originally developed in research on nicotine abuse (Ockene et al., 1991; Richmond & Heather, 1990) and in alcoholism treatment outcome studies conducted in Europe (Orford & Edwards, 1977; cf. Bien, Miller, & Tonigan, 1993). The latter research used a brief intervention as a minimal-treatment control condition and found that it produced positive behavior change similar to more intensive treatment. Brief interventions have since developed into a viable alternative to more intensive treatments. The approach is consistent with trends in the U.S. health care system to curb costs by shifting service delivery away from expensive, hospital-based treatments toward briefer, outpatient interventions. The development of cost-effective services is thus a high priority.

Brief interventions are a low-cost, effective treatment alternative for alcohol and drug problems that use time-limited, self-help, and preventive strategies to promote reductions in substance use in nondependent clients and, in the case of dependent clients, to facilitate their referral to specialized treatment programs. The primary goal in all cases to increase motivation for behavior change. Brief interventions do not teach specific cognitive or behavioral skills, nor do they attempt to change a client's social environment.

This chapter summarizes the conceptual and empirical foundations of brief interventions and describes components of the approach and the range of application in different health care and community settings. Key areas covered include applications with nondependent and dependent substance abusers, and the importance of increasing motivation for behavior change, with the goals for change being tied to clients' presenting circumstances and status. The chapter ends with a consideration of unresolved issues in the development and delivery of brief interventions, and with an illustration of the use of brief interventions in nonspecialized, primary health care settings.

## CONCEPTUAL FRAMEWORK
## FOR BRIEF INTERVENTIONS

Drawing upon the principles of motivational psychology and self-regulation theory, brief interventions were designed to stimulate the capacities of individuals to self-evaluate, self-monitor, and self-regulate behaviors in order to induce change (Miller & Rollnick, 1991; Miller, Zweben,

DiClemente, & Rychtarik, 1992; Orford, 1985; Prochaska, & DiClemente, 1984; Zweben & Barrett, 1993; Zweben, Pearlman, & Li, 1988). The brief intervention model assumes that the processes of change are activated when the perceived benefits of drinking and drug use are outweighed by the perceived costs of maintaining the behaviors. The benefits of drug or alcohol use may entail enhancing pleasurable activities and improving coping capacities, while the costs may involve family, legal, and employment problems.

Individuals presumably are placed in a state of disequilibrium when the benefits of drinking or drug use can no longer be sustained without interfering with valued relationships or performance in areas of life functioning. If substance use is reduced or eliminated in favor of adaptive behaviors that yield benefits unavailable from substance use, then equilibrium is restored. For example, needs for companionship may be satisfied by spending weekends with one's spouse and children at a vacation cottage rather by drinking excessively with soccer "buddies."

Brief interventions are seen as a vehicle to direct or facilitate this naturally occurring process of change (Bien et al., 1993). The approach helps raise an individual's awareness of the problems created by substance misuse, which in turn helps to create or enhance the dissonance about it. The intervention provides an opportunity for individuals to consider whether feasible, acceptable alternatives exist to their current drug-abusing lifestyle. These decision-making activities involve affective and cognitive processes (Orford, 1985). For example, persons may variously decide to abstain from alcohol or drug use because of the pain and harm it has caused their family, because they have lost a job due to substance use, or because they are ashamed of their behavior.

A critical issue in brief interventions centers on whether individuals possess sufficient self-efficacy to make and implement decisions necessary to change their behavior. Self-efficacy refers to one's expectation that there are alternatives available to the current lifestyle and that one can reasonably implement the changes necessary to realize them (Bandura, 1977). Persons with high self-efficacy presumably will be more motivated to take the necessary actions to modify their drug-abusing lifestyle and believe that they possess the requisite skills and resources to make the required changes (Miller & Rollnick, 1991).

Another aspect of brief interventions is the emphasis it places on client choice with respect to planning and implementing behavior change goals. The process of problem resolution presumably is facilitated by seeking client input regarding how to change the problem behavior patterns (Rollnick, Heather, & Bell, 1992). This process typically involves a negotiation of differences between the therapist and client concerning matters such as planning activities that are incompatible with drinking or drug use and determining the role of the family or marital partner in resolving the problem. Successful negotiation of a treatment contract means that the client and therapist have reached an agreement about the nature of the problems and how they will be addressed (Zweben & Barrett, 1993).

Recently, attempts have been made to involve a significant other, such as a spouse, in the brief intervention (Sobell & Sobell, 1993; Zweben & Barrett, 1993). Having significant others involved in more conventional alcohol and drug treatments has been associated with better retention rates and with more favorable outcomes, particularly if positive ties existed between the clients and their partners prior to the start of treatment (Longabaugh, Beattie, Noel, Stout, & Malloy, 1993; Sisson & Azrin, 1986; Sobell & Sobell, 1993; Zweben, Pearlman, & Li, 1983). In the context of brief interventions, emphasis is placed on having the significant other be an active participant in treatment sessions, especially if the relationship with the client is largely positive. The partner can provide valuable input, feedback, and support while the client is attempting to change behavior patterns. In some cases, having the significant other involved in the sessions can help minimize negative effects that he or she may otherwise have on the behavior change process.

In summary, the aims of brief interventions are to (1) increase the person's awareness of the costs and consequences of substance use, (2) strengthen beliefs about his or her ability to change (i.e., enhancing self-efficacy), (3) utilize the natural helping system to support change, (4) encourage the person to accept responsibility for change, and (5) promote commitment to change.

## COMPONENTS OF BRIEF INTERVENTIONS

A basic approach to conducting brief interventions, developed by the National Institute on Alcohol Abuse and Alcoholism (NIAAA) Working Group on Screening and Brief Intervention, is presented in Figure 9.1. For illustrative purposes, the strategies are described for individuals with alcohol problems, but they are readily generalizable to other types of substance abuse. Brief intervention procedures typically include assessment and feedback, contracting and goal setting, behavior modification techniques, and self-directed bibliotherapy (Babor, 1990; Edwards et al., 1977; Fleming, 1995; Heather, 1995a; Miller & Sovereign, 1989; Sanchez-Craig, 1990). These methods are particularly applicable in general health care delivery settings where interventions for substance abuse must fit into the context of a busy, high-volume practice with multiple treatment and prevention goals. The techniques can be used effectively by numerous health care and mental health care providers, including prima-

**STEPS FOR ALCOHOL SCREENING AND BRIEF INTERVENTION**

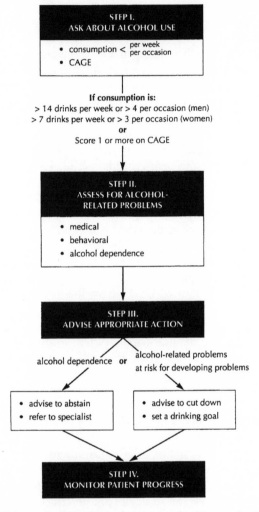

**FIGURE 9.1.** Schematic illustration of steps involved in conducting a brief intervention for alcohol problems (developed by the NIAAA Working Group on Screening and Brief Intervention).

ry care physicians, medical specialists, nurses and nurse practitioners, physicians' assistants, dentists, social workers, psychologists, and marriage and family therapists. Issues to consider in using brief interventions in settings that do and do not offer specialized treatment for alcohol and drug problems are discussed next, followed by a description of the intervention components.

## Applications in Nonspecialized Health Care Settings

Brief interventions are a "family" of interventions that can be utilized in a variety of health care and health promotion settings that are not affiliated with specialized substance abuse treatment programs (Heather, 1995a). In primary care settings, such as physician offices and hospital emergency departments, brief interventions have been employed opportunistically with individuals who have mild to moderate alcohol problems, as well as with smokers and overweight persons. Brief interventions also have become part of health promotion programs implemented by health care practitioners in primary care settings (Fleming, Barry, Manwell, Johnson, & London, 1997).

In such nonspecialized treatment settings, the components of the brief intervention typically consist of a 15–30 minute interview that involves a brief screening and assessment, feedback on personal risk, advice about how to change the problem behavior, a self-help pamphlet, and a referral for further counseling if warranted and desired (Anderson & Scott, 1992; Fleming et al., 1997; Heather, 1995a; National Institute on Alcohol Abuse and Alcoholism, 1995; Wallace, Cutler, & Haines, 1988). Booster sessions are sometimes offered (Fleming, 1997; Elvy, Wells, & Baird, 1988).

As applied to drinking problems, which are the most common form of substance abuse encountered in general medical practice, treatment goals are mostly geared toward cutting down on drinking rather than on abstaining completely. Feedback is aimed at increasing clients' awareness of the negative consequences of drinking (Fleming, 1997), which helps to change any misperceptions about the severity of their alcohol-related problems. Advice is focused on identifying actions aimed at changing the drinking pattern to reduce risk. This is followed by formulating goals about the drinking pattern (e.g., establishing stop points for daily and weekly consumption) and making plans for achieving them. Together, these strategies are aimed at mobilizing clients' motivation and coping resources in order to stimulate positive behavior change.

## Applications in Specialized Substance Abuse Treatment Programs

Brief interventions have been not been routinely incorporated into the menu of treatment options offered to individuals in the United States who present for alcohol or drug treatment services. Most studies of the utility of brief interventions in such specialized settings have been conducted outside of the United States in the United Kingdom and British Commonwealth countries (Chick, Ritson, Connaughton, Stewart, & Click, 1988; Orford &

Edwards, 1977; Zweben et al., 1988). In specialized settings, brief interventions have been employed as a stand-alone treatment (Chick et al., 1988; Drummond, Thom, Brown, Edwards, & Mullan, 1990; Edwards & Taylor, 1994; Zweben et al., 1988) or as an adjunct to conventional treatment (e.g., in methadone maintenance programs; Saunders, Wilkinson, & Phillips, 1995). Unlike primary health care practitioners, individuals who conduct the interventions in specialized settings are identified as "specialists" having expertise in treating alcohol and drug disorders.

Differences exist in the way brief interventions are delivered in specialized and nonspecialized treatment settings. Because persons with more serious substance-related problems typically seek help from specialized programs, the brief intervention usually is conducted over four to six sessions. This gives the practitioner sufficient opportunity to address motivational issues, thereby enabling clients to derive optimal benefits from the intervention. The assessment interview usually is more comprehensive (3 hours total in some cases) than the interview conducted in nonspecialized settings (Zweben et al., 1988; Orford & Edwards, 1977). The assessment interview is ordinarily conducted in separate sessions before the feedback and advice sessions. Information is obtained on a variety of life areas that may be affected by substance use (e.g., family relations, employment, and interpersonal matters), along with information on consumption patterns and related symptoms. The feedback and advice session (usually 90 minutes) also is more detailed and comprehensive. In accordance with the circumstances and status of clients, specialists typically are more interactive and exploratory compared to brief interventions delivered by providers in primary health care settings.

During the sessions, a great deal of attention is devoted to assessing and mobilizing clients' motivations and coping resources relevant to changing their drinking or drug use. Much emphasis is placed on facilitating their commitment to change and entails an examination of impediments to and incentives for change. Efforts are made to modify any misperceptions or misunderstandings about alcohol or drug use, to increase clients' awareness about the severity of their problems, and to help them express concerns about changing substance use practices. They also are asked to make a tentative commitment to change (e.g., "eliciting self-motivational statements"), which is a technique used throughout the intervention (Miller & Rollnick, 1991).

Despite variations in brief interventions across settings (e.g., in terms of intensity, goals, targeted groups, and intervention components), the basic orienting principles remain the same (Bien et al., 1993; Heather, 1995a). All versions place great emphasis on taking personal responsibility for change, client choice, increasing self-efficacy, and promoting optimism for change (Donovan et al., 1994; Zweben & Rose, in press).

## Implementation Steps

### Screening

The NIAAA physician guide recommends the use of the four (CAGE) questions (Ewing, 1984), which assess whether individuals (1) have tried to *cut down* on drinking, (2) others have been *annoyed* by their drinking, (3) they have felt *guilty* about drinking, or (4) they ever had an *eye-opener* in the morning, along with three questions concerned with drinking practices:

1. On average, how many days do you drink per week?
2. On a typical day when you drink, how many drinks do you have?
3. What is the maximum number of drinks you have had on a single occasion in the last month?

Cutoff limits for these questions are based on studies (National Institute on Alcohol Abuse and Alcoholism, 1995) that examined the relationship between levels of alcohol use and health problems. Women who consume more than seven drinks per week or three drinks per occasion and men who consume more than 14 drinks per week or four drinks per occasion, are considered a positive screen and should be further assessed.

### Assessment

Once a person has screened positive, practitioners need to assess for the presence of physical dependence, other medical and psychiatric problems, harmful drinking patterns, both with respect to the quantity and frequency of consumption and circumstances surrounding consumption, use of other mood altering drugs, and psychosocial problems in important areas of life functioning.

The assessment usually starts by asking clients whether their use of alcohol or drugs has caused any problems in their life. Practitioners may want to ask specifically about alcohol-related family, work, legal, social, and health problems, as well as any other medical and psychiatric problems. While most clients with alcohol use disorders (including at-risk users, problem drinkers, and dependent drinkers) have minimal health problems related to alcohol use, early identification may prevent future damage from drinking. Another area of assessment is to ask about symptoms of alcohol dependence, such as loss of control over drinking, tolerance, and withdrawal symptoms. Persons who show evidence of alcohol dependence should always be asked about suicidal ideation and symptoms of depression. If the problem is complex or serious, practitioners may want to refer a client to a substance use or mental health specialist for further assessment and possible intervention.

## Advice Giving

This is probably the key component of brief interventions. A simple, clear message from the provider expressing concern about the individual's drinking or other drug use can have a powerful effect on motivating the client to reduce consumption. The provider states concern about substance use, provides personalized feedback about how drinking or drug use affects health (e.g., disrupted sleeping patterns, family problems, headaches, injuries, and accidents), and advises the client about the need for change. Some clients will need to cut down on drinking, while others will need to abstain (e.g., for reasons related to health problems, pregnancy, use of prescription or illicit drugs, or symptoms of alcohol or drug dependence).

## Assessing Motivation for Change

Many clients are not ready or prepared to change their drinking or drug use. Therefore, it is important to assess their readiness for change, with a goal of placing them in one of five categories patterned after the transtheoretical stages of change model (e.g., Prochaska, DiClemente, & Norcross, 1992; see Chapter 6, this volume): (1) not interested in changing, (2) considering change, (3) ready for action, (4) initiating action, or (5) already acting. Such categories are useful for determining what kinds of steps need to be taken in relation to the substance use. For example, clients uninterested in changing may be asked to "think about" the consequences of drinking rather than to cut down. Those who are ready to change can set goals and make a plan of action, as discussed next.

## Establishing Drinking or Other Drug Use Goals

Providers can help clients establish reasonable substance use goals based on the (1) nature and severity of their problems, (2) life circumstances that may support or contraindicate one goal or another (e.g., being employed as a bus driver would suggest an abstinence goal), and (3) clients' personal and social resources (e.g., having a social network that supports moderation). Picking an unrealistic goal sets clients up to fail and may have countertherapeutic effects, including withdrawal from treatment. In this component, the provider negotiates a specific drinking or drug use goal, develops a written contract, and offers the client a self-help manual or other reading materials. Dates are scheduled for modifying the substance use pattern, and maximum amounts, or stop points, are negotiated. Clients are asked to sign the contract at the end of the session. A workbook is provided that includes homework exercises such as maintaining a diary of daily alcohol or drug use.

## Follow-Up Procedures

Providers can play a more significant role in supporting behavior change than previously appreciated by offering continued support and ongoing monitoring of clients' behavior. Strategies include follow-up phone calls by a member of the office staff to support a client's change effort. The phone call can be used to review the client's drinking and other goals, assess any problems, and offer further assistance as needed, such as additional office visits or phone calls. In addition to encouraging continued behavior change, return office visits may include a physical examination or laboratory testing when appropriate.

## Strategies for Dealing with Ambivalence

It is not unusual for clients to remain ambivalent about changing their substance use, and such ambivalence should be acknowledged and discussed as part of the intervention. With clients who remain ambivalent or uncertain about changing their alcohol or drug use, motivational counseling techniques can be applied, such as those described in the motivational enhancement therapy manual employed in Project MATCH (Miller, Zweben, DiClemente, & Rychtarik, 1992). These include strategies such as deploying discrepancy, delaying commitment to change, and eliciting self-motivational statements. For example, with regard to deploying discrepancy, the practitioner attempts to differentiate for clients "where they are" versus "where they say they want to be" to mobilize them to take the necessary actions to change. Involving a significant other in the behavior change effort is another option offered to clients to help facilitate the change process (Zweben, 1991).

Trials of abstinence or controlled substance use may help resolve ambivalence and help the clinician and client to identify appropriate behavior change strategies and goals (Miller & Page, 1991). If the client is unable to adhere to the plan or has difficulty doing so, a referral for specialized treatment, or at least evaluation for it, may be in order. Prior to the trial, the provider solicits the client's agreement that failure to adhere to the plan will indicate that such steps are necessary. The provider may negotiate for sources of verification about the client's compliance with the plan, preferably from family members, or may use blood, breath, or urine tests to check for substance use.

Encouraging involvement in the local recovering community of substance abusers is another resource that may help some, but not all, clients who are ambivalent about changing their behavior. In addition to the use of AA or other mutual-help groups, providers can identify individuals in their practice who have resolved their substance use problems and are

262 EXPANDING THE RANGE OF BEHAVIOR CHANGE INITIATIVES

willing to meet with ambivalent clients to help them understand risky substance use practices and to offer methods that they have found helpful.

## Strategies for Helping Dependent Drinkers

The style and format of sessions for dependent drinkers are similar to those for nondependent drinkers. However, due to their more severe problems, the content of the therapeutic communication needs to be different. First, the rationale for abstinence is clearly stated. The individual is advised that symptoms of alcohol dependence indicate that abstinence is the safest approach at this time. Detoxification procedures are reviewed if the individual is experiencing withdrawal. Since the prospect of entering more intensive alcohol treatment may be distressing, the client and his or her family members are given an opportunity to process the feedback. They may be asked to think about the recommendations and to come back in a few days to discuss any questions or concerns.

Once a dependent client is ready to change his or her substance use, several issues can be emphasized to facilitate referral to a specialized treatment program. It can be explained that substance abuse is a complex health problem with genetic, neurochemical, social, and behavioral components. The relationship between neurochemical changes and cravings, and loss of control over substance use can be discussed. Emphasis is placed on the idea that lack of control over use has nothing to do with weakness and that many individuals would like to stop but cannot do it on their own. Labels such as "alcoholic" and "addict" usually are avoided, as are arguments about the veracity of clients' self-reports of substance use and related events. Scare tactics and threats are avoided, such as comparing the client with individuals who have died from alcohol or drug misuse. Rather, the risks of alcohol or drug misuse are stated in an objective, neutral, and professional manner whenever feasible. Efforts are made to minimize the client's guilt and self-blame, and the stigma associated with substance abuse and its treatment, by framing the alcohol or drug problem as a health concern similar to other chronic medical problems such as hypertension or diabetes. If the client remains ambivalent about entering treatment, the motivational counseling techniques described earlier may be employed.

With dependent drinkers, the goal of brief interventions often is to motivate behavior change and to facilitate entry into a specialized treatment program. Brief interventions alone may not be sufficient to resolve these individuals' more complex problems. Depression, suicidal ideation, anxiety, sleep disorders, and relationship issues often are exacerbated in early abstinence and require closer monitoring than can be provided in the brief intervention format. Other medical concerns such as lipid problems, poor nutrition, risk of sexually transmitted diseases (including HIV), lack of exercise, cigarette use, and illicit drug use often are observed during the initial recovery period. Such individuals would likely benefit from a more intensive treatment that begins with medical detoxification and is followed by effective therapy for substance abuse, such as self-control and skills training as provided in cognitive-behavioral therapy. Other clients may require the help of an extensive support system such as an AA fellowship or a halfway house program. Pharmacotherapy (e.g., Antabuse, Rivia, Prozac, and desipramine) may be needed as an adjunct to behavior therapy for some clients.

For those requiring specialized help, a referral appointment usually is scheduled before the client leaves the office. Ideally, the referral will be made directly to the substance abuse specialist who will take over the client's care to increase communication and treatment planning. A client's decision to accept or reject a particular treatment is honored and, when a referral is rejected, it is essential that the sources of the rejection be discussed and, if appropriate, another referral be arranged. If treatment is rejected completely, the brief intervention may still be beneficial by laying a positive foundation for future action and treatment seeking. Overly coercive attempts to force treatment entry when clients are not ready may taint their perceptions of the treatment system and reduce their future use of it.

## Optimism Is Critical

Providers need to maintain a sense of optimism about the prospects for eventual problem resolution. Alcohol and drug problems are chronic, relapsing, and remitting problems. Some individuals are amenable to treatment and some are not and, even among those who are, stable behavior change often does not occur immediately or within the context of a single treatment episode. Changing addictive behavior patterns is a long-term process, and many persons with problems need to hear concerns from several people or experience further negative consequences before they see the need for and become committed to change (Miller & Rollnick, 1991). Expressions of concern may lead to problem resolution many months or years later.

The attitudes and beliefs of service providers can have a profound effect on their ability to identify and treat persons affected by substance use. Clinicians often feel helpless in dealing with these problems. Many have worked hard to help clients with alcohol and drug problems only to find that many of them do not improve. Teaching clinicians effective methods such as brief interventions empowers them to deal with substance-abusing clients and helps to change their attitudes and beliefs.

## STATE OF KNOWLEDGE ABOUT
## BRIEF INTERVENTIONS: WHAT WE DO
## AND DO NOT KNOW

### Brief Interventions for Nondependent Drinkers

The majority of the randomized clinical trials testing the efficacy of brief interventions have been conducted in primary care settings outside of the United States (reviewed by Bien et al., 1993; Kahan, Wilson, & Becker, 1995). Several trials are currently in progress in the United States and are expected to add to understanding of the potential role of brief interventions in the U.S. health care system (Fleming, Barry, Manwell, Johnson, & London, 1997). Major studies of brief interventions carried out in primary care settings in Europe and in North America are summarized in Table 9.1.

The sample size of the trials ranged from 1,661 in the World Health Organization (WHO) trial (Babor & Grant, 1992) to 47 in the Maheswaran, Beevers, and Gareth (1992) study. Women were included in most studies. The brief intervention procedures varied somewhat across studies, although most consisted of a single, brief, 5–20 minute counseling session with a variable number of booster sessions. Physicians were the primary service providers in many trials. Most studies limited follow-up to 12 months and attrition rates over the follow-up periods varied from 3% to 40%.

The majority of trials found reductions in alcohol use in both the intervention and control groups, with many observing significantly greater reductions in the brief intervention groups. Three trials that included men and women found reduced alcohol use in both genders following brief interventions (Babor & Grant, 1992; Fleming, Barry, Maxwell, Johnson, & London, 1997; Wallace, Cutler, & Haines, 1988), two trials found decreased utilization of other health services (Fleming, Barry, Manwell, Johnson, & London, 1996; Kristenson et al., 1983), and one trial found decreased mortality 5 years after treatment (Kristenson et al., 1983).

Overall, the available research suggests that brief interventions delivered in primary care settings promote reductions in drinking in both genders, may facilitate entry into specialized alcohol treatment programs (cf. Cooney et al., 1995), and reduce utilization of other health care services. More studies are needed, however, because of methodological limitations in many trials, including small sample sizes, modest follow-up rates, variations in the quality of clinician-delivered interventions, and lack of blinding of the control participants.

**TABLE 9.1. Brief Intervention Trials in Primary Care Settings**

| Authors | Location | Selection process | Sample size | Sample characteristics | Intervention protocol | Follow-up assessments | Results |
|---|---|---|---|---|---|---|---|
| | | | | European and Australian trials | | | |
| Anderson & Scott (1992) | 8 group medical practices in the Oxford, England, Regional Health Authority | Mailed and in-office questionnaires; selected if cosuming >350 g/week | BI = 80 C = 74 | Males aged 17–69 | BI: Physician advice for 10 minutes and self-help book C: No advice | 12-month follow-up; attrition: BI = 31%, C = 39% | BI group showed significant decreases in drinking compared to controls. |
| Chick et al. (1985) | Medical wards, Royal Edinburgh Hospital, Scotland | Consecutive admissions of ≥ 48 hours' duration | BI = 78 C = 78 | Males aged 18–65 | BI: Counseling with nurse up to 1 hour plus self-help booklet C: Nurse assessment only | 12-month follow-up; attrition: BI = 12%, C = 18% | BI group had reduced GGT levels. |
| Drummond et al. (1990) | Hospital alcohol clinic, United Kingdom | Consecutive patients seen in the clinic | BI 1 = 20 BI 2 = 20 | Male problem drinkers | BI 1: Counseling and advice with routine follow-up in alcohol clinic BI 2: Initial counseling and advice and return visit to physician | 6-month follow-up; attrition: 3% | Both groups reduced drinking and showed improved status. |
| Heather et al. (1987) (DRAMS project) | General practices, Scotland | In-office questionnaire; males selected if consuming > 35 drinks/week; females > 20 drinks/week | BI 1 = 34 BI 2 = 32 C = 38 | Males and females aged 18–65 | BI 1: DRAMS leaflet for general practitioner, medical record card, checklist of complications, drinking diary card, self-help booklet BI 2: Simple advice, no follow-up C: No intervention | 6-month follow-up; attrition: BI 1 = 15%, BI 2 = 6%, C = 16% | No significant group differences. All showed decreased drinking and improved well-being. |

(continued)

**TABLE 9.1.** (cont.)

| Authors | Location | Selection process | Sample size | Sample characteristics | Intervention protocol | Follow-up assessments | Results |
|---|---|---|---|---|---|---|---|
| | | | | *European and Australian trials (cont.)* | | | |
| Kristenson et al. (1983) | Community health centers, Malmö, Sweden | Screening invitation for cardiovascular disease, diabetes, and heavy drinking | BI = 317<br>C = 268 | Males aged 46–53 | BI: Physician consultation every 3 months, monthly GGT, and monthly contact with nurse<br>C: Informed of GGT results by letter, told to cut down, further liver tests in 2 years | 2-, 4-, and 5-year follow-ups; attrition not reported | GGT values reduced in both groups. Reduced sick days, hospital days, and mortality in BI group compared to control group. Alcohol use not measured. |
| Persson & Magnuson (1989) | Outpatient medical clinics, Sweden | Questionnaires and GGT levels; males selected if consuming > 200 g/week; females > 150 g/week; or GGT greater than 0.6 | BI = 36<br>C = 42 | Males and females aged 15–70 | BI: Doctor interview, monthly follow-up visit with nurse, quarterly visit with doctor, advice to cut down<br>C: Initial questionnaire only; no discussion about alcohol consumption and no blood sample at 12 months | 12-month follow-up; attrition = 0% | Drinking, triglycerides, GGT, and sick days decreased in BI group. Sick days increased in control group, but no follow-up alcohol data reported for controls. |
| Richmond et al. (1995) | 40 GP outpatient practices in Sydney, Australia | Questionnaires administered in physician offices; males > 35 drinks/week; females > 21 drinks/week | BI 1 = 96<br>BI 2 = 96<br>Assessment only = 93<br>C = 93 | Males and females in general medical settings | BI 1: 1–5 sessions<br>BI 2: 5 minutes of advice | 6- and 12-month follow-ups; attrition = 31% | No significant group differences. |

266

| Study | Setting | Screening method | N | Sample | Intervention | Follow-up/attrition | Results |
|---|---|---|---|---|---|---|---|
| Wallace et al. (1988) (MRC Trial) | Rural and small urban general practices, England | Mailed and in-office questionnaires; males selected if consuming > 35 drinks/week; females > 20 drinks/week | BI = 319 males, 131 females; C = 322 males, 137 females | Males and females aged 17–69 | BI: Physician assessment, booklet, told to cut down. C: No advice unless patient requested it or if there was impairment | 6- and 12-month follow-ups; attrition at 12 months: males = 19% females = 17% | At 6 and 12 months, both genders in BI group showed reduced drinking compared to controls. Male BI participants only had reduced GGT levels and lower blood pressure. |
| WHO (1996) | WHO 10-nation study; multiple settings | Interviews at ERs, hospitals, clinics, workplaces, and health screening agency; males selected if consuming > 350 g/week; females > 225 g/week | Males = 1260 Females = 299 | Cross-cultural sample | BI 1: Interview, 5-minute advice, pamphlet. BI 2: 5-minute advice, 15-minute counseling, self-help manual. C: 20-minute interview | Follow-ups varied from 6–19 months with average of 9 months; attrition: mean of 25%, varied by center | Significant reductions in alcohol use in both BI groups, which did not differ. |

### North American trials

| Study | Setting | Screening method | N | Sample | Intervention | Follow-up/attrition | Results |
|---|---|---|---|---|---|---|---|
| Buchsbaum (1994) | University of Virginia primary care clinic | Interviewed using the Diagnostic Interview Schedule | N = 110 | Adults who attended a university teaching hospital | BI: 15-minute counseling session with physician or nurse. C: Health booklet | 12-month follow-up; attrition = 40% | No group differences on any outcome measures. |
| Burge et al. (1997) | University-based primary care clinics, San Antonio, TX | Patients screened at regular appointments | BI 1 = 45 BI 2 = 23 BI 3 = 25 C = 53 | Males and females aged 18–65, primarily Mexican Americans | BI 1: Physician intervention with brochure and follow-up checklist. BI 2: Six 1-hour patient education sessions. BI 3: Physician intervention and patient education sessions (BI 1 and BI 2). C: Routine medical care | 12- and 18-month follow-ups; attrition = 30% | All groups improved; no group differences in drinking, GGT levels, and Addiction Severity Index variables. |

*(continued)*

**TABLE 9.1. (cont.)**

| Authors | Location | Selection process | Sample size | Sample characteristics | Intervention protocol | Follow-up assessments | Results |
|---|---|---|---|---|---|---|---|
| | | | | *North American trials (cont.)* | | | |
| Fleming et al., 1997 (Project TrEAT) | 64 primary care practices in 10 southern Wisconsin counties | In-office questionnaires; males selected if consuming > 15 drinks/week; females > 12 drinks/week, plus binge drinking, positive CAGE | BI = 392 C1 and C2 = 382 | Males and females aged 18–65 attending primary care clinics | BI: Two 15-minute physician visits, self-help pamphlet, drinking contract and diary cards, 2 nurse follow-up calls<br>C: General health booklet<br>C2: No health booklet, no intervention | 6- and 12-month follow-ups; attrition = 7% | Significant reduction in 7-day alcohol use, binge drinking, hospital days, in BI group compared to control groups. |
| Israel (1996) | Primary care practices, Toronto, Canada | TRAUMA screening instrument given to 15,686 patients | BI = 52 C = 53 | Adults aged 30–60 who attended family medicine clinics | BI: 20-minute counseling session with nurse educator every 2 months for 1 year, self-help pamphlet<br>C: Brief advice and self-help pamphlet | 12-month follow-up; attrition = 30% | Both groups showed reduced alcohol consumption but did not differ significantly. BI group showed a significant reduction in psychosocial problems, physician visits, and GGT levels. |
| Senft (1994) | Kaiser Permanente primary care clinics, Oregon | AUDIT given to patients receiving routine care | N = 220 | Adults who attended family medicine clinics | BI 1: 15-minute physician visit<br>BI 2: Multiple contacts with counselor<br>C: No treatment | 12-month follow-up; attrition = 31% | No group difference on any outcome measures. |

*Note.* BI, brief intervention group; C, control group (numbered if more than one BI or C group); 1 standard drink or unit = 12 grams of 190-proof ethanol; AA, Alcoholics Anonymous; AUDIT, Alcohol Use Disorders Identification Test; GGT, gamma-glutamyltransferase; DRAMS Project, Drinking Reasonably and Moderately with Self-Control Project; GP, general practice; MRC Trial, Medical Research Council Trial; TrEAT, Trial of Early Treatment; WHO, World Health Organization.

# Brief Interventions for Dependent Drinkers

Brief interventions appear to be as effective as more intensive alcoholism treatments for alcohol-dependent clients who seek help in specialized treatment settings. A meta-analysis of relevant studies found that brief interventions produced drinking outcomes that were similar to those observed following more intensive or conventional treatments (Bien et al., 1993). For example, several studies showed no differences in drinking outcomes between intensive treatment and a single session of brief advice (Chick et al., 1988; Orford & Edwards, 1977; Zweben et al., 1988). However, Chick et al. (1988) found that the more intensive treatment produced greater reductions in negative consequences of drinking (e.g., marital conflict), even though the brief and more extensive interventions resulted in similar abstinence rates.

The recent findings of Project MATCH also underscore the utility of brief interventions for alcohol-dependent clients who seek help. The Project MATCH brief intervention, termed motivational enhancement therapy (MET), included several motivational counseling techniques and was compared to two more intensive treatment modalities, cognitive-behavioral therapy (CBT) and 12-step facilitation (TSF) (Donovan et al., 1994). The 1-year outcome data from Project MATCH showed similar reductions in drinking and drinking-related problems across the three interventions, which suggest that MET could be used in lieu of more extensive outpatient treatments (Project MATCH Research Group, 1997). Importantly, despite differences in philosophy, theoretical orientation, and intensity, the three MATCH treatments had equivalent efficacy with participants who had more serious alcohol problems.

The Project MATCH findings are consistent with other brief intervention studies that included alcohol-dependent samples who sought treatment (Drummond et al., 1990; Edwards & Taylor, 1994; Zweben et al., 1988). In these studies, however, questions have been raised about the integrity of the brief interventions, the selection of therapists who provided the different treatments, and differences in sample characteristics (Bien et al., 1993; Heather, 1995b; Mattick & Jarvis, 1994). At issue is whether individuals in the brief intervention actually received more treatment than indicated, while those in the conventional intervention received less (Mattick & Jarvis, 1994). Another issue is whether the lack of differences between brief and more intensive interventions can be attributed to nonspecific factors such as the attributes of the therapist (e.g., empathy) rather than to the potency of the brief intervention modality. Despite these concerns, no convincing basis exists to refute the conclusions drawn by Bien et al. (1993) in their seminal review of brief interventions. They concluded that there is no evidence (1) that extensive treatments were superior to brief interventions across a broad range of individuals who sought help for alcohol problems, or (2) that brief interventions were more effective with individuals who had relatively less severe problems.

## Brief Interventions for Drug Problems

As indicated earlier, most clinical trials of brief interventions have been conducted using individuals with alcohol or tobacco problems (cf. Ockene et al., 1991). Studies of brief interventions with individuals who misuse illicit drugs have been marred by methodological deficiencies, such as not verifying client reports, lack of random assignment, short follow-up periods, and high attrition rates during the follow-ups (Alterman et al., 1996; Roffman, Stephens, & Simpson, 1989; Rosenblum et al., 1995; Saunders et al., 1995; Van Bilsen & Whitehead, 1994). These limitations make it difficult to interpret the inconsistent findings.

For example, Saunders et al. (1995) compared a brief motivational and an educational intervention with heroin users seen in a methadone clinic. Participants who received the brief intervention fared relatively better on measures of opiate-related problems, readiness to change, length of time in treatment, and time to first relapse. However, participants were only followed for 6 months and, by then, 40% had withdrawn from the study.

Alterman and colleagues (1994, 1996) conducted two studies that investigated the effectiveness of cocaine treatments that varied in intensity. The first study compared inpatient and outpatient treatment for cocaine dependence, and the second compared two outpatient treatments that involved either 6 or 12 hours of treatment per week. Neither study found significant differences between treatments, and clients tended to improve regardless of their treatment condition.

In contrast to these findings suggesting that brief interventions are equally or more effective than other treatments, Rosenblum et al. (1995) found that session attendance in an outpatient cocaine treatment program was inversely related to cocaine use, with clients who attended the most sessions showing the greatest reductions in use. However, this correlational study provides only weak evidence for a possible dose–response relationship between treatment intensity and outcomes. More convincing evidence comes from two studies by Baker et al. (Baker, Heather, Wodale, Dixon, & Holt, 1993; Baker, Kochan, Dixon, Heather, & Wodak, 1994), who evaluated three interventions aimed at reducing HIV risk-taking behaviors among intravenous drug users. Results showed that a more intensive cognitive-behavioral intervention provided certain benefits beyond what was observed in a brief intervention and in a usual methadone treatment condition. Individuals who received the cognitive-behavioral intervention evidenced relatively lower rates of needle risk-taking behaviors.

The inconsistent findings and methodological limitations of these studies preclude clear conclusions. Further evaluation of brief interventions are necessary before recommendations can be offered about their utility with drug abusers.

## UNRESOLVED ISSUES IN BRIEF INTERVENTIONS

### Number of Sessions

The length and number of sessions necessary to maximize favorable outcomes remain unclear. For example, Wallace et al. (1988) found a positive correlation between additional follow-up interventions and reductions in alcohol use. In a comparison of brief advice versus extended treatment of clients in an alcohol treatment clinic (Chick & Ritson, 1989), fewer alcohol-related problems were noted in the extended treatment group, but no group differences were found for alcohol use, liver function tests, or dependency symptoms.

Whereas these studies suggested a treatment dose–response effect, at least on some outcome measures, studies by Babor and Grant (1992), Romelsjo et al. (1989), and Zweben et al. (1988) did not find any added benefit of additional sessions beyond a single, brief intervention session. For example, Romelsjo et al. (1989) compared a single, brief advice session to a series of physician visits and found small, statistically insignificant reductions in gamma-glutamyltransferase (GGT) levels, alcohol use, and alcohol-related problems in the extended intervention group. Zweben et al. (1988) compared a single session of counseling advice to a series of eight conjoint therapy sessions with problem drinkers and their spouses. No group differences were found for drinking or other outcome measures.

The negative results of the latter studies are in sharp contrast with studies of brief advice for smoking cessation (e.g., Richmond & Heather, 1990; Richmond & Webster, 1985; Wilson, Wood, Johnston, & Sicurella, 1982), which reported much higher abstinence rates when follow-up booster sessions were combined with the initial brief intervention. Recent meta-analyses of the relevant smoking studies (Agency for Health Care Policy Research, 1996) found a clear dose–response effect between the number of interventions and the frequency of abstinence. The marked differences between the smoking and alcohol literatures may be related to the greater addictive properties of nicotine and to the higher prevalence of physical dependence in smokers compared to drinkers. Another explanation for the discrepant findings may be related to methodological weaknesses in the alcohol studies (Fleming, 1995; Gallant, 1988; Hore, 1988). Thus, the most effective length and number of brief intervention sessions has yet to be determined for treating alcohol problems.

## Population Differences

Another question of importance is whether different demographic groups respond differently to brief interventions. Sanchez-Craig (1990) studied the role of gender using male and female problem drinkers who received one of three interventions that consisted of (1) a two-page booklet and three counseling sessions with a health care provider; (2) a 40-page self-help booklet and three counseling sessions; or (3) six 1-hour sessions with a therapist. Participants in all groups reduced their heavy drinking days ($\geq$ 5 drinks/day) an average of 23 days over the 12-month follow-up period. Moreover, females had significantly greater reductions in drinking than did males (75% vs. 35%) in the two self-help intervention groups, but not in the therapist intervention group. Project TrEAT (Fleming et al., 1997; see Table 9.1) similarly found greater reductions in alcohol use in women than in men in both the intervention and control groups. These finding tentatively suggest that brief interventions may be especially beneficial for women problem drinkers and merit replication.

Studies with ethnic minority groups are generally lacking but warrant attention, since they may be less likely to access conventional substance abuse treatment programs. Their needs may be more widely served by offering brief interventions in nonspecialized settings. It also is unknown whether brief interventions are as effective with adolescents or older adults as they are with young and middle-aged adults, who are the main age groups that have been studied.

## Relative Effectiveness of Intervention Components

Studies that investigated the effectiveness of individual components of brief interventions have focused primarily on bibliotherapy. Several studies examined the effectiveness of bibliotherapy alone (Glascow & Rosen, 1978; Heather, Kissoon-Singh, & Fenton, 1990; Heather, Whitton, & Robertson, 1986; Miller & Taylor, 1980), which may involve mailing self-help booklets to individuals who respond to newspaper advertisements, random mailings to heads of households, or distributions in health care or community settings.

Heather et al. (1990) conducted a clinical trial with hazardous drinkers who were randomized into four groups: (1) no-intervention controls, (2) booklet only, (3) booklet plus unscheduled telephone support, and

(4) booklet plus scheduled telephone contact. The booklet (*So You Want to Cut Down on Your Drinking?: A Self Help Guide to Sensible Drinking*) (Heather et al., 1990) was a modification of one developed for the DRAMS project (Heather, Campion, Neville, & MacCabe, 1987; see Table 9.1) and focused on methods to reduce drinking. At the 6-month follow-up, there was a 10% reduction in the number of hazardous drinkers in the control group and a 35% reduction in the three treatment groups combined, which did not differ significantly. Thus, the addition of telephone contacts did not increase the effectiveness of bibliotherapy. This study replicated previous research by Harris and Miller (1990) and suggests that bibliotherapy alone can be an effective brief intervention for heavy drinkers who are not dependent. However, because these studies followed clients for only 3–12 months, the long-term effects of bibliotherapy remain unknown.

The relative contributions to the effectiveness of brief interventions of other motivational counseling components, such as advice, feedback, deploying discrepancy, delaying compliance, and immunization, also remain unclear (Miller et al., 1992). And is it necessary to employ the full array of these strategies in order to obtain positive outcomes? A recently funded study by the NIAAA will answer these questions concerning the incremental effectiveness of adding individual motivational counseling components to brief interventions (Maisto, 1994).

## Significant Other Involvement

Several studies of brief interventions with problem drinkers (Chick, Lloyd, & Crombie, 1985; Edwards et al., 1977; Zweben et al., 1988) involved the nondrinking partner in the sessions with positive results. Zweben et al. (1988), for instance, found that 60% of their problem drinker participants demonstrated significant improvements in the brief treatment condition; similar outcomes were found in an extended treatment condition, which also involved the nondrinking partner. These data, along with clinical observation, suggest that having the significant other (SO) actively involved in the brief intervention helps enhance the client's motivation. However, none of these studies were designed to test explicitly the relative contribution of SO involvement to treatment outcomes, and it is unknown whether similar results would be obtained if the nondrinking partner were absent from the sessions (Zweben & Barrett, 1993).

## Summary

Areas that need further investigation include examining (1) optimal length and number of brief advice sessions; (2) gender, age, and other population differences; (3) relative contributions of key components of brief interventions, such as the use of verbal and written contracts, completion of weekly self-monitoring forms, and advice alone versus advice and motivational counseling; (4) hospital-based intervention and referral programs; and (5) the utility of SO involvement in treatment. Also, while many studies demonstrated efficacy during the first year posttreatment, little is known about the long-term impact of brief interventions on substance use and other health-related outcome measures. For example, does the treatment help reduce health care utilization and costs, and improve health status through a reduction in substance-related health problems (e.g., liver disease, injuries, HIV)? Are there characteristics of providers that can be linked to intervention success? Can brief interventions be used effectively with dependent and nondependent drug users? Answers to these questions await further research.

# A SYSTEMS PERSPECTIVE ON INTEGRATING BRIEF INTERVENTIONS INTO NONSPECIALIZED TREATMENT SETTINGS: PRIMARY HEALTH CARE AS AN EXAMPLE

Screening procedures and brief intervention programs should be expanded in primary care settings for several reasons. They can be applied to communities and populations with minimal resources and can be implemented by numerous doctoral and subdoctoral health care professionals as part of routine clinical care. Since the main focus of brief intervention programs is on nondependent alcohol abusers, the potential exists to decrease significantly alcohol use and associated problems in the 20% or more of the U.S. adult population who are at risk for, or who are experiencing, alcohol-related problems but are not reached by conventional treatment programs. Brief interventions are inexpensive, much less costly than a single emergency department visit for an alcohol-related injury.

The implementation of screening and brief intervention protocols needs to be approached as a systems issue. Health care settings are complex systems with multiple, competing agendas. Funding brief interventions depends on convincing employers, governmental agencies, insurance companies, and MCOs that the prevention and treatment of substance abuse will improve the health of their population and will reduce health care and social costs. Ongoing U.S. clinical trials should provide the empirical foundation needed to support the widespread application of the technology in the U.S. health care system.

Primary care settings should incorporate screening and brief interventions for substance abuse into the wide range of clinical and prevention services that they routinely offer. Strategies could include the use of self-administered screening tests such as the AUDIT (Saunders, Aasland, Babor, de la Fuenta, & Grant, 1993), including questions about alcohol or drug use as part of routine vital signs, or setting up computerized reminder systems to cue clinicians to screen clients for alcohol and drug problems. Reminders can be attached to the front of clients' medical records or in another prominent location, and clinical protocols such as the one illustrated in Figure 9.1 can be displayed in clinical care areas. Self-help booklets, alcohol diary cards, lists of AA and other mutual-help group meetings, and referral information with phone numbers and names of local substance abuse specialists can assist clinicians and clients in establishing referral plans and strategies.

Providers require skills training workshops and incentives to make brief interventions for alcohol, tobacco, and related problems an essential clinical activity. The NIAAA has supported the development of a number of skills training curricula that have been shown to increase the clinical skills of providers (Murray & Fleming, 1996). Incentives include financial reimbursement for this clinical activity, paid education time to attend training workshops, and quality improvement peer review programs.

Currently, it is often difficult, however, for providers to receive compensation for providing alcohol and drug abuse screenings and brief interventions. Behavioral health contracts in MCOs tend to carve out substance abuse and mental health services to specialized providers and are an impediment to general medical providers and therapists receiving compensation for routine screenings for substance abuse and for conducting brief interventions. Yet these health professionals are more likely than specialized treatment programs to come into contact with individuals with mild to moderate problems. Quality improvement programs are now being implemented throughout the health care system and provide an opportunity to change provider practice behavior and reimbursement policies. The establishment of monitoring systems to examine rates of alcohol screening in persons being treated for hypertension, depression, or anxiety disorders could exert positive effects on practice patterns.

Another issue in a systems perspective concerns the need to better coordinate specialized substance abuse treatment with general medical care. Substance abuse treatment programs have long been segregated outside the medical care system, often in freestanding, community-based programs. Lack of communication between these specialized treatment programs and clients' health care providers can have negative effects on clients' potential for long-term sobriety. In contrast to referrals for medical specialty services (e.g., to surgical practices), alcohol and drug programs do not routinely send copies of assessments, treatment plans, or discharge summaries to referring providers, or call them to develop and coordinate long-term plans of care. Referring providers could aid communication by sending referral letters to the alcohol and drug specialists.

One way to facilitate an integrated treatment process and increase communication between providers is to locate alcohol and drug treatment programs in close physical proximity to general medical care facilities and to "carve-in," rather than to "carve-out," behavioral health care. Providers are more likely to refer clients to a trusted colleague whose office is located down the hall than to a stranger located many miles away in a different system of care. Clients also will find it easier to accept and follow through with referrals. Confidentiality concerns about sharing information between health care and substance abuse treatment providers can be handled through informed consent procedures that ask clients to release relevant information. Ideally, health care providers and substance abuse specialists should be part of the same interdisciplinary treatment team to provide clients with coordinated, comprehensive care.

## CONCLUSIONS

Clinicians from many professions increasingly must address the needs of persons with alcohol and drug problems of varying severity. At the same time, clinicians are encouraged to utilize cost-effective methods to treat these problems. Employing extensive, conventional treatment is inconsistent with the latter goal and with the related principle of "parsimony," which guides practitioners to use the least intensive but effective treatment for a given health or behavioral problem. Brief interventions represent a valuable clinical resource that can enable practitioners to treat persons with alcohol and drug problems of mild to moderate severity. The approach also may help reduce health care utilization and costs associated with substance misuse, and has wide potential applicability in managed health care systems, where individuals with substance use problems are increasingly seen.

Brief interventions can be used in specialized and nonspecialized settings in a number of ways. In nonspecialized settings, they have been successfully incorporated into health promotion programs for alcohol, tobacco, and other addictive behaviors. They also have been used to facilitate referrals in non-health-care settings (e.g., by child protection agencies), particularly with individuals who have more severe problems. Although less common, brief interventions can be included in the menu of treatment options offered in specialized treatment settings and used as needed with other procedures (e.g., methadone maintenance) to help individuals derive the maximum benefits of treatment. Finally, brief interventions may serve as a treatment of "last resort" for individuals who may be suitable for extensive treatments but who, for a variety of reasons, reject them (Heather, 1995b).

Findings to date strongly support the use and further evaluation of brief interventions in specialized and nonspecialized health care settings. A major challenge is to devise methods to facilitate their incorporation into routine health care that is increasingly governed by the managed care movement.

## REFERENCES

Agency for Health Care Policy Research. (1996). *Smoking cessation: Clinical practice guidelines* (No .18) (U.S. DHHS Publication No. 96-0692). Washington, DC: U.S. Government Printing Office.

Alterman, A., Snider, E., Caccioia, J., May, D., Parikh, G., Maany, I., & Rosenbaum, P. (1996). A quasi-experimental comparison of the effectiveness of 6-versus 12-hour per week outpatient treatments for cocaine dependence. *Journal of Nervous and Mental Disease, 184,* 54–56.

Alterman, A. I., O'Brien, C. P., McLellan, A. T., August, D. A., Snider, E. C., Drobra, M., Corrish, J. W., Hall, C. P., Raphaelson, A. H., & Schrode, F. X. (1994). Effectiveness and costs of inpatient versus day hospital cocaine rehabilitation. *Journal of Nervous and Mental Disease, 182*(3), 157–163.

Anderson, P., & Scott, E. (1992). The effect of general practitioners' advice to heavy drinking men. *British Medical Journal, 87,* 891–900.

Babor, T. (1990). Brief intervention strategies for harmful drinkers: New directions for medical education. *Canadian Medical Association Journal, 143,* 1070–1074.

Babor, T., & Grant, M. (Eds.). (1992). *Project on identification and management of alcohol-related problems, report on phase II: A randomized clinical trial of brief interventions in primary health care.* Geneva, Switzerland: World Health Organization.

Baker, A., Heather, N., Wodak, A., Dixon, J., & Holt, P. (1993). Evaluation of a cognitive-behavioral intervention for HIV prevention among injecting drug users. *AIDS, 7,* 247–256.

Baker, A., Kochan, J., Dixon, N., Heather, N., & Wodak, A. (1994). Controlled evaluation of a brief intervention for HIV prevention among injecting drug users not in treatment. *AIDS Care, 6,* 559–570.

Bandura, A. (1977). Self-efficacy: Toward a unifying theory of behavioral change. *Psychological Review, 84,* 191–215.

Bien, T. H., Miller, W. R., & Tonigan, J. S. (1993). Brief interventions for alcohol problems: A review. *Addiction, 88,* 315–336.

Buchsbaum, D. G. (1994, January). *A brief intervention trial in a primary care sample of dependent drinkers.* Paper presented at the NIAAA Working Group on Screening and Brief Intervention, Rockville, MD.

Burge, S. K., Amodei, N., Elkin, B., Catala, S., Andrew, S. R., Lane, P. A., & Seale, J. P. (1997). An evaluation of two primary care interventions for alcohol abuse among Mexican-American patients. *Addiction, 92*(12), 1705–1716.

Chick, J., Lloyd, G., & Crombie, E. (1985). Counseling problem drinkers in medical wards: A controlled study. *British Medical Journal, 290,* 965–967.

Chick, J., & Ritson, E. (1989). Alcoholism: Advice versus extended treatment. *British Journal of Addiction, 84,* 817–819.

Chick, J., Ritson, B., Connaughton, J., Stewart, A., Chick, J. (1988). Advice versus extended treatment for alcoholism: A controlled study. *British Journal of Addiction, 83*(2), 159–170.

Cooney, N. L., Zweben, A., & Fleming, M. F. (1995). Screening for alcohol problems and at-risk drinking in healthcare settings. In R. K. Hester & W. R. Miller (Eds.), *Handbook of alcoholism treatment approaches* (2nd ed., pp. 45–60). Boston: Allyn & Bacon.

Donovan, D. M., Kadden, R. M., DiClemente, C. C., Carroll, K. M., Longabaugh, R. H., Zweben, A., & Rychtarik, R. (1994). Issues in selection and development of therapies in alcoholism treatment matching research. *Journal of Studies on Alcohol* (Suppl. 12), 101–111.

Drummond, D. C., Thom, B., Brown, C., Edwards, G., & Mullan, M. J. (1990). Specialist versus general practitioner treatment of problem drinkers. *Lancet, 336,* 915–918.

Edwards, G., Orford, J., Egert, S., Guthrie, S., Hawker, A., Hensmen, C., Mitcheson, M., Oppenheimer, E., & Taylor, C. (1977). Alcoholism: A controlled trial of "treatment" and "advice." *Journal of Studies on Alcohol, 38,* 1004–1031.

Edwards, G., & Taylor, C. (1994). A test of the        matching hypothesis: Alcohol dependence, intensity of treatment and 12 month outcome. *Addiction, 89,* 553–561.

Elvy, G. A., Wells, J. E., & Baird, K. A. (1988). Attempted referral as intervention for problem drinking in the general hospital. *British Journal of Addiction, 83,* 83–89.

Ewing, J. A. (1984). Detecting alcoholism. The CAGE questionnaire. *Journal of the American Medical Association, 252,* 1905–1907.

Fleming, M. F. (1995, November). *What we know and what we don't about brief intervention treatment.* Paper presented at the annual meeting of Addiction Medicine Research on Substance Abuse, Association for Medical Education and Research in Substance Abuse (AMERSA), Washington, DC.

Fleming, M. F., Barry, K. L., Manwell, L. B., Johnson, K., & London, R. (1997). A trial of early alcohol treatment (Project TrEAT): A randomized trial of brief physician advice in community-based primary care practices. *Journal of American Medical Association, 277,* 1039–1045.

Gallant, D. (1988). A controlled study of advice versus extended treatment [Editorial]. *Alcoholism: Clinical and Experimental Research, 12,* 725–726.

Glascow, R., & Rosen, G. (1978). Behavioral bibliotherapy: A review of self-help behavior therapy behaviors manual. *Psychological Bulletin, 85,* 1–23.

Harris, K. B., & Miller, W. R. (1990). Behavioral self-control training for problem drinkers: Components of efficacy. *Psychology of Addictive Behaviors, 4,* 82–90.

Heather, N. (1995a). Brief intervention strategies. In R. H. Hester & W. R. Miller (Eds.), *Handbook of alcoholism treatment approaches: Effective alternatives* (pp. 105–122). Needham Heights, MA: Allyn & Bacon.

Heather, N. (1995b). Interpreting the evidence on brief intervention: The need for caution. *Alcohol and Alcoholism, 30,* 287–296.

Heather, N., Campion, P. D., Neville, R. G., & MacCabe, D. (1987). Evaluation of a controlled drinking minimal intervention for problem drinkers in general practice (the DRAMS Scheme). *Journal of Royal College General Practitioners, 37*(301), 358–363.

Heather, N., Kissoon-Singh, J., & Fenton, G. (1990). Assisted natural recovery from alcohol problems: Effects of a self-help manual with and without supplementary telephone contact. *British Journal of Addiction, 85*, 1177–1185.

Heather, N., Whitton, B., & Robertson, I. (1986). Evaluation of a self-help manual for media-recruited problem drinkers: Six-month follow-up results. *British Journal of Clinical Psychology, 25*, 19–34.

Higgins-Biddle, J., & Babor, T. F. (1996). *Reducing risky drinking: A report on early identification and management of alcohol problems through screening and brief intervention.* Unpublished manuscript.

Hore, B. (1988). Advice versus extended treatment for alcoholism [Letter to the Editor]. *British Journal of Addiction, 83*, 969.

Institute of Medicine, National Academy of Sciences. (1990). *Broadening the base of treatment for alcohol problems.* Washington, DC: National Academy Press.

Israel, Y., Hollander, O., Sanchez-Craig, Booker, S., Miller, V., Gingrich, R., & Rankin, J. (1996). Screening for problem drinking and counseling by the primary care physician–nurse team. *Alcoholism: Clinical and Experimental Research, 20*, 1443–1450.

Kahan, M., Wilson, L., & Becker, L. (1995). Effectiveness of physician based interventions with problem drinkers: A review. *Canadian Medical Journal, 152*, 851–857.

Kristenson, H., Ohlin, H., Hulten-Nosslin, M., Hood, B., & Trell, E. (1983). Identification and intervention of heavy drinking middle aged men: Results and follow-up of 24–60 months on long-term studies with randomized centers. *Alcoholism: Clinical and Experimental Research, 7*, 203–209.

Longabaugh, R., Beattie, M., Noel, N., Stout, R., & Malloy, P. (1993). The effect of social investment on treatment outcome. *Journal of Studies on Alcohol, 54*, 465–478.

Maheswaran, R., Beevers, M., & Gareth, D. (1992). Effectiveness of advice to reduce alcohol consumption in hypertensive patients. *Hypertension, 19*, 79–84.

Maisto, S. A. (1994). *Education for Lifestyle Modification (ELM study).* Rockville, MD: National Institute on Alcohol Abuse and Alcoholism (Funded grant proposal).

Marlatt, G. A., Larimer, M. E., Baer, J. S., & Quigley, L. A. (1993). Harm reduction for alcohol problems: Moving beyond the controlled drinking controversy. *Behavior Therapy, 24*, 461–504.

Mattick, R. P., & Jarvis, T. (1994). Brief or minimal intervention for "alcoholics"? The evidence suggests otherwise. *Drug and Alcohol Review, 13*, 137–144.

Miller, W. R., Brown, J. M., Simpson, T. L., Handmaker, N. S., Bien, T. H., Luckie, L. F., Montgomery, H. A., Hester, R. K., & Tonigan, J. S. (1995). What works?: A methodological analysis of the alcohol treatment literature. In R. K. Hester & W. R. Miller (Eds.), *Handbook of alcoholism treatment approaches* (2nd ed., pp. 12–44). Boston: Allyn & Bacon.

Miller, W. R., & Page, A. C. (1991). Warm turkey: Other routes to abstinence. *Journal of Substance Abuse Treatment, 8*, 227–232.

Miller, W. R., & Rollnick, S. (1991). *Motivational interviewing: Preparing people to change addictive behavior.* New York: Guilford Press.

Miller, W. R., & Sovereign, R. (1989). The check-up: A model for early intervention in addictive behaviors. In T. Loberg, W. R. Miller, P. Nathan, & G. A. Marlatt (Eds.), *Addictive behaviors: Prevention and early intervention* (pp. 219–231). Amsterdam: Swets & Zeitlinger.

Miller, W. R., & Taylor, C. A. (1980). Relative effectiveness of bibliotherapy, individual and group self-control training in the treatment of problem drinkers. *Addictive Behaviors, 5,* 13–24.

Miller, W. R., Zweben, A., DiClemente, C. C., & Rychtarik, R. G. (1992). *Motivational enhancement therapy (MET): A clinical research guide for therapists treating individuals with alcohol abuse and dependence* (DHHS Publication No. ADM 92-1894). Washington, DC: U.S. Government Printing Office.

Murray, P., & Fleming, M. F. (1996). Prevention and treatment of alcohol-related problems: An international medical education model. *Academic Medicine, 71*(11), 1204–1210.

National Institute on Alcohol Abuse and Alcoholism. (1995). *The physicians' guide to helping patients with alcohol problems* (NIH Publication No. 95-3769, National Institute on Alcohol Abuse and Alcoholism, National Institutes of Health). Washington, DC: U.S. Government Printing Office.

Ockene, J. K., Kristeller, J., Goldberg, R., Amick, T. L., Pekow, L., Hosmer, P. S., Quirk, M., & Kalan, K. (1991). Increasing the efficacy of physician-delivered smoking interventions: A randomized clinical trial. *Journal of General Internal Medicine, 6,* 1–8.

Orford, J. (1985). *Excessive appetites: A psychological view of addictions.* New York: Wiley.

Orford, J., & Edwards, G. (1977). *Alcoholism: A comparison of treatment and advice, with a study of the influence of marriage* (Institute of Psychiatry, Maudsley Monograph No. 26). New York: Oxford University Press.

Persson, J., Magnusson, P. H. (1989). Early intervention in patients with excessive consumption of alcohol: A controlled study. *Alcohol, 6,* 403–408.

Prochaska, J. O., & DiClemente, C. C. (1984). *The transtheoretical approach: Crossing traditional boundaries of therapy.* Homewood, IL: Dow Jones-Irwin.

Prochaska, J. O., DiClemente, C. C., & Norcross, J. C. (192). In search of how people change: Applications to addictive behaviors. *American Psychologist, 47,* 1102–1114.

Project MATCH Research Group. (1997). Matching alcoholism treatments to client heterogeneity: Project MATCH posttreatment during outcomes. *Journal of Studies on Alcohol, 58*(1), 7–29.

Richmond, R., & Heather, N. (1990). General practitioners intervention for smoking cessation: Past results and future prospects. *Behavioral Change, 7,* 110–119.

Richmond, R., Heather, N., Wodak, A., Kehoe, L., & Webster, I. (1995). Controlled evaluation of a general practice-based brief intervention for excessive drinking. *Addiction, 90,* 119–132.

Richmond, R., & Webster, I. (1985). Evaluation of general practitioners use of smoking intervention program. *International Journal of Epidemiology, 14,* 396–401.

Roffman, R. A., Stephens, R. S., & Simpson, E. (1989). Relapse prevention with adult chronic marijuana smokers. In D. C. Daley (Ed.), *Relapse: Conceptual, research and clinical perspectives* (pp. 241–257). Binghamton, NY: Haworth Press.

Rollnick, S., Heather, N., & Bell, A. (1992). Negotiating behavior change in medical settings: The development of brief motivational interviewing. *Journal of Mental Health, 1,* 25–37.

Romelsjo, A., Anderson L., Barrner, H., Borg, S., Granstand, C., Hultman, O., Hassler, A., Kallqvist, A., Magnusson, P., Morgell, R., Nyman, K., Olofsson, A., Olsson, E., Rhedin, A., & Wikblad, W. (1989). A randomized study of secondary prevention of early stage problem drinkers in primary health care. *British Journal of Addiction, 84,* 1319–1327.

Rose, S., Zweben, A., & Stoffel, G. (in press). Interface between substance abuse treatment and other health and social systems. In B. McCrady & E. Epstein (Eds,), *Addiction: A comprehensive guidebook for practitioners.* New York: Guilford Press.

Rosenblum, A., Magura, S., Foote, J., Palij, M., Handelsman, L., Lovejoy, M., & Stimmel, B. (1995). Treatment intensity and reduction in drug use for cocaine-dependent methadone patients: A dose–response relationship. *Journal of Psychoactive Drugs, 27,* 151–159.

Sanchez-Craig, M. (1990). Brief didactic treatment for alcohol and drug-related problems: An approach based on client choice. *British Journal of Addiction, 85,* 169–170.

Saunders, B., Wilkinson, C., & Phillips, M. (1995). The impact of a brief motivational intervention with opiate users attending a methadone program. *Addiction, 90,* 415–424.

Saunders, J., Aasland, O., Babor, T., de la Fuenta, J., & Grant, M. (1993). WHO collaborative project on early detection of persons with harmful alcohol consumption: II. Development of the screening instrument "AUDIT." *British Journal of Addiction, 88,* 349–362.

Senft, R. (1994, March). *Brief intervention in an HMO.* Paper presented at the National Institute of Alcohol Abuse and Alcoholism Research Symposium, Rockville, MD.

Single, E. (1995). Defining harm reduction. *Drug and Alcohol Review, 14,* 287–290.

Sisson, R. W., & Azrin, N. H. (1986). Family-member involvement to initiate and promote treatment of problem drinkers. *Journal of Behavior Therapy and Experimental Psychiatry, 17,* 15–21.

Skinner, H. A., & Allen, B. S. (1982). Alcohol dependence syndrome: Measurement and validation. *Journal of Abnormal Psychology, 91,* 199–209.

Sobell, M. B., & Sobell, L. C. (1993). *Problem drinking: Guided self-change treatment.* New York: Guilford Press.

Van Bilsen, H., & Whitehead, B. (1994). Learning controlled drugs use: A case study. *Behavioral and Cognitive Psychotherapy, 22,* 87–95.

Wallace, P., Cutler, S., & Haines, A. (1988). Randomized controlled trial of general practitioner intervention in clients with excessive alcohol consumption. *British Medical Journal, 297,* 663–668.

Wilson, D., Wood, G., Johnston, N., & Sicurella, J. (1982). Randomized clinical trial of supportive follow-up for cigarette smoking in a family practice. *Canadian Medical Association Journal, 126,* 127–129.

World Health Organization Brief Intervention Study Group. (1996). A cross-national trial of brief interventions with heavy drinkers. *American Journal of Public Health, 86*(7), 948–955.

Zweben, A. (1991). Motivational counseling with alcoholic couples. In W. R. Miller & S. Rollnick, *Motivational interviewing: Preparing people to change addictive behavior* (pp. 225–235). New York: Guilford Press.

Zweben, A., & Barrett, D. (1993). Brief couples treatment for alcohol problems. In T. J. O'Farrell (Ed.), *Treating alcohol problems: Marital and family interventions* (pp. 353–380). New York: Guilford Press.

Zweben, A., & Barrett, D. (1997). Facilitating compliance in alcoholism treatment. In B. Blackwell (Ed.), *Treatment compliance and the therapeutic alliance* (pp. 277–293). New York: Gordon & Breach.

Zweben, A., & Cisler, R. (1996). Composite outcome measures in alcoholism treatment research: Problems and potentialities. *Substance Use and Misuse, 31,* 1783–1805.

Zweben, A., Pearlman, S., & Li, S. (1983). Reducing attrition from conjoint therapy with alcoholic couples. *Drug and Alcohol Dependence, 11,* 321–331.

Zweben, A., Pearlman, S., & Li, S. (1988). A comparison of brief advice and conjoint therapy in the treatment of alcohol abuse: The results of the marital system study. *British Journal of Addiction, 83,* 899–916.

Zweben, A., & Rose, S. J. (1998). Innovations in treating alcohol problems. In C. D. Biegel & A. Blum (Eds.), *Innovations in practice and service delivery* (pp. 197–217). New York: Oxford University Press.

# 10

## Potential Contributions of the Community Reinforcement Approach and Contingency Management to Broadening the Base of Substance Abuse Treatment

### STEPHEN T. HIGGINS

The purpose of this chapter is to discuss some potential contributions of the community reinforcement approach (CRA) and contingency management to broadening the base for substance abuse treatment. In so doing, I describe the conceptual foundations of CRA and results of clinical trials supporting its efficacy in treating alcohol dependence. More recently, CRA was combined with contingency-management procedures to treat cocaine and, to a more limited extent, opioid dependence. Those innovations and the results of clinical trials supporting their efficacy are described as well. Last, I suggest some additional ways that CRA and contingency-management interventions might be used to increase treatment utilization in clinic settings and extend services to other settings and populations.

## CONCEPTUAL FRAMEWORK

CRA was developed within the conceptual framework of behavior analysis. Within that framework, drug use and abuse are considered operant behavior that is maintained, in part, by the reinforcing effects of the drugs involved (Goldberg & Stolerman, 1986). The reliable empirical observation that abused drugs function as reinforcers in humans and laboratory animals provides sound scientific support for that position (Henningfield, Lukas, & Bigelow, 1986). Psychomotor stimulants, ethanol, opioids, nicotine, and sedatives serve as reinforcers and are voluntarily self-administered by a variety of species (Young & Herling, 1986). Neither a prior history of drug exposure nor physical dependence is necessary for these drugs to support ongoing and stable patterns of voluntary drug use in otherwise normal laboratory animals. Commonalities do not end there. Effects of alterations in drug availability, drug dose, schedule of reinforcement, and other environmental manipulations on drug use are orderly and have generality across different species and types of drug abuse (Griffiths et al., 1980; Henningfield et al., 1986; Higgins, 1997). These commonalities support a theoretical position that reinforcement is a fundamental determinant of drug use and abuse.

Within this conceptual framework, drug use is considered a normal, learned behavior that falls along a continuum ranging from patterns of little use and few problems to excessive use and many untoward effects, including death. The same processes and principles of learning are assumed to operate across the continuum. All physically intact humans are assumed to possess the necessary neurobiological systems to experience drug-produced reinforcement and hence to develop patterns of drug use, abuse, and dependence. Said differently, individuals need not have any exceptional or pathological characteristics in order to develop drug abuse or dependence. No doubt, genetic or acquired characteristics (e.g., family history of alcohol dependence, other psychiatric disorders) affect the probability of developing drug abuse or dependence, but they are not necessary conditions for the problems to emerge.

If we are all biologically capable of operating at any point along this continuum with regard to drug use, then what factors regulate one's position on it? Here is where the influence of social or community factors becomes very important. First, drug availability and the social acceptability of drug use are important factors. No matter how biologically or psychologically prepared one is to develop drug abuse or dependence, if drugs are unavailable, then the problems will not emerge. Unfortunately, abused drugs are readily available in most segments of our society and use of licit drugs such as tobacco and alcohol is widely accepted. To get a glimpse of the impact of availability and acceptability on drug use, consider the differences in the prevalence of licit and illicit drug use in the United States. For example, based on 1994 figures, approximately 59.9 million members of U.S. households aged 12 or older reported current use (i.e., past month) of cigarettes, and approximately 112.8 million reported current use of alcohol (Substance Abuse and Mental Health Services Administration,

1995). Comparable figures for cocaine and heroin were 1.3 and 0.2 million, respectively, and 12.5 million for any illicit drug including marijuana, cocaine, heroin, hallucinogens, inhalants, and nonmedical use of therapeutics. Consider also estimates that more than 400,000 people in the United States die annually from smoking-related causes, and more than 100,000 from alcohol-related causes, while comparable numbers for cocaine and heroin abuse combined are estimated to be less than 10,000 (Centers for Disease Control and Prevention, 1993; Crowley, 1988; Substance Abuse and Mental Health Services Administration, 1996). There is little doubt that the wider availability and social acceptability of licit drug use are important determinants of the higher prevalence rates and attendant problems associated with them.

Recent scientific advances in the study of drug use and other forms of reinforced responding have conceptualized them in terms of consumer–demand theory (see Chapter 7, this volume; Bickel & DeGrandpre, 1996; Bickel, DeGrandpre, & Higgins, 1993; Higgins, 1996; Vuchinich & Tucker, 1988). Issues of availability are subsumed under the concept of supply. The economic principle of price is another important principle. Price is defined more broadly than monetary cost. Price subsumes all of the resources directly expended as well as the physically, socially, or psychologically adverse events experienced in purchasing, consuming, and recovering from drug use. In communities where drug use is widely accepted, the social price associated with use will be lower. Again, consider the different monetary and social prices associated with use of tobacco and alcohol versus cocaine or heroin in most middle-class communities. Both licit and illicit drug use occur at some level in most communities, but the relative frequencies are disproportionately in favor of the licit types. There seems to be little question that price, both monetary and social, is an important determinant of those differences.

Another very important economic concept in conceptualizing drug use is opportunity cost; that is, the alternative opportunities that are lost by choosing to consume drugs rather than spending time doing something else (Bickel et al., 1993). Sound scientific evidence from controlled experiments with humans and laboratory animals illustrates that the frequency of drug use can be significantly modified by varying opportunity cost (Higgins, 1996, 1997). For example, laboratory animals with well-established patterns of intravenous cocaine use engage in that behavior significantly less when it results in the loss of an essential food substance (Nader & Woolverton, 1991). Similarly, cocaine use in humans, including cocaine-dependent individuals, decreases as an orderly function of increases in the opportunity cost (e.g., monetary loss) associated with drug use (Higgins, Bickel, & Hughes, 1994; Higgins, Budney, Bickel, et al., 1994). Although deceptively simplistic, the learning principle of reinforcement in combination with the economic principles of supply, price, and opportunity cost can contribute much to our understanding of location and movement along this continuum of drug use.

Of particular relevance to this chapter is that these principles form the cornerstone of CRA and contingency-management procedures. These interventions attempt to reduce drug use and its attendant problems by systematically altering cost–benefit ratios between drug use and abstinence to favor the latter. How those ratios are altered is described in the following chronological review of studies that have examined the efficacy of CRA and, more recently, CRA plus contingency management. Please note that this chapter was not written to instruct the interested clinician in the implementation of these procedures. Those with such interests can consult alternative sources (e.g., Budney & Higgins, 1998; Meyers, Dominguez, & Smith, 1996; Meyers & Smith, 1995).

# TREATMENT OF ALCOHOL DEPENDENCE

## Seminal Study

The seminal CRA study was conducted with 16 men admitted to a state hospital for severe alcohol dependence who were randomly assigned to receive CRA plus standard hospital care or standard care alone (Hunt & Azrin, 1973). Standard hospital care consisted of 25 1-hour didactic sessions involving lectures and audiovisuals focused on the workings of Alcoholics Anonymous (AA), basic descriptive information about alcoholism, and examples of alcohol-related medical problems and related topics.

CRA was designed to rearrange and improve the quality of patients' vocational, family, social, and recreational reinforcers. The goal was for these reinforcers to be operational and of high quality when the patient was sober and to be unavailable if drinking was resumed. In economic terms, the opportunity cost of drinking was the usual price of drinking plus short-term forfeiture of these improved naturalistic sources of reinforcement.

Plans for rearranging these reinforcers were individualized to conform with the specifics of each patient's situation. Immediate barriers to treatment participation, such as pending legal matters or other crises, were addressed first. The next priority was vocational counseling. Hospital discharge was dependent on obtaining employment, which provided a powerful incentive for patients to participate in this treatment component. Marital and family therapy was also initiated during hospitalization and continued after discharge. Patients and significant others were taught to negotiate contracts for reciprocally reinforcing changes in each other's behavior. Social counseling was implemented to develop or reinstate social interactions with other friends, relatives, and community groups who had low tolerance for drinking, and to discourage interactions with heavy drinkers (i.e., attempts were made to decrease the availability and acceptability of drinking opportunities). To further facilitate this process, staff renovated a former tavern to serve as an alcohol-free social club and encouraged patients and their wives to attend for social activities. Last, patients were taught how to solve problems that had previously resulted in drinking.

As shown in Figure 10.1, during a 6-month follow-up period after hospital discharge, time spent drinking was 14% for CRA versus 79% for the standard treatment; time unemployed was 5% for CRA versus 62% for standard treatment; time away from family was 16% for CRA versus 36% for standard treatment; and time institutionalized was 2% for CRA versus 27% for the standard treatment.

## Improvements in CRA

In the next report (Azrin, 1976), CRA was expanded to include disulfiram therapy with monitoring by a significant other to ensure medication com-

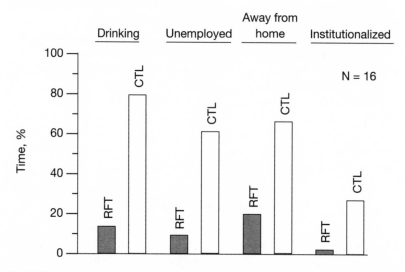

**FIGURE 10.1.** Comparison of the CRA and control groups on key dependent measures during the 6 months of follow-up following hospital discharge: Mean percentage of time spent drinking, unemployed, away from home, and institutionalized. From Hunt and Azrin (1973). Copyright 1973 by Elsevier Science, Ltd. Reprinted with kind permission of Elsevier Science, Ltd.

pliance, additional counseling directed toward anticipating and avoiding potential crises, a "buddy" system wherein individuals in the patient's neighborhood were available to give assistance with practical issues such as repairing cars, and a switch from individual to group counseling to reduce the total number of counselor hours needed to implement the treatment.

Twenty matched pairs of men hospitalized for severe alcohol dependence were randomly assigned to receive CRA or a standard hospital program similar to the one described earlier but that also included providing patients a prescription for disulfiram. During the 6 months after hospital discharge, outcomes achieved with CRA were significantly better than with the standard treatment for time spent drinking, employed, out of home, and institutionalized, thereby replicating and improving upon the differences noted in the first study. During the 2 years following discharge, the CRA group spent 90% or more time abstinent; comparable data were not reported for the standard treatment group.

## Efficacy of the Social Club

Next, effects of adding the social club described in Hunt and Azrin (1973) to a standard regimen of outpatient counseling for patients with less severe alcohol dependence were examined (Mallams, Godley, Hall, & Meyers, 1982). The social club was designed to provide the social atmosphere and, presumably, the social reinforcement associated with taverns, but without alcohol consumption being involved. Individuals had to be abstinent to attend. Forty male and female alcoholics were randomly assigned to receive systematic encouragement to attend the social club (experimental group), or were informed about it's existence without being systematically encouraged to attend (control group). At the 3-month follow-up point, only the experimental group showed significant improvements from intake on measures of drinking quantity and frequency, behavioral impairment, and time spent in heavy-drinking situations.

## Monitored Disulfiram Therapy

A fourth study was designed to dissociate the effects of monitored disulfiram therapy from the other aspects of CRA (Azrin, Sisson, Meyers, & Godley, 1982). This study continued the process of extending CRA to less severely impaired outpatients and to women. Forty-three male and female alcohol-dependent outpatients were randomly assigned to receive traditional treatment and traditional disulfiram therapy with no attempt to influence compliance, traditional therapy plus disulfiram therapy involving significant others to monitor compliance, or CRA in combination with disulfiram therapy and significant-other monitoring. At the 6-month follow-up, CRA in combination with disulfiram and compliance procedures produced the greatest reductions in drinking; disulfiram in combination with compliance procedures but without CRA produced intermediate results; and traditional treatment and disulfiram therapy produced the poorest results. Interestingly, as shown in Table 10.1, married patients did equally well with the full CRA treatment package or disulfiram plus compliance procedures alone. Only single patients appeared to need the package of CRA treatment and monitored disulfiram to achieve abstinence, perhaps because they lacked the level of social support for abstinence that was available to married individuals.

## Treating Significant Others

CRA was later adapted for use with the significant others (SOs) of treatment-resistant individuals (Sisson & Azrin, 1986). Twelve SOs of alcohol-dependent individuals who refused to enter treatment were randomly assigned to receive the CRA intervention or a standard program that involved group instruction about alcohol and the disease model of alcoholism. The adapted CRA intervention included education about alcohol problems, information and discussion of the positive consequences of abstinence, assistance in involving the alcohol-abusing family member in activities that might compete with drinking, increasing the involvement of SOs in social/recreational activities, and training SOs in how to respond to drinking episodes and how to recommend treatment entry.

There was no evidence of improvement in the control group during a 3-month follow-up, in that none of the abusing family members entered treatment and their drinking remained unchanged. In the CRA group, by contrast, 6 of the 7 abusing family members entered treatment and their frequency of drinking decreased significantly. This promising area of in-

**TABLE 10.1. Mean Number of Days Abstinent during the 30 Days Preceding the 6-Month Follow-Up (N = 43)**

| Intervention | Singles | Couples |
|---|---|---|
| Standard care and disulfiram without compliance monitoring | 6.8 | 17.4 |
| Standard care and disulfiram with compliance monitoring | 8.0 | 30.0 |
| CRA and disulfiram with compliance monitoring | 28.3 | 30.0 |

*Note.* Adapted from Azrin et al. (1982). Copyright 1982. Adapted with permission from Elsevier Science.

quiry is currently being pursued with SOs of severely dependent and less impaired abusers of alcohol and other drugs (Kirby et al., 1998; Meyers et al., 1996).

## Other Empirical Support

Another, sometimes overlooked source of empirical support for CRA comes from the alcohol treatment literature on coping/social skills training and behavioral marital and family therapy. Recall that coping/social skills training and marital and family therapy are core elements of CRA. The efficacy of training in these and related skills in decreasing drinking and drinking-related problems has been demonstrated in a series of controlled trials conducted after and independent of the CRA studies described in this section (e.g., Monti, Rohsenow, Colby, & Abrams, 1995; O'Farrell, 1995).

## TREATMENT OF COCAINE DEPENDENCE

During the past 7 years or so, a series of studies were completed at the University of Vermont demonstrating the efficacy of CRA combined with contingency-management procedures in the outpatient treatment of cocaine dependence (Budney, Higgins, Delaney, Kent, & Bickel, 1991; Higgins, Budney, Bickel, Hughes, Foerg, et al., 1993; Higgins, Budney, Bickel, et al., 1994; Higgins et al., 1991, 1995). CRA was implemented as described in earlier alcohol studies, minus the social club and buddy system. The primary contingency-management procedure used in these studies was one in which patients earned vouchers exchangeable for retail items contingent on documentation via urinalysis testing that they recently had abstained from cocaine. The voucher system was in effect for weeks 1–12 of treatment, and the average amount earned was approximately $6.00 per day.

The rationale for combining the voucher system with CRA was as follows: Many cocaine-dependent individuals arrive in treatment with their lives in disarray. A reasonable assumption is that some time will be needed to assist these individuals in stabilizing and restructuring their lives so that naturalistic sources of reinforcement for abstinence can exert some influence over their behavior. Hospitalization is an option, but the voucher program was deemed a less expensive alternative. The plan was to have this incentive program play a major role during the initial 12 weeks of treatment, during which time CRA therapy would be ongoing as well. Ideally, sufficient progress could be made with CRA so that naturalistic reinforcers would be in place to sustain drug abstinence when the vouchers were discontinued.

In an effort to facilitate naturalistic sources of support, patients were encouraged to include SOs in treatment. This was not limited to spouses or romantic partners. Any SO who was not a drug abuser, excepting nicotine, was eligible. All SOs were encouraged to develop behavioral contracts with patients wherein the former contracted to do something potentially reinforcing contingent on the latter abstaining from cocaine use. So that this contingency-management intervention could be implemented with precision, clinic staff notified SOs of the results of all urinalysis testing.

## Seminal Studies

Two controlled trials examined the efficacy of this combined CRA and contingency-management treatment by comparing it against standard outpatient drug abuse counseling based on the disease-model approach (Higgins et al., 1991; Higgins, Budney, Bickel, Hughes, Foerg, et al., 1993). The first of these two trials assigned consecutive clinic admissions to the respective treatment groups, whereas the second trial used random assignment. In both trials, the CRA plus contingency-management treatment retained patients significantly longer in treatment and was associated with longer periods of cocaine abstinence than standard counseling. For example, in the randomized trial, 58% of patients assigned to the behavioral treatment completed 24 weeks of treatment compared to 11% of those assigned to standard counseling. Across time, 68% and 42% of patients in the behavioral group were documented to have achieved 8 and 16 weeks of continuous cocaine abstinence, respectively, versus 11% and 5% of those in the counseling group.

## Efficacy of Vouchers

In a third trial, patients were randomly assigned to receive CRA with or without the voucher program (Higgins, Budney, Bickel, et al., 1994). Treatment was 24 weeks in duration and the voucher versus no-voucher difference was in effect during weeks 1–12 only. Vouchers significantly improved treatment retention and cocaine abstinence. Seventy-five percent of patients in the group with vouchers completed 24 weeks of treatment versus 40% in the group without vouchers and, based on data presented in Figure 10.2, average duration of continuous cocaine abstinence documented via urinalysis in the two groups were 11.7 ± 2.0 weeks in the vouchers group versus 6.0 ± 1.5 in the no-vouchers group.

Follow-up results at 6, 9, and 12 months after treatment entry were described in a separate report based on the randomized controlled trials comparing the CRA plus contingency-management treatment to drug

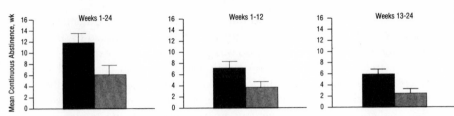

**FIGURE 10.2.** Mean durations of continuous cocaine abstinence documented via urinalysis testing in each treatment group during weeks 1–24, 1–12, and 13–24 of treatment. Solid and shaded bars indicate the voucher and no-voucher groups, respectively. Error bars represent + standard error of measurement. From Higgins, Budney, Bickel, et al. (1994). Copyright 1994–1996 by the American Medical Association. Reprinted by permission.

abuse counseling and to CRA without vouchers (Higgins et al., 1995). In the trial comparing CRA and contingency-management to drug abuse counseling, significantly greater cocaine abstinence was documented via urinalysis at 9- and 12-month follow-ups in the former; both groups showed comparable and significant improvements on the Addiction Severity Index (ASI). In the trial comparing CRA with and without vouchers, no differences were observed in urinalysis results, but the magnitude of improvement throughout the follow-up on the ASI composite drug scale was significantly greater in the voucher group, and only the voucher group showed significant improvement on the ASI psychiatric scale.

## Social Support

In a retrospective analysis conducted to identify predictors of cocaine abstinence during treatment with this intervention, participants who had a SO involved in treatment were significantly more likely to achieve sustained periods of cocaine abstinence than were those without an SO involved (Higgins, Budney, Bickel, & Badger, 1994). However, that finding was not supported in a subsequent prospective clinical trial (Higgins, Budney, & Badger, 1994).

## Monitored Disulfiram Therapy

While these trials were focused on treatment of cocaine dependence, approximately 60% of the cocaine-dependent individuals met diagnostic criteria for alcohol dependence, and a great percentage met criteria for alcohol abuse. Disulfiram therapy is a core component of CRA; thus it was offered to all individuals who reported evidence of concurrent alcohol problems. As a first step toward assessing the contribution of this element of treatment to outcome, a chart review was conducted with 16 individuals who met DSM III-R criteria for cocaine dependence and alcohol abuse/dependence (Higgins, Budney, Bickel, Hughes, & Foerg, 1993). Disulfiram therapy was associated with significant decreases in drinking and, unexpectedly, in cocaine use. The ability of monitored disulfiram therapy to decrease alcohol and cocaine use in patients who abuse both substances was replicated in subsequent controlled trials conducted in the absence of the other CRA components (Carroll, Nich, Ball, McCance, & Rounsaville, 1998; Carroll et al., 1993).

## Assessing Generality to Other Populations of Cocaine Abusers

Because the studies described here involving CRA plus vouchers were conducted in Vermont, important questions were raised about the generality of those findings to inner-city cocaine abusers. The studies cited above by Carroll and colleagues with disulfiram were completed in New Haven, Connecticut, demonstrating the generality of the monitored disulfiram component to inner-city cocaine abusers. To address this issue regarding vouchers, controlled trials were conducted with methadone maintenance patients in clinics located in Baltimore (Silverman et al., 1996a) and San Francisco (Tusel et al., 1995).

In the Baltimore study, intravenous cocaine abusers were randomized to an experimental group ($n = 19$) in which vouchers exchangeable for retail items were received contingent upon cocaine-negative urinalysis tests or to a control group ($n = 18$) in which vouchers were received independent of urinalysis results (Silverman et al., 1996a). Both groups received a standard form of outpatient drug and alcohol abuse counseling. As shown in Figure 10.3, during a 12-week treatment period, cocaine use was substantially reduced in the experimental group and remained relatively unchanged in the control group.

In the San Francisco study, 100 opioid addicts enrolled in a 180-day methadone-based detoxification program were randomly assigned to an adaptation of the voucher program described here or to usual care (Tusel et al., 1995). Significantly greater periods of sustained abstinence from illicit drugs were observed in the voucher group.

## TREATMENT OF OPIOID DEPENDENCE

In a randomized trial completed recently at the University of Vermont, CRA in combination with the voucher program was compared to standard drug abuse counseling in 39 opioid-dependent individuals undergoing opioid detoxification (Bickel, Amass, Higgins, Badger, & Esch, 1997).

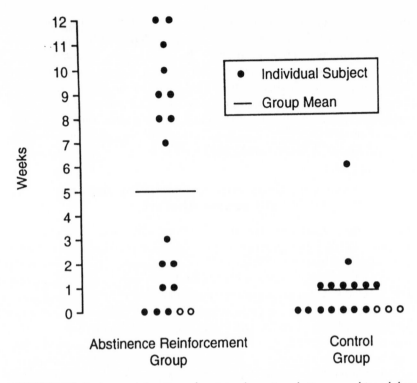

**FIGURE 10.3.** Longest duration of sustained cocaine abstinence achieved during the 12-week voucher condition. Each data point indicates data from an individual subject, and the lines represent group means. Subjects in the reinforcement and control conditions are displayed in the left and right columns, respectively. Open circles represent early study dropouts. From Silverman et al. (1996a). Copyright 1994–1996 by the American Medical Association. Reprinted by permission.

CRA generally was delivered in the same manner as in the studies with cocaine-dependent individuals described earlier. The voucher program was modified so that one-half of the available vouchers could be earned via drug-free urinalysis test results and the other half by participating in activities specified as part of CRA therapy. Participants assigned to the CRA plus vouchers group were significantly more likely to complete the 24-week detox and had longer durations of continuous opioid abstinence during the detox than did participants assigned to the standard treatment.

Similarly, in a within-subject study conducted with 13 inner-city methadone maintenance patients, a voucher-based incentive program significantly decreased illicit-opiate abuse (Silverman et al., 1996b).

## NATURALISTIC VERSUS CONTRIVED
## REINFORCEMENT CONTINGENCIES

The combined use of CRA and contingency management in the studies on cocaine and opioid dependence raise questions regarding the use of naturalistic versus contrived reinforcers. I have suggested previously in discussing this issue that it might be fruitful to conceptualize contingencies as running along a continuum from contrived to naturalistic (Higgins, 1996). Contingency-management interventions typically fall more along the contrived end and CRA along the naturalistic end of that continuum. Considering that, in most instances, naturalistic contingencies ultimately must maintain any therapeutic changes made, treatments that rely more on that end of the continuum would seem to have advantages over those on the contrived end, although that is an empirical question that has not been thoroughly tested. A likely disadvantage of interventions falling on the naturalistic end is that the contingencies cannot be managed as precisely as those located on the more contrived end. Because operant behavior is generally sensitive to the precision with which such factors are managed, this drawback is likely to decrease treatment efficacy.

A reasonable assumption is that the greater the reinforcing effects being exerted by the drugs involved, the more important precise contingency-management issues are likely to be. To take an example from basic research, simply making a palatable alternative available in laboratory studies with rats can significantly retard the acquisition of cocaine-reinforced responding despite the absence of any programmed contingencies between drug use and access to the alternative (Carroll, Lac, & Nygaard, 1989). However, when the same alternative is introduced after cocaine use is well established, effects on drug use are relatively weak; that is, once cocaine use is established, explicit contingencies between cocaine use and gaining access to alternative reinforcers appear to be necessary to produce robust decreases in drug use. Relating this information back to the clinical situation, the need for precise management of the various factors contributing to the price of drug use is likely to vary as a positive function of the reinforcing effects that the drug(s) is exerting. As such, the importance of managing the contingencies precisely is likely to increase progressively as one moves from primary prevention through treatment of mildly impaired abusers and perhaps be most important when dealing with initial efforts at abstinence or reduced drug use by severely dependent individuals.

These observations underscore the potential utility in combined use of contrived and naturalistic contingencies, especially during the early stages of treatment for severely dependent individuals. In the CRA studies with alcohol-dependent individuals, disulfiram therapy can be considered to fall more along the contrived end and the other aspects of CRA along the naturalistic end. In the studies with cocaine-dependent individuals, both disulfiram therapy and the voucher program fall along the contrived end, while other aspects of CRA treatment fall more along the naturalistic end. No comparisons of CRA with and without disulfiram therapy in the treatment of alcohol dependence have yet been reported. Results from the one study by Azrin et al. (1982) suggested that married individuals may achieve positive outcomes with only monitored disulfiram therapy. The experiment comparing CRA with and without vouchers in the treatment of cocaine dependence indicated that adding the contrived reinforcement contingencies resulted in greater reductions in drug use for as long as 9 months after termination of the voucher program (Higgins, Budney, Bickel, & Foerg, 1994; Higgins et al., 1995). These studies illustrate the feasibility and efficacy of combining interventions based on naturalistic and contrived contingencies. As is illustrated next, both types of contingency-based interventions have contributions to make to broadening the base of substance abuse treatment services. The important challenge is to determine the conditions under which one, the other, or both are effective.

## BROADENING THE BASE OF TREATMENT

The preceding sections addressed applying CRA and contingency management with alcohol- and drug-dependent individuals in clinic and hospital settings, which will remain an important element of any reconfiguration of substance abuse treatment services. However, a comprehensive effort to reduce substance abuse and its attendant problems must also include interventions aimed at (1) reaching and treating dependent individuals who fail to seek formal substance abuse treatment, (2) assisting less impaired treatment seekers with appropriately circumscribed and focused interventions, and (3) preventing substance-related problems in general and at-risk populations. Below I have listed some possible contributions that CRA and contingency management may make to such an effort. By no means is the list exhaustive. Instead, it is meant to share the tremendous potential that I see in the CRA and contingency-management interventions discussed in this chapter for making significant and varied contributions to the important goal of expanding the base of substance abuse treatment services.

### Working with Significant Others

The study by Sisson and Azrin (1986) illustrating the efficacy of CRA in assisting SOs to motivate alcohol-dependent individuals who were initially uninterested in treatment to enroll and in facilitating positive treatment outcomes is very promising. Only seven SOs received CRA in that study; thus the ongoing efforts to replicate and extend these findings to less impaired drinkers and to illicit drug abusers are very important (Kirby et al., 1998; Meyers et al., 1996). Should those efforts prove successful, which is suggested by preliminary evidence, this intervention could contribute significantly to broadening the base of treatment by increasing the number of individuals who enroll in treatment.

## Monitored Disulfiram Therapy

Should the observation by Azrin et al. (1982) that more socially stable alcohol-dependent patients (e.g., married individuals) need only monitored disulfiram therapy for a positive outcome prove reliable, it, too, has great potential for broadening the base of treatment. Monitored disulfiram therapy is a straightforward protocol that could easily be administered in settings other than formal substance abuse treatment clinics (e.g., employee assistance programs, community health centers) and, in that way, could be made available to individuals who are reluctant to enroll in formal treatment. Our work and that of Carroll and colleagues suggests that this protocol also has the potential to reduce concurrent cocaine abuse (Carroll et al., 1993, 1998; Higgins, Budney, Bickel, Hughes, & Foerg, 1993).

## Alcohol-Free Social Clubs

The observation by Mallams et al. (1982) that encouraging participation in an alcohol-free social club was effective in reducing drinking is promising and merits further investigation, including studies using abusers of other drugs. Should the finding prove to be reliable, similar clubs could be established in communities and presumably would not need to have any formal affiliation with a substance abuse treatment program. Some communities already have alcohol-free social clubs in place, but perhaps their numbers would be increased if they were demonstrated to be efficacious. Employee assistance programs would seem to be a good source of support for such programs, both financially and in terms of encouraging employee participation in them.

## Criminal Justice System

Licit and illicit drug dependence are prevalent at alarming levels in newly arrested and other criminal offenders (National Institute of Justice, 1995). Cocaine use in particular is contributing immensely to the high U.S. incarceration rates and attendant escalating costs associated with prison con-struction and maintenance. A plausible alternative for cases involving nonviolent crimes related to cocaine use are programs similar to the voucher program described here (Higgins, 1996). Instead of vouchers, in-dividuals in these programs might earn progressively greater reductions in their level of criminal justice supervision by continuously abstaining from cocaine use. Objective evidence of cocaine use would reset supervision back to a stricter level. Important features of such programs would be reg-ular and sensitive urinalysis monitoring, so that cocaine use is readily de-tected, consistent consequences for cocaine use and abstinence delivered with minimal delay, and consequences set at an intensity and duration that permit clients to interact repeatedly with the contingencies, so that they may learn from the consequences of their behavior. Many states currently have programs that approximate this suggestion, but, based on my experi-ence, they generally lack the important contingency-management features just mentioned. I know of no controlled trials examining the efficacy of such a program in reducing cocaine use among criminal offenders. Con-sidering the relatively robust evidence supporting the sensitivity of cocaine use to contingency-management interventions, this approach seems to of-fer a reasonable and cost-effective alternative to current practices. Com-bining such programs with drug refusal, vocational, and other skills train-ing might further increase efficacy and decrease the probability of relapse once the contrived contingencies are terminated. Comparable programs involving monitored disulfiram therapy and naltrexone (opioid antagonist) therapy for alcohol-related and opioid-related nonviolent crimes, respec-tively, should be evaluated as well. Such programs have great potential for extending treatment services to large numbers of incarcerated drug abusers that otherwise might never enroll in treatment.

## Supported Employment

Innovative programs that make greater use of vocational opportunities are another way to broaden the base of treatment. For example, a new project for pregnant, drug-dependent women funded by the National In-stitute on Drug Abuse will examine use of a modification of the voucher program to decrease drug use and improve vocational skills (Silverman & Robles, in press). The program will be conducted in phases, with the ini-tial phases involving voucher-based reinforcement of abstinence as de-scribed earlier. The women will then move into a second phase wherein voucher-based reinforcement will continue to be available, but the contin-gencies will be expanded to reinforce both drug abstinence and participa-tion in a structured vocational training program. The goal is eventually to transition the women into gainful employment. Employment settings that involve regular employee drug testing might be the best arrangement for these individuals.

A family reunification program described recently in *The New York Times* also makes creative use of incentives to integrate parental responsibility, employment, and drug abstinence (Rabinovitz, 1996). In this program, young fathers who have children on welfare are offered a $22/hour demolition and asbestos-abatement job in a housing project, along with housing and other incentives. In return, the fathers agree to remove their children from welfare and participate in urinalysis monitoring of drug use. According to the report, the U.S. Department of Housing and Urban Development (HUD) is encouraging housing authorities nationwide to develop similar incentive programs.

## Entitlement Programs

Cocaine and other drug abuse are serious problems among a subset of individuals receiving Veterans and Social Security Insurance disability income (Satel, 1995). A recent study that examined the relationship between cocaine use and disability payments among schizophrenics provides an interesting example (Shaner et al., 1995). The severity of psychiatric symptoms, hospitalization rates, and cocaine urine toxicology screens were assessed for 15 consecutive weeks in 105 veterans who met diagnostic criteria for schizophrenia and cocaine dependence. On average, these individuals reported spending half their total income on illegal drugs. Cocaine use, psychiatric symptoms, and hospital admissions peaked during the first or second week of the month, coincident with delivery of the disability payment. Citing the efficacy of voucher-based incentives in reducing cocaine use, the investigators raised the possibility of using similar incentive programs that could be implemented in some manner through use of the disability payments. Obviously, such a program would need to be designed with great sensitivity to individual rights and could not legally involve withholding entitlements. Those concerns notwithstanding, at least two programs for the dually diagnosed are currently implementing and evaluating such an approach (Shaner et al., 1995; Ries, 1995, cited in Satel, 1995). The programs are being conducted in the same mental health clinics in which patients are receiving their other psychiatric care, thereby expanding the base of substance abuse services.

## Helping Substance Abusers
## with Mild to Moderate Problems

There is a clear need for interventions targeting the population of persons with mild to moderate alcohol- and drug-related problems. Estimates related to alcohol abuse, for example, indicate that these less impaired abusers outnumber the severely dependent by a ratio of approximately 4:1 (Institute of Medicine, 1990). The potential utility of CRA as an intervention approach for persons with less severe problems is suggested by the fact that it has been successfully modified from initially being a treatment for hospitalized, severely alcohol-dependent males to an approach for use with less severely dependent male and female outpatients and their SOs, and then has been generalized to cocaine- and opioid-dependent outpatients and their SOs. A reasonable next step is to evaluate its efficacy as an intervention for relatively less impaired substance abusers. These individuals would need a less intense version of CRA, but there is no logical reason why that should be a problem, since CRA is delivered according to the special needs and circumstances of the individual. Some have argued that those with milder substance abuse problems mostly need interventions that focus on increasing their motivation for change (Sobell & Sobell, 1993), which is an integral feature of CRA that could be further adapted to address the needs of less impaired substance abusers. A successful adaptation of this sort would increase the number of empirically based, effective interventions available for use with the many individuals who experience significant, but more circumscribed, problems related to substance abuse.

## Prevention Efforts

Last, sufficient epidemiological information is available from the National Household Survey to identify specific neighborhoods that foster illicit drug use and abuse (Lillie-Blanton, Anthony, & Schuster, 1993). These at-risk neighborhoods should be targeted for prevention programs that are strategically designed and scheduled to increase the availability of healthy and effective alternatives to cocaine and other illicit drug use (Higgins, 1996, 1997). Well-conducted, basic research studies have demonstrated the efficacy of alternative, nondrug reinforcers in preventing the acquisition of cocaine and other drug use. They can do so in the absence of any explicit contingencies between drug use and access to the alternatives. The fact that more contrived contingencies are unnecessary is important, because it means that the efficacy of such interventions need not depend on objective monitoring of illicit drug use (e.g., through urinalysis), which can be costly and is impractical in community-based prevention efforts. Considering the tremendous need for effective strategies to prevent cocaine and other illicit drug use, and the strong empirical support for the influence of alternative reinforcers on the acquisition of drug use, such strategies merit careful evaluation. Evaluating the use of similar programs for prevention of alcohol use and abuse would also be prudent. The epidemiological data on at-risk neighborhoods might be less relevant to alcohol use because of its wide-scale prevalence in most U.S. communities, but the importance of alternative reinforcers should be of the same fundamental importance.

## CONTINUUM OF CARE

Within the Institute of Medicine's (1990) recommendations for broadening the base of treatment for alcohol problems, the treatment services system was conceptualized as including two parts: community agencies (e.g., health care, social service, workplace, education, and criminal justice agencies) and specialized, comprehensive substance abuse treatment centers. Community agencies would focus on screening and providing brief interventions for those with mild or moderate problems and referring those with severe problems to more intensive treatment programs. Those with severe problems, and those who failed to improve with the brief interventions, would be treated in the specialized centers. This framework seems reasonable for conceptualizing a service delivery system for the treatment of illicit-drug abuse as well.

Within such a framework, the CRA and contingency-management interventions researched thus far are of the specialty clinic variety save for the social club intervention reported by Mallams et al. (1982). I have outlined a number of other possibilities for extending CRA and contingency management into community agencies. There is nothing inherent in CRA or contingency management that must restrict them to the specialized clinic setting, although their efficacy in other settings will need to be evaluated. A possible difference between my suggestions for extending CRA and contingency management to community agencies and the system outlined in the Institute of Medicine report is that some of my proposed interventions would be of longer duration rather than brief and would include individuals with severe problems rather than being restricted to those with mild to moderate problems. I see no reason to presume that community agencies (e.g., criminal justice agencies) cannot or should not participate in the provision of longer-term services directed at reducing substance abuse and attendant problems among their more severely dependent clientele.

Any discussion of the continuum of care must address matters of cost. As is the case with most treatment modalities, limited information is available regarding the cost-effectiveness of CRA and contingency-management interventions. The information that is available is based exclusively on alcohol treatment outcome studies. CRA was included in the seminal study by Holder and colleagues examining the cost-effectiveness of treatments for alcohol problems (Holder, Longabaugh, & Miller, 1991).

Contingency management was included as well, but under the heading of behavioral contracting. To assess effectiveness, Holder and colleagues assigned each of 33 treatment modalities a weighted score based on a ratio of the number of controlled clinical trials that did and did not support their efficacy. The weighted scores were then used to rank the treatments into five categories (i.e., "no evidence," "insufficient evidence," "indeterminate evidence," "fair evidence," and "good evidence." CRA and contingency-management were ranked in the "good evidence" and "fair evidence" categories, respectively. Treatments were also divided into five categories based on estimated costs to deliver them (i.e., "minimum," "low," "medium-low," "medium-high," and "high"). CRA and contingency management were placed in the "medium-low" and "low" categories, respectively. Finally, cost effectiveness was summarized in a 5 × 5 table contrasting cost and effectiveness rankings. Cost-effectiveness rankings for CRA and contingency management equaled or exceeded 91% and 81%, respectively, of the other treatment modalities assessed. A more recent review of treatment effectiveness (Miller et al., 1995) that incorporated Holder et al.'s earlier cost analyses provided comparable relative rankings for CRA and behavioral contracting.

Overall, CRA and contingency management appear to fare well in terms of relative cost-effectiveness for treating alcohol problems. In the two reviews, brief intervention and motivational enhancement interventions were the modalities ranked equal to or above CRA and contingency management in terms of effectiveness and lower in terms of cost. Interestingly, the Mallams et al. (1982) study that assessed the efficacy of the CRA social club as an adjunct to drug abuse counseling was included under the heading of motivational enhancement interventions rather than CRA in the Miller et al.(1995) review of treatment effectiveness. Nevertheless, the important question appears to be whether briefer or more circumscribed interventions can produce comparable positive outcomes to CRA and contingency management with more severely dependent individuals. If they can, then there would be little justification for continuing with CRA or contingency management in specialized substance abuse treatment centers. Only randomized clinical trials comparing these interventions with more severely impaired populations can provide a satisfactory answer to that question.

I know of no comprehensive evaluations of the cost-effectiveness of CRA or contingency-management interventions with illicit drug abusers. Given the relatively extensive empirical support for their efficacy in the treatment of illicit drug abuse compared to other psychosocial interventions (Stitzer & Higgins, 1995), however, it seems likely that results comparable to those noted earlier for the alcohol treatment outcome literature would be obtained.

In addition to relative cost-effectiveness, there is the question of cost–benefit; that is, whether the reductions in substance use and attendant problems produced by CRA or contingency management result in sufficient individual and societal cost savings to offset fully or partly the costs of providing those services. I know of no such cost–benefit studies specifically addressing CRA or contingency-management interventions, which is the case for most substance abuse treatment modalities. Answers to those questions will be extremely important arbiters of the future of CRA, contingency management, and all other substance abuse treatment modalities.

## ACKNOWLEDGMENT

Preparation of this chapter was supported by Grants Nos. R01 DA09378 and R01 DA08076 from the National Institute on Drug Abuse.

## REFERENCES

Azrin, N. H. (1976). Improvements in the community-reinforcement approach to alcoholism. *Behaviour Research and Therapy, 14*, 339–348.

Azrin, N. H., Sisson, R. W., Meyers, R., & Godley, M. (1982). Alcoholism treatment by disulfiram and community reinforcement therapy. *Journal of Behavior Therapy and Experimental Psychiatry, 13*, 105–112.

Bickel, W. K., Amass, L., Higgins, S. T., Badger, G. J., & Esch, R. A. (1997). Effects of adding behavioral treatment to opioid detoxification with buprenorphine. *Journal of Consulting and Clinical Psychology, 65*, 803–810.

Bickel, W. K., & DeGrandpre, R. J. (1996). Modeling drug abuse policy in the behavioral economics laboratory. In L. Green & J. H. Kagel (Eds.), *Advances in behavioral economics: Substance use and abuse* (Vol. 3, pp. 69–95). Norwood, NJ: Ablex.

Bickel, W. K., DeGrandpre, R. J., & Higgins, S. T. (1993). Behavioral economics: A novel experimental approach to the study of drug dependence. *Drug and Alcohol Dependence, 33*, 173–192.

Budney, A. J., & Higgins, S. T. (1998). *A community reinforcement plus vouchers approach: Treating cocaine addiction* (National Institute on Drug Abuse Therapy Manuals for Drug Addiction, Manual 2; NIH Publication No. 98:4309). Rockville, MD: National Institute on Drug Abuse.

Budney, A. J., Higgins, S. T., Delaney, D. D., Kent, L., & Bickel, W. K. (1991). Contingent reinforcement of abstinence with individuals abusing cocaine and marijuana. *Journal of Applied Behavior Analysis, 24*, 657–665.

Carroll, K. M., Nich, C., Ball, S. A., McCance, E., & Rounsaville, B. J. (1998). Treatment of cocaine and alcohol dependence with psychotherapy and disulfiram. *Addiction, 93*, 713–727.

Carroll, K., Ziedonis, D., O'Malley, S., McCance-Katz, E., Gordon, L., & Rounsaville,

B. (1993). Pharmacologic interventions for alcohol- and cocaine-abusing individuals: A pilot study of disulfiram vs. naltrexone. *American Journal on Addictions, 2,* 77–79.

Carroll, M. E., Lac, S. T., & Nygaard, S. L. (1989). A concurrently available nondrug reinforcer prevents the acquisition or decreases the maintenance of cocaine-reinforced behavior. *Psychopharmacology, 97,* 23–29.

Centers for Disease Control. (1993). Cigarette smoking—attributable mortality and years of potential life lost—1990. *Mortality and Morbidity Weekly Report, 42,* 37–39.

Crowley, T. J. (1988). Learning and unlearning drug abuse in the real world: Clinical treatment and public policy. In B. A. Ray (Ed.), *Learning factors in substance abuse* (NIDA Research Monograph No. 84, DHHS Publication No. ADM 90-1576, pp. 100–121). Washington, DC: U.S. Government Printing Office.

Goldberg, S. R., & Stolerman, I. P. (Eds.). (1986). *Behavioral analysis of drug dependence.* Orlando, FL: Academic Press.

Griffiths, R. R., Bigelow, G. E., & Henningfield, J. E. (1980). Similarities in animal and human drug taking behavior. In N. K. Mello (Ed.), *Advances in substance abuse: Behavioral and biological research* (pp. 1–90). Greenwich, CT: JAI Press.

Henningfield, J. E., Lukas, S. E., & Bigelow, G. E. (1986). Human studies of drugs as reinforcers. In S. R. Goldberg & I. P. Stolerman (Eds.), *Behavioral analysis of drug dependence* (pp. 69–122). Orlando FL: Academic Press.

Higgins, S. T. (1997). The influence of alternative reinforcers on cocaine use and abuse: A brief review. *Pharmacology Biochemistry and Behavior, 57,* 419–427.

Higgins, S. T. (1996). Some potential contributions of reinforcement and consumer-demand theory to reducing cocaine use. *Addictive Behaviors, 21,* 803–816.

Higgins, S. T., Bickel, W. K., & Hughes, J. R. (1994). Influence of an alternative reinforcer on human cocaine self-administration. *Life Science, 55,* 179–187.

Higgins, S. T., Budney, A. J., & Badger, G. J. (1994). [Effects of contingent reinforcement from significant others on cocaine use]. Unpublished raw data.

Higgins, S. T., Budney, A. J., Bickel, W. K., Foerg, F. E., Ogden, D., & Badger, G. J. (1995). Outpatient behavioral treatment for cocaine dependence: One-year outcome. *Experimental and Clinical Psychopharmacology, 3,* 205–212.

Higgins, S. T., Budney, A. J., Bickel, W. K., & Badger, G. J. (1994). Participation of significant others in outpatient behavioral treatment predicts greater cocaine abstinence. *American Journal of Drug and Alcohol Abuse, 20,* 47–56.

Higgins, S. T., Budney, A. J., Bickel, W. K., Foerg, F. E., Donham, R., & Badger, G. J. (1994). Incentives improve treatment retention and cocaine abstinence in ambulatory cocaine-dependent patients. *Archives of General Psychiatry, 51,* 568–576.

Higgins, S. T., Budney, A. J., Bickel, W. K., Hughes, J. R., Foerg, F., & Badger, G. (1993). Achieving cocaine abstinence with a behavioral approach. *American Journal of Psychiatry, 150,* 763–769.

Higgins, S. T., Budney, A. J., Bickel, W. K., Hughes, J. R., & Foerg, F. (1993). Disulfiram therapy in patients abusing cocaine and alcohol. *American Journal of Psychiatry, 150,* 675–676.

Higgins, S. T., Delaney, D. D., Budney, A. J., Bickel, W. K., Hughes, J. R., Foerg, F., & Fenwick, J. W. (1991). A behavioral approach to achieving initial cocaine abstinence. *American Journal of Psychiatry, 148,* 1218–1224.

Holder, H., Longabaugh, R., & Miller, W. R. (1991). The cost-effectiveness of treatment for alcoholism: A first approximation. *Journal of Studies on Alcohol, 52*, 517–540.

Hunt, G. M., & Azrin, N. H. (1973). A community-reinforcement approach to alcoholism. *Behaviour Research and Therapy, 11*, 91–104.

Institute of Medicine. (1990). *Broadening the base of treatment for alcohol problems.* Washington, DC: National Academy Press.

Kirby, K. C., Festinger, D. S., Garvey, K., Firely, M., Follis, A., Marlowe, R. J., Lamb, R. J., & Iguchi, M. Y. (1998). Effects of drug abuse on the family: Family members, the problems, and treatment outcomes. In L. S. Harris (Ed.), *Proceedings of the 59th Annual Meeting of the College on Problems of Drug Dependence, Inc.* (p. 247). Rockville, MD: National Institute on Drug Abuse.

Lillie-Blanton, M., Anthony, J., & Schuster, C. R. (1993). Probing the meaning of racial/ethnic group comparisons in crack smoking. *Journal of the American Medical Association, 269*, 993–997.

Mallams, J. H., Godley, M. D., Hall, G. M., & Meyers, R. J. (1982). A social-systems approach to resocializing alcoholics in the community. *Journal of Studies on Alcohol, 43*, 1115–1123.

Meyers, R. J., Dominguez, T. P., & Smith, J. E. (1996). Community reinforcement training with concerned others. In V. B. Van Hasselt & M. Hersen (Eds.), *Sourcebook of psychological treatment manuals for adult disorders* (pp. 257–294). New York: Plenum.

Meyers, R. J., & Smith, J. E. (1995). *Clinical guide to alcohol treatment: The community reinforcement approach.* New York: Guilford Press.

Miller, W. R., Brown, J. M., Simpson, T. L., Handmaker, N. S., Bien, T. H., Luckie, L. F., Montgomery, H. A., Hester, R. K., & Tonigan, J. S. (1995). What works? A methodological analysis of the alcohol treatment outcome literature. In R. K. Hester & W. R. Miller (Eds.), *Handbook of alcoholism treatment approaches: Effective alternatives* (2nd ed., pp. 12–44). Boston: Allyn & Bacon.

Monti, P. M., Rohsenow, D. J., Colby, S. M., & Abrams, D. B. (1995). Coping and social skills training. In R. K. Hester & W. R. Miller (Eds.), *Handbook of alcoholism treatment approaches: Effective alternatives* (2nd ed., pp. 221–241). Boston: Allyn & Bacon.

Nader, M. A., & Woolverton, W. L. (1991). Effects of increasing the magnitude of an alternative reinforcer on drug choice in a discrete-trials choice procedure. *Psychopharmacology, 105*, 169–174.

National Institute of Justice. (1995). *Drug use forecasting: 1994 annual report on adult and juvenile arrestees.* Washington, DC: National Criminal Justice Reference Service.

O'Farrell, T. J. (1995). Marital and family therapy. In R. K. Hester & W. R. Miller (Eds.), *Handbook of alcoholism treatment approaches: Effective alternatives* (2nd ed., pp. 195–220). Boston: Allyn & Bacon.

Rabinovitz, J. (1996, June 16). A Hartford program to put fathers back in the family. *The New York Times*, pp. 1, 28.

Satel, S. L. (1995). When disability benefits make patients sicker. *New England Journal of Medicine, 333*, 794–796.

Shaner, A., Eckman, T. A., Roberts, L. J., Wilkins, J. N., Tucker, D. E., Tsuang, J. W., &

305

Mintz, J. (1995). Disability income, cocaine use, and repeated hospitalization among schizophrenic cocaine abusers. *New England Journal of Medicine, 12,* 777–783.

Silverman, K., Higgins, S. T., & Brooner, R. K., Montoya, I. D., Cone, E. J., Schuster, C. R., & Preston, K. L. (1996a). Sustained cocaine abstinence in methadone maintenance patients through voucher-based reinforcement therapy. *Archives of General Psychiatry, 53,* 409–415.

Silverman, K., & Robles, E. (in press). Employment as a drug abuse treatment intervention: A behavioral economic analysis. In F. J. Chaloypka, W. K. Bikel, M. Grossman, & H. Safer (Eds.), *The economic analysis of substance use and abuse: An integration of econometric and behavioral economic research.* Chicago, IL: University of Chicago Press.

Silverman, K., Wong, C. J., Higgins, S. T., Brooner, R. K., Montoya, I. D., Contoregi, C., Umbricht-Schneiter, A., Schuster, C. R., & Preston, K. L. (1996b). Increasing opiate abstinence through voucher-based reinforcement therapy. *Drug and Alcohol Dependence, 41,* 157–165.

Smith, J. E., & Meyers, R. J. (1995). The community reinforcement approach. In R. K. Hester & W. R. Miller (Eds.), *Handbook of alcoholism treatment approaches: Effective alternatives* (2nd ed., pp. 251–266). Boston: Allyn & Bacon.

Sobell, M. B., & Sobell, L. C. (1993). *Problem drinkers: Guided self-change treatment.* New York: Guilford Press.

Stitzer, M. L., & Higgins, S. T. (1995). Behavioral treatment of drug and alcohol abuse. In F. E. Bloom & D. J. Kupfer (Eds.), *Psychopharmacology: The fourth generation of progress* (pp. 1807–1819). New York: Raven Press.

Substance Abuse and Mental Health Services Administration. (1995). *National household survey on drug abuse: Population estimates 1994* (DHHS Publication No. SMA 95-3063). Washington, DC: U.S. Government Printing Office.

Substance Abuse and Mental Health Services Administration. (1996). *Annual medical examiner data 1994: Data from the Drug Abuse Warning Network (DAWN)* (Series 1, No. 14-B, DHHS Publication No. SMA 95-3063). Washington, DC: U.S. Government Printing Office.

Tusel, D. J., Piotrowski, N. A., Sees, K. L., Reilly, P. M., Banys, P., Meek, P., & Hall, S. M. (1995). Contingency contracting for illicit drug use with opioid addicts in methadone treatment. In L. S. Harris (Ed.), *Problems of drug dependence 1994: Proceedings of the 56th annual scientific meeting* (NIDA Research Monograph No. 153, pp. 155). Washington, DC: U. S. Government Printing Office.

Vuchinich, R. E., & Tucker, J. A. (1988). Contributions from behavioral theories of choice as a framework to an analysis of alcohol abuse. *Journal of Abnormal Psychology, 97,* 181–195.

Young, A. M., & Herling, S. (1986). Drugs as reinforcers: Studies in laboratory animals. In S. R. Goldberg & I. P. Stolerman (Eds.), *Behavioral analysis of drug dependence* (pp. 9–67). Orlando FL: Academic Press.

# 11

# Increasing the Impact of Nicotine Dependence Treatment: Conceptual and Practical Considerations in a Stepped-Care Plus Treatment-Matching Approach

DAVID B. ABRAMS
MATTHEW M. CLARK
TERESA K. KING

Research on tobacco and nicotine dependence (primarily cigarette smoking) spans more than 30 years of concerted interdisciplinary efforts to reduce the overall population prevalence of tobacco use and its health-damaging consequences (U.S. Department of Health and Human Services, 1989, 1990). Intervention opportunities include primary prevention directed at youth, self-help and clinical treatments directed at smokers who are motivated to quit, and public health interventions directed at all tobacco users and that include mass media, informational, educational, legislative, and policy approaches (Abrams, Emmons, Niaura, Goldstein, & Sherman, 1991). The enormous breadth and depth of knowledge on tobacco use provides a unique opportunity to examine the potential for developing more comprehensive, populationwide models to further reduce tobacco liability. At the center of this opportunity is the need to integrate individual and public health perspectives in order to optimize the use of limited societal resources in a cost-effective manner.

Despite steady reductions in population smoking prevalence since the 1964 Surgeon General's Report, the reduction in prevalence has recently begun to level off (Centers for Disease Control and Prevention, 1994) and youth adoption is once more on the rise. Smoking remains the leading preventable cause of chronic disease, morbidity, mortality, and unnecessary expense to society (U.S. Department of Health and Human Services, 1990). Traditional clinical treatment models are limited in that they reach only a small minority of highly motivated and generally more educated smokers with efficacious but costly treatments, requiring face-to-face meetings over weeks or months (Shiffman, 1993). New strategies are needed to (1) proactively reach and motivate the vast majority of those adults who are still smoking; (2) provide access to appropriate treatments, including addressing the needs of the uninsured and less educated; and (3) enhance the likelihood of successful cessation and long-term maintenance of cessation. The shift from predominantly clinical models to population or public health approaches requires concomitant changes in conceptual, methodological, and practical perspectives (Abrams, 1995; Abrams et al., 1991; Lichtenstein & Glasgow, 1992).

This chapter focuses on strategies to move beyond traditional clinical approaches to smoking cessation among adults by employing a hypothetical or ideal model, namely, a combined stepped-care and patient treatment–matching approach (Abrams et al., 1993, 1996). The chapter explores conceptual and methodological issues that underlie an integrated model that bridges clinical and public health perspectives; reviews selected interventions that primarily lie at the public health end of the spectrum of interventions, and discusses computer applications made possible by technological advances. The more intensive clinical (i.e., cognitive-behavioral and pharmacological) treatments have been reviewed elsewhere (e.g., Fiore, Smith, Jorenby, & Baker, 1994; Shiffman, 1993; Silagy, Mant, Fowler, & Lodge, 1994) and are mentioned only briefly to complete the range of intervention options. Primary prevention of smoking initiation among youth and public health strategies, including tax disincentives and restrictive smoking policies, also are part of a comprehensive approach to renewing the stalled rate of smoking prevalence reduction in the United States, but are beyond the scope of the chapter (see Abrams et al., 1991).

## CONCEPTUAL AND METHODOLOGICAL CONSIDERATIONS

Despite the lessons learned from decades of research on tobacco dependence, the field still needs a better theoretical integration of knowledge derived from the disciplines that embrace basic biobehavioral mechanisms (e.g., individual differences in dependence severity, comorbidity of mood disorders), behavioral and pharmacological clinical trials, and larger scale public health interventions directed at defined populations (e.g., community or work-site settings, members of a group health plan). The conceptual challenge for the year 2000 and beyond is to integrate knowledge to reach the largest number of people at the most reasonable cost, with the best possible quality of care and range of treatments.

The target population for a comprehensive approach to adult smoking prevalence reduction within society is often given insufficient consideration. Ideally, the population should be viewed as including all current smokers. The vast majority of smokers, however, may be unmotivated to quit or reluctant to volunteer for an intervention. Thus, achieving a reduction in the population smoking prevalence is a conservative outcome measure of overall impact, since it includes all adult smokers in the denominator, not simply the participants who were recruited reactively or who volunteered for treatment programs.

The evaluation of a comprehensive intervention strategy requires a new measure of outcome that includes the concept of overall population impact, which is a combination of three related factors: (1) treatment efficacy; (2) degree of "reach" or penetration into the target population; and (3) cost and feasibility of intervention delivery. Clinical treatments have the greatest efficacy, but they are the most costly and reach only a very small minority of smokers (e.g., 3–5%) who are highly motivated, have higher incomes, are more educated, and who self-select into the clinical treatment (Abrams & Biener, 1992; Biener & Abrams, 1991). Large-scale public health interventions usually employ low-cost treatments, such as self-change booklets, in their education campaigns and generally can proactively reach a much larger proportion of the target population. Treatment efficacy is low when using educational booklets, and the vast majority of smokers who are reached by them will be low in motivation to quit (Abrams & Biener, 1992; Lichtenstein & Glasgow, 1992; Velicer et al., 1995). However, large-scale public health interventions can still have a moderate impact due to a combination of low efficacy and high reach. Many interventions fall somewhere in between the extremes of the clinical to public health continuum. Generally, the cost of an intervention is related to its intensity and its efficacy, with the most intensive programs (e.g., inpatient or outpatient clinical, pharmacological, and cognitive behavioral treatments) being the most costly and the public health interventions (e.g., self-change brochures, booklets) being the least costly.

Clearly, an index of "impact" that combines measures of efficacy, cost, and reach permits a more level playing field to compare different interventions that vary in their intensity, mode and method of delivery, and degree of penetration into a population (Abrams et al., 1993, 1996). The impact variable permits a direct comparison of qualitatively different interventions along the clinical through the public health continuum, and it avoids the confounding of treatment components with recruitment or self-selection bias in the defined population. Intervention research that adopts this standardized measure of impact will permit a more rational and empirically based planning process for optimal delivery of a range of interventions.

The rapidly changing medical care systems in the United States (managed care) and the broader public health arena, where the emphasis is on health promotion and disease prevention, provide an extraordinary opportunity to consider an expanded definition of intervention and outcome. At a time when society demands more accountability, smoking intervention strategies need to move beyond clinical and therapist-assisted interventions that are intensive, costly, and time-consuming to provide a range of intervention options, while at the same time ensuring that all individuals receive the proper level and intensity of treatment that they need (i.e., based on individual differences and past history of quit attempts). Such an approach requires a theoretical integration of (1) research knowledge concerning etiological and biobehavioral mechanisms of tobacco dependence; (2) "best practice" guidelines (e.g., Fiore et al., 1996); and (3) knowledge concerning ways to increase motivation and methods of overcoming barriers to access, especially for hard-to-reach populations of smokers. Three related conceptual categories are useful in identifying an optimal range of intervention possibilities. These dimensions include individual smoker characteristics; treatment characteristics; and the channels, modes, and methods of intervention delivery that range from individuals to small groups, organizations, communities, and societal levels of social structure.

Smoker characteristics include individual differences at the biobehavioral level, as well as sociodemographics and group characteristics such as cultural and ethnic background. The major factors relevant to behavior change appear to be the smoker's level of motivation and interest in cessation, the degree of severity of nicotine dependence, the degree of comorbidity of a substance use disorder, mood disorder (especially depression), and medical disorders that are complicated or exacerbated by smoking (Hughes, 1994; Ockene et al., 1992). Other important considerations include smoking and social learning history, coping skills in high-risk situations, social supports, sociodemographics, and socioeconomic status (SES) (Shiffman, 1993). Poverty is a common barrier that limits access to treatment of any kind and especially to the more intensive and costly treatments. There is an overrepresentation of ethnic minorities in the lower SES groups, and lower SES groups have a higher prevalence of smoking (Fiore et al., 1989). Special populations such as pregnant women also are important. The individual and group characteristics of smokers must be considered when developing an optimal approach to adult smoking cessation, and interventions tailored to them are likely to be more effective than generic cessation programs (Gritz, Kristeller, & Burns, 1993; Ockene et al., 1992; Orleans, Rotberg, Quade, & Lees, 1990; Taylor, Houston-Miller, Killen, & DeBusk, 1990; Windsor et al., 1885). If such characteristics are ignored, an intervention's overall impact and cost-effectiveness can be diminished, either by reducing its efficacy or by limiting its reach into the target population.

Along with the smoker's characteristics, treatment components will also influence the impact, outcome, and cost-effectiveness of interventions. The Agency for Health Care Policy and Research (AHCPR) recently conducted a meta-analysis of the essential elements in effective treatment (Fiore et al., 1996). In general, a dose–response relationship exists between treatment intensity and positive outcomes. Although this relationship is more tenuous for other addictive behaviors (e.g., the treatment of alcohol dependence), the dose–response relationship for smoking cessation interventions provides suggestive support for a stepped-care approach to treatment matching. Treatments can range from minimal self-change and self-help programs to moderate interventions such as brief advice, with or without pharmacological aid delivered in a primary care physician's office, to more traditional and intensive clinical treatment programs such as 8- to 24-week behavior therapy programs or behavior therapy plus nicotine replacement pharmacotherapy. Treatments can vary in mode and methods of delivery, as well as in their intensity, complexity, and cost. In general, treatments can be arranged along a continuum from the least to the most intensive, complex, and costly. Typically, the more intensive interventions will employ highly trained specialist providers (e.g., doctoral psychologists or psychiatrists with expert training in nicotine dependence), and such treatments will also combine pharmacological and behavioral components to yield the enhanced effectiveness observed in the more intensive randomized clinical trials (Fiore et al., 1996). For example, the 6- to 12-month abstinence rates range from 5% to 15% for self-change programs, from 8% to 25% for moderately intense programs (brief advice and nicotine replacement), and from 20% to 40% for intensive clinical treatments (Lichtenstein & Glasgow, 1992; Schwartz, 1985; Shiffman, 1993).

Different treatment settings and modes of delivery will have implications for cost and ease of dissemination and, therefore, for impact. The options include telephone, direct mail, television, interactive computer, primary care physician offices, substance abuse programs, hospitals, worksites, schools, other community organizations, visiting nurses, health insurance plans, volunteer agencies (e.g., American Lung, Cancer, or Heart Associations) and for-profit commercial programs. Treatment programs also usually assume that the smoker is motivated to quit and ready to acquire skills for cessation and relapse prevention. Yet the vast majority of smokers (over 70%) in a defined population are not interested in quitting (Abrams & Biener, 1992; Velicer et al., 1995), which results in a serious mismatch between treatment goals and smoker needs. In order to evaluate progress toward cessation among the majority of smokers who are not motivated to quit, measures that are precursors to active behavior change need to be considered as intermediate outcomes. Measures of intermediate outcomes usually include the number of 24-hour quit attempts made during the past year, movement along the stages of readiness to change as conceptualized by the transtheoretical model (Prochaska, Redding, & Evers, 1996), or increases in the continuous measure of motivational readiness as conceptualized from the social learning theory perspective (Biener & Abrams, 1991).

In both the alcohol and nicotine dependence research literatures, the notion of client treatment matching is neither new nor without strong intuitive and conceptual appeal (Institute of Medicine, 1990). Empirical studies of basic genetic, biological, and cognitive-behavioral mechanisms; human and animal laboratory studies; treatment outcome trials; and, recently, prevention and early intervention trials with a more population or public health focus can be used to develop promising matching hypotheses (Abrams et al., 1996; Longabaugh, Wirtz, DiClemente, & Litt, 1994; Mattson et al., 1994). Yet surprisingly few adequately powered, controlled trials of matching hypotheses have been conducted, and we are not aware of any in the smoking literature. Thus, the stepped-care plus matching model outlined here is speculative and heuristic. Moreover, in the alcohol literature, Project MATCH (Project MATCH Research Group, 1997), the largest and most rigorous matching trial conducted to date, generally did not support the matching hypotheses, and 1-year outcomes were similar across the study's three psychosocial treatments (cognitive behavioral skills training, motivational enhancement therapy, and 12-step facilitation).

For several reasons, the negative results of Project MATCH should be interpreted cautiously within the context of alcohol treatment (see Chapter 2, this volume) and should not be generalized prematurely to nicotine dependence treatment or to other therapies for other addictive behaviors. With respect to the dimensions of treatment variables and patient characteristics, Project MATCH researchers had to make compromises that potentially truncated the range of options tested. This truncation is most evident concerning the more "macro" dimensions of matching. First, the qualitatively different levels of complexity of treatments were not tested in the MATCH trial. For example, Project MATCH did not test the full range of intensity of treatment options, from minimal self-help materials to moderate, brief interventions, to the most intensive combined multicomponent treatments (e.g., group therapy, phamacotherapy, individual therapy, medical education, and support groups). Second, the treatment sample was a clinical, self-selected, and reactively recruited sample that severely truncated the range of several key patient characteristics that may influence treatment engagement (e.g., motivational readiness to change) and outcomes (e.g., individuals with more severe psychiatric problems were excluded, as were those who lacked a social network contact who could serve as a collateral informant). Third, the use of a clinical sample skewed the sample in the direction of overrepresenting the minority of problem drinkers with the means and motivation to seek formal treatment. As is the case for smoking treatment, the vast majority of problem drinkers do not present for formal treatment. In the smoking literature, such smokers tend to be very low in motivation for treatment, or they lack access to clinical care due to barriers such as cost and lack of health insurance. Finally, all treatments in Project MATCH were psychosocial in nature and may have shared common elements that overshadowed their differences, and no pharmacotherapies were used, even though they are a common, effective component in smoking cessation programs.

Clearly, various components of nicotine dependence treatment can interact with smoker characteristics to produce a number of ways to conceptualize treatment matching, as well as to optimize intervention impact and cost-effectiveness. The potential for improving outcomes by matching smoker characteristics to intervention components is conceptually appealing at both a macro and micro level. The macro level of matching involves tailoring interventions to group-level characteristics, including the degree of motivational readiness to quit; demographics such as age, gender, education, and income; and the needs of special populations, such as cultural factors for ethnic minorities or materials designed for low literacy groups. Micro-level matching involves biobehavioral factors at the individual level, such as the severity of nicotine dependence, past history of quit attempts, and comorbid mood or substance use disorders. A comprehensive algorithm for smoking prevalence reduction using a concept such as the assessment (triage) of selected individual differences and the assignment of smokers to interventions (matching) is needed, but its precise parameters remain to be determined. Few studies have explicitly evaluated promising matching hypotheses in a rigorous fashion, which requires (1) the inclusion of smokers with a full range of differences in individual characteristics (e.g., smokers with low, moderate, and high dependence on nicotine); (2) development of assessment instruments with reasonable sensitivity and specificity; and (3) treatments that include random assignment to both matched and mismatched conditions.

In summary, recent literature reviews (e.g., Lichtenstein & Glasgow, 1992) indicate a movement away from individual clinical treatments toward brief interventions delivered by generalists, rather than by specialists, and toward more broadscale public health interventions. Other reviews (Abrams et al., 1991; Shiffman, 1993) suggest that increasing smoking cessation rates through further improvements in clinical cognitive-behavioral treatments is unlikely and that further reductions in cessation rates will likely come from distributing available interventions over a broader segment of the smoking population. A paucity of data exists, however, about the essential elements required for optimal intervention strategies that combine knowledge of biobehavioral mechanisms, clinical trials, and public health models; identify how best to match smoker characteristics with treatment research on "best practice" guidelines for both pharmacotherapy and cognitive behavioral therapy; and take into account issues of program cost, treatment delivery, motivation, reach, and access to treatment among underserved segments of the smoking population. The major dimensions of smoker characteristics, standardized measures, modes and methods of delivery, and types of treatment components must be better integrated to bridge the gap between individual clinical treatments and population or public health interventions for adult smoking cessation. As discussed next, numerous empirical studies and recent reviews suggest the utility of a stepped-care patient treatment-matching approach that spans the clinical to public health continuum of interventions. While this approach is not new (Abrams et al., 1993, 1996; Hughes, 1994; Orleans, 1993), it remains to be empirically evaluated in a systematic way.

## A STEPPED-CARE PLUS
## TREATMENT-MATCHING MODEL

The stepped-care plus treatment-matching model has been presented in detail elsewhere (Abrams et al., 1993, 1996) and is summarized here. The model assumes that the goal is to intervene to reduce overall smoking prevalence in the entire population of smokers within a society. The model takes a proactive approach of reaching out to make contact with all smokers, regardless of their current interest in or motivational readiness for cessation. Any proactive intervention must overcome barriers to access and then must reach and begin to motivate the majority of smokers who are not ready to quit. This initial assessment and treatment of motivational readiness ensure that more costly pharmacological or behavioral treatments for cessation are not prematurely provided to smokers who are not ready for them. Since change in motivation becomes the target of the intervention, the variables that influence motivation (e.g., environmental factors, cognitive-behavioral processes; see Chapter 5, this volume) need to be better understood and measured. In order to measure progress with unmotivated smokers, an appropriate time frame must also be established to allow for changes to take place. The time frame is likely to be on the order of years, rather than the weeks or months used in clinical outcome studies to measure initial cessation.

Cognitive-behavioral interventions to enhance motivation are used, such as those described by Miller and Rollnick (1991). Motivational interventions are based on social learning theory (Bandura, 1986, 1995) and share variables and processes with other theories, such as those described in the health belief model (see Strecher & Rosenstock, 1996) and the transtheoretical model (e.g., Prochaska et al., 1996). Interventions to enhance motivation are provided to smokers with low motivation to quit and employed until such time as the assessment of motivational readiness (Biener & Abrams, 1991; Prochaska, et al., 1996) reveals that the smoker is ready to consider cessation.

There is controversy concerning how best to conceptualize and measure change in motivational readiness, that is, either as a series of stages (e.g., Prochaska et al., 1996) or as a continuous variable or set of mediating mechanisms involving nicotine dependence and cognitive social learning constructs such as proximal goal setting and outcome expectations (Abrams & Biener, 1992; Bandura, 1986, 1995; Farkas et al., 1996; Sutton, 1996). This debate notwithstanding, consensus exists about the importance of the concept of motivational readiness and the need to develop sensitive measures of change in motivation. Thus, the first phase in the stepped-care plus matching model involves tailoring motivation-enhancing interventions to smokers who can be reached but are not ready to consider cessation (see Figure 11.1). Those smokers who cannot be reached require an intervention that examines the barriers to the utilization of interventions (e.g., social, cultural, financial, or educational issues; see Chapters 3 and 4, this volume). These factors can sometimes be addressed only at a policy or regulatory level.

As shown in Figure 11.1, once a smoker is motivated to quit, then the model has three broad levels of intervention in the stepped-care component. There is also an assessment and subsequent matching component in the model that is based on smoker characteristics (described later). The stepped-care levels of intervention are as follows:

Step 1—Minimal, self-change or self-help approaches
Step 2—Moderate, brief counseling
Step 3—Maximal, specialized intensive clinical treatments in outpatient and inpatient settings.

The three-step distinction is arbitrary; therefore, consensus on the boundaries between steps can be difficult to achieve. For example, a more intensive Step 1 intervention begins to overlap with a less intensive Step 2 inter-

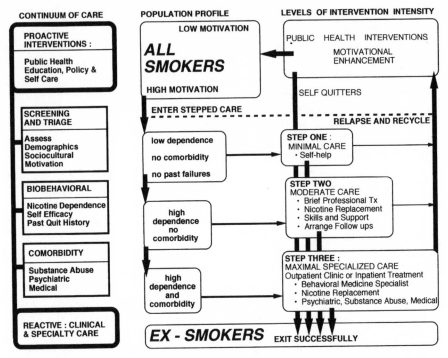

**FIGURE 11.1.** Schematic overview of the stepped-care plus treatment-matching model for smoking cessation. From Abrams et al. (1996). Reprinted by permission of the *Annals of Behavioral Medicine.*

vention. These three steps represent a simplified heuristic classification based on possible interventions that range from the least to the most intensive and costly.

The primary goal of the stepped-care component of the model is to ensure that the largest possible percentage of the population of smokers is reached with the least costly and most easily disseminated intervention that is nevertheless sufficiently intensive to promote smoking cessation. The model presumes that most of the smokers who have never tried to quit before, and especially those who fall within the light range of severity of nicotine dependence (the relatively uncomplicated smoker), should be treated sequentially, beginning with Step 1, and should be "stepped up" only if they fail to quit or show emerging complications (e.g., withdrawal symptoms, depression) during a serious quit attempt. There is some empirical justification for this strategy in that lighter smokers (≤ 20 cigarettes/day) are 2.1 times more likely to succeed with minimal interventions than are heavier smokers (Cohen et al., 1989). In contrast, smokers with serious complications such as comorbid psychiatric or substance use disorders can bypass the stepped-care part of the model and be assigned directly to more intensive treatment to avoid potential failure experiences (see triage system below).

Smokers who fail to achieve cessation at a lower level of intervention intensity are then stepped up to a moderate level of treatment (Step 2) that includes one or all of the following: brief behavioral counseling, a support group such as those offered by voluntary agencies (American Lung Association or American Cancer Society), and pharmacological interventions such as nicotine replacement. Pharmacological interventions can be delivered by a primary care physician and include brief face-to-face counseling and telephone follow-ups, usually with a health educator or nurse (Hollis, Lichtenstein, Vogt, Stevens, & Biglan, 1993).

Finally, a smaller number of smokers will require the most specialized and intensive treatment (Step 3) either on an outpatient or inpatient basis. Recent reports suggest consideration of inpatient treatment for smokers with severe levels of nicotine dependence and comorbid complications such as psychiatric or substance use disorders (Hurt et al., 1992). Inpatient treatment could be viewed as the maximal level of a Step 3 intervention or as a distinct, new category (Step 4). The AHCPR guidelines and meta-analyses (Fiore et al., 1994, 1996) provide empirical support for Steps 2 and 3, suggesting that nicotine replacement boosts the quit rates of all smokers (approximately a doubling effect), and especially the rates for heavy smokers (> 25 cigarettes/day), and that treatment intensity and efficacy are positively related.

To ensure that smokers with a history of repeated, failed quit attempts, known complications such as severe withdrawal symptoms during past quit attempts, or comorbid mood or substance use disorders, receive the appropriate level of care, a triage system is included in the stepped-care model by adding a patient treatment-matching component. Each smoker is evaluated for individual differences that can range from the needs of the least complicated smoker (e.g., low dependence, no comorbidity) to the needs of the smoker with severe complications, who is likely to be at high risk of failure to quit (e.g., a smoker with severe nicotine dependence, past difficulty quitting, and comorbid substance abuse). Based on this assessment, a smoker with complications can be directly assigned to a more intensive (Step 2 or 3) level of intervention, rather than first going through the sequential stepped-care process beginning with Step 1, which is the appropriate starting point for smokers with few complications and may be all that is necessary.

Recalcitrant smokers are included in the treatment model on an ongoing and repeated basis. Smoking at any level is harmful, and continued engagement in interventions should eventually lead to sustained motivation to quit, higher efficacy expectations, and periods of abstinence. The model considers smoking as a chronic disease, requiring continued monitoring over many years, as necessary. The chronic disease concept is the equivalent of treating diabetes or hypertension in medical practice where pharmacological, cognitive-behavioral, and social support interventions are required for a lifetime. For some recalcitrant smokers, the emphasis of interventions may have to change from abstinence to a harm reduction (Marlatt & Tapert, 1993) counseling approach. The client may be unable to quit for many reasons, for example, because of severe nicotine dependence, a comorbid psychiatric or substance use disorder, lack of health insurance or limited financial resources, or demoralization due to repeated failed attempts to quit. Harm reduction as an alternative to repeated attempts at smoking cessation could be considered, but only if abstinence-oriented alternatives have been tried and failed. Therefore, individuals who have repeatedly failed to quit on their own or with minimal interventions, but have lacked access to a credible Step 3 treatment that offers state-of-the-art behavioral and pharmacotherapy, should not be considered candidates for harm reduction until the Step 3 treatment has been given and has also failed.

A harm reduction approach is controversial because it can be misinterpreted as accepting lesser levels of smoking rather than total abstinence. Any level of smoking is harmful, as is exposure to secondhand smoke. However, given the ready availability of effective and safe alternative nicotine delivery systems (e.g., nicotine gum, transdermal patches, nasal spray), harm reduction for recalcitrant smokers becomes attractive if it employs one of these safer, alternative forms of nicotine delivery. Harm reduction involves a client-centered approach to intervention, beginning with meeting the client's needs and accepting small steps that reduce the health damaging effects of smoking. Although some may view reduced rates of smoking as "harm reduction," this is arguable because of evidence that smoking topography (e.g., rate and depth of inhalation) may change to compensate for reductions in the number of cigarettes smoked or in the nicotine level in cigarettes (Kozlowski & Ferrence, 1990; Kozlowski, Pope, & Lux, 1988). These changes could increase harm to the smoker. Nicotine replacement using one of the alternative delivery systems thus is preferable to reduced cigarette smoking as a means of reducing harm.

Nicotine dependence is approached within a stepped-care matching model like a chronic disease, such as diabetes or hypertension, rather than an acute illness. Physical and psychological dependence may be severe. The basic craving for nicotine may remain for a lifetime. Encouragement to quit and continued support after cessation to prevent relapse (Marlatt & Gordon, 1985) can be made available over the lifespan. Fiore et al. (1994)

suggested that smoking status and treatment be made a "vital sign" to be assessed routinely at every contact with a health care provider. The "best practice" guidelines of the AHCPR (Fiore et al., 1996) have adopted this position, and it also has been proposed as part of the "report card" for quality assurance of managed care organizations by the National Committee on Quality Assurance.

The chronic disease concept also provides for flexibility of care, rather than an "all or nothing" approach that implies failure on the part of both the provider and the smoker unless cessation occurs immediately (Marlatt & Tapert, 1993). It also requires changes at the systems level, in terms of national health care policy and the alignment of practice guidelines and incentives within existing health care delivery systems.

There are certain essential elements of treatment that form a common core for all three levels of intervention within and across steps (for details, see Orleans & Slade, 1993). Cognitive-behavioral treatment strategies (Schwartz, 1985; Shiffman, 1993; U.S. Department of Health and Human Services, 1988, 1990) include the following: during the early phase of treatment, behavioral strategies such as contingency contracting, nicotine fading, stimulus control, choosing a quit date, and self-monitoring of smoking are useful (Abrams & Wilson, 1986; Brown, Goldstein, Niaura, Emmons, & Abrams, 1993). Once the quit day has been reached, the other major social-cognitive learning techniques are typically introduced, such as relapse prevention strategies (Brown et al., 1993; Marlatt & Gordon, 1985). These include developing skills to cope with high-risk emotional and social situations and enhancing social support (Lichtenstein, Glasgow, & Abrams, 1986). Two decades of research suggest that this basic cognitive-behavioral approach can provide the components for a high-quality treatment program at any level of intensity, such as a self-help manual or an inpatient treatment program (Abrams et al., 1991; Lichtenstein & Glasgow, 1992; Orleans, 1988; Orleans & Slade, 1993; Schwartz, 1985), and will produce good outcomes in the range of 25–40% cessation at 6- to 12-month follow-ups (Abrams & Wilson, 1986; Hughes, 1993; Schwartz, 1985). These elements can also form the basis for developing best practice guidelines, standards for certification and training of service providers (both generalists and specialists), and for developing "report cards" (Health Plan Employer Data & Information Set, 1994) to evaluate the quality of programs for consumers and purchasers of health insurance plans (see Chapter 13, this volume).

In summary, the stepped-care plus matching model takes into account the lessons learned from the basic biobehavioral and biomedical sciences, individual differences, psychosocial and motivational factors in clinical and public health interventions, and the need to be accountable and cost-effective to society. The remainder of the chapter focuses on selected practical examples of stepped care, with emphasis on self-change and other less intensive interventions that form the backbone of Step 1 and low-level Step 2 interventions. These interventions are likely to be more easily disseminated and less costly, but they typically are less effective at the individual level compared to clinical treatments. A more complete review of all three steps (minimal, moderate, and maximal) may be found in Abrams et al. (1996).

## SELF-CHANGE AND SELF-HELP

Self-change can be viewed as reflecting the background quit rate in the population in the absence of formal interventions. Smokers may perceive themselves as having "quit on their own," and the level of intervention intensity is by definition close to zero. Self-change is hard to define because smokers may have been exposed to some behavior-change communications on an informal basis. Few smokers (less than 5%) per year successfully quit without an intervention, and self-changers can make many quit attempts before they attain maintenance of cessation (American Psychiatric Association, 1996; Cohen et al., 1989). Research is needed to investigate whether the natural process of self-change can be accelerated and whether key elements of it can be incorporated into or facilitated by interventions.

Self-help programs are interventions that smokers can obtain without having to see a professional or attend a clinic. Materials can be sent (proactively) or a smoker can initiate brief contact (reactively) with whatever system provides the materials. Programs typically involve the use of standardized self-help manuals using the latest research (Curry, 1993; Glynn, Boyd, & Gruman, 1990). These self-help programs can be widely disseminated and produce 5–15% cessation rates at 12-month follow-up (Curry, 1993; Curry, Wagner, & Grothaus, 1991; Fiore et al., 1989, 1990; Glynn et al., 1990; Velicer, Prochaska, Rossi, & Snow, 1992). One limitation of self-help programs is that standardized materials may not be effective for underserved minority or other hard-to-reach populations. Two questions, therefore, need to be addressed: First, are there different outcomes among minority and majority population groups, and, second, can efficacious, tailored, self-help materials be designed for underserved groups? Unfortunately, because of a lack of research, these questions cannot be answered definitely at this time, but experts have noted that tailoring is sometimes necessary for interventions to be effective, especially for minority populations (Smoking Cessation Clinical Practice Guideline Panel and Staff, 1996).

In support of this consensus statement, evidence suggests that programs that specifically target a particular group increase smoking cessation rates (e.g., Gritz et al., 1993; Orleans, 1993; Rimer et al., 1994; Windsor et al., 1985). Rimer and colleagues (1994), for example, conducted focus groups with older adults to create a self-help guide entitled *Clear Horizons* for older smokers. *Clear Horizons* included state-of-the-art advice about quitting and continued abstinence, and photo vignettes using older, multiracial smokers and health messages that highlighted the benefits of quitting for older smokers. Smokers aged 50–74 ($N$ = 1,867) were then randomly assigned to one of three conditions: (1) a control group that received a standard self-help packet, *Clearing the Air*, published by the National Cancer Institute; (2) an experimental group that received *Clear Horizons*; or (3) an experimental group that received *Clear Horizons* plus two brief (10- to 15-minute) telephone counseling sessions. At a 12-month follow-up, self-reported quit rates were 15%, 20%, and 19%, respectively. The experimental groups achieved significantly higher quit rates, providing support for the continued development and design of tailored self-help material. Similar quit rates (14–18%) have been reported by other researchers (e.g., Orleans et al., 1991).

## APPLICATIONS INVOLVING COMPUTER TECHNOLOGY

A stepped-care approach recognizes the need to minimize intrusions in individuals' lives, the importance of containing costs at all levels of the health care system, and the importance of interventions that can be applied to the community at large. Interventions using computer applications are uniquely capable of achieving these goals and have been developed and implemented for smoking cessation (e.g., Curry et al., 1991; Orlandi, Dozier, & Marta, 1990; Velicer et al., 1993). For example, Curry and colleagues (1991) found that computer-generated personalized feedback, which was designed to increase smokers' confidence in utilizing a self-help smoking cessation program, significantly increased both utilization and quit rates. Computer technology also has been used to simulate consumer preferences for different smoking cessation interventions. Spoth (1992) described the use of computer simulations to illustrate how adding or deleting a specific element of a smoking cessation program affected consumer responses. The methodology could be used to modify existing programs to increase acceptability among subgroups of smokers.

The more general challenge is how to deliver such interventions in a cost-effective manner. Until the advent of computer technology, tailoring interventions to subgroup, much less individual, characteristics appeared daunting, if not impossible, except on a small scale. Once developed, computer programs can deliver interventions that are tailored to the subgroup or individual level at low cost. For example, interventions can be tailored according to participants' educational level and other demographic characteristics and also to their individual level of motivation. Such interventions are increasingly available, although the number of well-controlled treatment outcome studies are few (Ramirez & Gallion, 1993).

In the past, Step 1 self-help smoking cessation materials contained costs by delivering the same generic intervention to all smokers, and no attempt was made to tailor the materials to the needs of individuals. Although such universal interventions have been a keystone of public health interventions that have decreased the prevalence of smoking, an important but unanswered question is whether the smoking materials used in these programs can be varied and then distributed in targeted ways that increase their utilization and efficacy (Ockene, 1992). Computer technology offers a dissemination vehicle for tailored interventions and can be used, for example, to deliver smoking cessation communications that are tailored to smokers' levels of motivation and personal risks of continued smoking.

Expert systems have proven to be an efficacious, cost-effective way to tailor smoking cessation materials and can be implemented on a large enough scale to reach significant segments of the population (e.g., Velicer et al., 1993). Expert systems are software applications that utilize a collection of facts and rules to mimic the reasoning of a human expert in order to solve problems and give advice (Jackson, 1986). Velicer and colleagues (1993) described an expert system they developed and implemented for smoking cessation that used the transtheoretical model as its conceptual base (Prochaska & DiClemente, 1983). Smokers first completed questionnaires concerning their smoking habits and cognitive-behavioral mediators of smoking cessation. This information was then used in the expert system to develop individualized baselines and progress reports that were mailed to the smokers. The baseline report compared each smoker's answers with normative data on smokers who had quit and suggested strategies to move the smoker toward taking action to quit. Subsequent reports used normative and individual data to provide feedback regarding progress and suggestions for improvement. Prochaska, DiClemente, Velicer, and Rossi (1993) compared this expert system intervention to three other interventions, including standardized self-help manuals, individualized self-help manuals matched to participants' stage of change, and the expert system augmented with personalized counselor calls. At all follow-up points for smokers at all stages of change, the expert system alone produced better outcomes than either self-help-manual intervention and produced outcomes that were equivalent to or better than the more costly expert system augmented by personalized calls.

Although expert systems appear promising, the initial investment of time and effort, and the necessary computer skills and equipment may discourage their widespread use. Continued improvement in commercial software will ease this impediment to application. For example, word-processing software exists to combine a data document of relevant characteristics of the smoker with a master document containing the structure of a tailored letter; tailored letters have been shown to increase smoking cessation rates among moderate to light smokers, more so than a generic letter (Strecher et al., 1994). This type of message tailoring can be easily accomplished by individuals who lack computer programming skills.

Step 2 interventions involve more interaction between health care providers and smokers, as well as greater intervention tailoring and social support, and are indicated for higher risk smokers with higher nicotine dependence. Trained clinicians typically deliver Step 2 interventions, but this labor-intensive approach is prohibitively expensive for use on a large scale. Given that at least one study (Prochaska et al., 1993) found that computer-generated feedback alone was as good as or better than feedback plus personalized counselor calls in promoting smoking cessation, computer applications may be a good way to reduce costs while providing personalized treatment. For example, personalized computer messages could be combined with use of a nicotine patch as a Step 2 intervention.

Step 3 interventions for smokers who have failed to quit smoking with Steps 1 and 2, or who have comorbid psychiatric or medical conditions, also can be computerized in part, but probably not in their entirety. For instance, depression is a significant barrier to smoking cessation (e.g., Anda et al., 1990) and may indicate the need for costly pharmacological and inpatient interventions. One less expensive alternative that shows promise is the use of "digital therapists" (Brandon, Copeland, & Saper, 1995). Providing smokers with computer-controlled audiotape players that present personalized therapeutic messages negates or reverses the usual association between negative affect and poor outcomes (Brandon et al., 1995).

Medical comorbidity suggests the need for a higher level of care, and medical conditions such as coronary artery disease can preclude the use of effective nicotine replacement agents. Thus, a need exists for effective smoking cessation protocols (e.g., nicotine fading) that are not contraindicated by medical conditions. Nicotine fading uses a standard schedule to reduce nicotine delivery by 30% each week for 3 weeks (Foxx & Brown, 1979). On the one hand, compensatory smoking (increased puffing) has been observed in some smokers who tried to quit with nicotine fading (Burling, Lovett, Frederiksen, Jerome, & Jonske-Gubosh, 1989), which attenuates its therapeutic impact. On the other hand, the precision of nicotine fading can be enhanced by the use of computer technology. Burling, Seidner, and Gaither (1994) recently described a program that used computer technology to measure puffing. A cigarette holder and pressure transducer were attached to a microcomputer, so that puffs taken through the holder were computer recorded. This information was used to individualize nicotine fading schedules for smokers based on their daily smoking behavior. Preliminary data indicated that computer-directed nicotine fading resulted in reductions in biological levels of nicotine, and it thus may provide a safe alternative for smokers who cannot use nicotine replacement products.

Overall, computer technology has numerous applications and may help contain costs while increasing intervention effectiveness and accessibility. Probably the greatest benefit is the opportunity that computers afford to individualize interventions in a manner akin to therapist-directed treatments, but at the low cost of traditional public health approaches. Computer applications can enhance interventions at every level of the stepped-care approach. They can be designed so that they are accessible to large segments of the smoking population and may prove to be more acceptable to the vast majority of smokers who do not enroll in formal cessation programs. Computer applications also can be combined with behavioral treatments and pharmacological agents for smokers who require more intensive treatment.

## CONCLUSIONS

Intervention strategies for nicotine dependence have ranged from primary prevention directed at youth, to public health approaches that involve media campaigns or legislative initiatives, to specialized clinical interventions that utilize pharmacotherapy and behavior therapy. From 1964 to 1990, the prevalence of smoking in the United States decreased, but since 1990, smoking rates have remained steady. New strategies are needed to reduce further the prevalence of smoking and the harm that it causes, and the stepped-care plus treatment-matching approach may prove useful. The model takes a proactive approach by reaching out to all smokers and then considers individual smoker characteristics when conceptualizing and delivering interventions that vary in cost, intensity, effectiveness, and reach. By distributing intervention resources in the manner suggested by the model, the total resource pool available for promoting smoking cessation is spread according to need and, in theory, should reach a greater portion of the population of smokers, including unmotivated smokers and smokers in vulnerable groups with limited access to health care.

Smoking cessation produces huge direct and indirect benefits, including improved health, reduced mortality, and reduced health care costs. Interventions are available that collectively form a continuum of care to promote cessation. The challenge is to distribute these interventions appropriately across the population of smokers, who vary in problem severity, motivation to change, and access to the health care system. The stepped-care plus treatment-matching model provides an approach to meet this challenge during a period when containing costs, while improving the quality and accessibility of care, are paramount.

## REFERENCES

Abrams, D. B. (1995). Integrating basic, clinical, and public health research for alcohol-tobacco interactions. In J. B. Fertig & J. P. Allen (Eds.), *Alcohol and tobacco: From basic science to clinical practice* (U.S. Department of Health and Human Services Publication No. NIH 9S-3931, pp. 3–16). Bethesda, MD: U.S. Department of Health and Human Services, National Institutes of Health, National Institute on Alcohol Abuse and Alcoholism, U.S. Government Printing Office.

Abrams, D. B., & Biener, L. (1992). Motivational characteristics of smokers at the workplace: A public health challenge. *Preventive Medicine, 21,* 679–687.

Abrams, D. B., Emmons, K. M., Niaura, R., Goldstein, M. G., & Sherman, C. B. (1991). Tobacco dependence: An integration of individual and public health perspectives. In P. Nathan, B. McCrady, J. Langenbucher, & W. Frankenstein (Eds.), *Annual review of addictions treatment and research* (Vol. 1, pp. 331–396). New York: Pergamon Press.

Abrams, D. B., Orleans, C. T., Niaura, R., Goldstein, M., Prochaska, J., & Velicer, W. (1996). Integrating individual and public health perspectives for treatment of tobacco dependence under managed health care: A combined stepped-care and matching model. *Annals of Behavioral Medicine, 18,* 290–304.

Abrams, D. B., Orleans, C. T., Niaura, R. N., Goldstein, M. G., Velicer, W., & Prochaska, J. O. (1993). Treatment issues: Towards a stepped-care model. *Tobacco Control, 2,* S17–S37.

Abrams, D. B., & Wilson, G. T. (1986). Clinical advances in treatment of smoking and alcohol addiction. In A. J. Frances & R. E. Hales (Eds.), *The American Psychiatric Association annual review: Psychiatric update* (pp. 606–626). Washington, DC: American Psychiatric Association Press.

American Psychiatric Association. (1996). Practice guideline for the treatment of patients with nicotine dependence. *American Journal of Psychiatry, 153*(Suppl. 10), 1–31.

Anda, R. F., Williamson, D. F., Escobedo, L. G., Mast, E. E., Giovino, G. A., & Remington, P. L. (1990). Depression and the dynamics of smoking: A national perspective. *Journal of the American Medical Association, 264,* 1541–1545.

Bandura, A. (1986). *Social foundations of thought and action: A social cognitive theory.* Englewood Cliffs, NJ: Prentice-Hall.

Bandura, A. (1995, March). *Moving in forward gear in health promotion and disease prevention.* Paper presented at the annual meeting of the Society of Behavioral Medicine, San Diego, CA.

Biener, L., & Abrams, D. B. (1991). The contemplation ladder: Validation of a measure of readiness to consider smoking cessation. *Health Psychology, 10,* 360–365.

Brandon, T. H., Copeland, A. L., & Saper, Z. L. (1995). Programmed therapeutic messages as a smoking treatment adjunct: Reducing the impact of negative affect. *Health Psychology, 14,* 41–47.

Brown, R. A., Goldstein, M. G., Niaura, R., Emmons, K. M., & Abrams, D. B. (1993). Nicotine dependence: Assessment and management. In A. Stoudemire & B. S. Vogel (Eds.), *Psychiatric care of the medical patient* (pp. 877–902). New York: Oxford University Press.

Burling, T. A., Lovett, S. B., Frederiksen, L. W., Jerome, A., & Jonske-Gubosh, L. (1989). Can across-treatment changes in cumulative puff duration predict treatment outcome during nicotine fading? *Addictive Behaviors, 14,* 75–82.

Burling, T. A., Seidner, A. L., & Gaither, D. E. (1994). A computer-directed program for smoking cessation treatment. *Journal of Substance Abuse, 6,* 427–431.

Centers for Disease Control and Prevention. (1994). Cigarette smoking among adults—United States, 1993. *Morbidity and Mortality Weekly Report, 43,* 925–930.

Cohen, S., Lichtenstein, E., Prochaska, J. O., Rossi, J. S., Gritz, E. R. Carr, C. R., Orleans, C. T., Schoenbach, V. J., Biener, L., Abrams, D., DiClemente, C., Curry, S., Marlatt, G. A., Cummings, K. M., Emont, S. L., Giovino, G., & Ossip-Klein, D. (1989). Debunking myths about self-quitting: Evidence from 10 prospective studies of persons who attempt to quit smoking by themselves. *American Psychologist, 44,* 1355–1365.

Curry, S. J. (1993). Self-help interventions for smoking cessation. *Journal of Consulting and Clinical Psychology, 61,* 790–803.

Curry, S. J., Wagner, E. G., & Grothaus, L.C. (1991). Evaluation of intrinsic and extrinsic motivation interventions with a self-help smoking cessation program. *Journal of Consulting and Clinical Psychology, 59,* 318–324.

Farkas, A. J., Pierce, J. P., Zhu, S.-H., Rosbrook, B., Gilpin, E. A., Berry, C., & Kaplan, R. M. (1996). Addiction versus stages of change models in predicting smoking cessation. *Addiction, 91,* 1271–1280.

Fiore, M. C., Bailey, W. C., Cohen, S. J., Fiore, M.C., Bailey, W. C., Cohen, S. J., Dorfman, S. F., Goldstein, M. G., Gritz, E. R., Heyman, R. B., Holbrook, J., Jaen, C. R., Kottke, T. E., Lando, H. A., Mecklenberg, R., Mullen, P. D., Nett, L. M., Robinson, L., Stitzer, M. L., Tommasello, A., & Villejo, L., & Wewers, M. E. (1996). *Smoking cessation* (Clinical Practice Guideline No. 18, AHCPR Publication No. 96-0692). Rockville, MD: U.S. Department of Health and Human Services, Public Health Service, Agency for Health Care Policy and Research.

Fiore, M. C., Novotny, T. E., Pierce, J. P., Giovino, G. A., Hatziandreu, E. J., Newcomb, P. A., Surawicz, T. S., & Davis, R. M. (1990). Methods used to quit smoking in the United States: Do cessation programs help? *Journal of the American Medical Association, 263,* 2760–2765.

Fiore, M. C., Novotny, T. E., Pierce, J. P., Hatziandreu, E., Patel, K. M., & Davis, R. (1989). Trends in cigarette smoking in the United States: The challenging influence of gender and race. *Journal of the American Medical Association, 261,* 49–55.

Fiore, M. C., Smith, S. S., Jorenby, D. E., & Baker, T. B. (1994). The effectiveness of the nicotine patch for smoking cessation: A meta-analysis. *Journal of the American Medical Association, 271,* 1940–1947.

Foxx, R. M., & Brown, R. A. (1979). Nicotine fading and self-monitoring for cigarette abstinence or controlled smoking. *Journal of Applied Behavior Analysis, 12,* 111–125.

Glynn, T., Boyd, G., & Gruman, J. (1990). Essential elements of self-help/minimal intervention strategies for smoking cessation. *Health Education Quarterly, 17,* 329–345.

Gritz, E. R., Kristeller, J., & Burns, D. M. (1993). Treating nicotine addiction in high-risk groups and patients with medical co-morbidity. In C. T. Orleans & J. Slade (Eds.), *Nicotine addiction: Principles and management* (pp. 279–309). New York: Oxford University Press.

Health Plan Employer Data & Information Set Indicators and Quality Report Cards. (1994). *Quality Letter, 6,* 24–27.

Hollis, J. F., Lichenstein, E., Vogt, T. M., Stevens, V. J., & Biglan, A. (1993). Nurse-assisted counseling for smokers in primary care. *Annals of Internal Medicine, 118,* 521–525.

Hughes, J. R. (1993). Pharmacotherapy for smoking cessation: Unvalidated assumptions, anomalies, and suggestions for future research. *Journal of Consulting and Clinical Psychology, 61,* 751–760.

Hughes, J. R. (1994). An algorithm for smoking cessation. *Archives of Family Medicine, 3,* 280–285.

Hurt, R. D., Dale, L. C., McClain, F. L., Eberman, K. M., Offord, K. P., Bruce B. K., & Lauger, G. G. (1992). A comprehensive model for the treatment of nicotine dependence in a medical setting. *Medical Clinics of North America, 76,* 495–514.

Institute of Medicine. (1990). *Broadening the base of treatment for alcohol problems.* Washington, DC: National Academy Press.

Jackson, P. (1986). *Introduction to expert systems.* Wokingham, UK: Addison-Wesley.

Kozlowski, L., & Ferrence, R. G. (1990). Statistical control in research on alcohol and tobacco mortality. *British Journal of Addiction, 85,* 271–278.

Kozlowski, L. T., Pope, M. A., & Lux, J. E. (1988). Prevalence of the misuse of ultra low tar cigarettes by blocking filter vents. *American Journal of Public Health, 78,* 694–695.

Lichtenstein, E., & Glasgow, R. E. (1992). Smoking cessation: What have we learned over the past decade? *Journal of Consulting and Clinical Psychology, 60,* 1–10.

Lichtenstein, E., Glasgow, R. E., & Abrams, D. B. (1986). Social support in smoking cessation: In search of effective interventions. *Behavioral Therapy, 17,* 607–619.

Longabaugh, R., Wirtz, P. W., DiClemente, C. C., & Litt, M. (1994). Issues in the development of client–treatment matching hypotheses. *Journal of Studies on Alcohol* (Suppl. 12), 46–59.

Marlatt, G. A., & Gordon, J. R. (Eds.) (1985). *Relapse prevention.* New York: Guilford Press.

Marlatt, G. A., & Tapert, S. F. (1993). Harm reduction: Reducing the risks of addictive behaviors. In J. S. Baer, G. A. Marlatt, & R. McMahon (Eds.), *Addictive behaviors across the lifespan* (pp. 243–273). Newbury Park, CA: Sage.

Mattson, M. E., Allen, J. P., Longabaugh, R., Nickless, C. J., Connors, G. J., & Kadden, R. M. (1994). A chronological review of empirical studies matching alcoholic clients to treatment. *Journal of Studies on Alcohol* (Suppl. 12), 16–29.

Miller, W. R., & Rollnick, S. (1991). *Motivational interviewing: Preparing people to change addictive behavior.* New York: Guilford Press.

Ockene, J. K. (1992). Are we pushing the limits of public health interventions for smoking cessation? *Health Psychology, 11,* 277–279.

Ockene, J., Kristeller, J., Goldberg, R., Ockene, J., Kristeller, J. L., Goldberg, R., Ockene, I., Merriam, P., Barrett, S., Pekow, P., Hosmer, D., & Gianelli, R. (1992). Smoking cessation and severity of disease: The coronary artery smoking intervention study. *Health Psychology, 11,* 119–126.

Orlandi, M. A., Dozier, C. E., & Marta, M. A. (1990). Computer-assisted strategies for substance abuse prevention: Opportunities and barriers. *Journal of Consulting and Clinical Psychology, 58,* 425–431.

Orleans, C. T. (1988). Smoking cessation in primary care settings. *Journal of the Medical Society of New Jersey, 85,* 116–125.

Orleans, C. T. (1993). Treating nicotine dependence in medical settings: A stepped care model. In C. T. Orleans & J. Slade (Eds.), *Nicotine addiction: Principles and management* (pp. 145–161). New York: Oxford University Press.

Orleans, C. T., Rotberg, H., Quade, D., & Lees, P. (1990). A hospital quit-smoking consult service: Clinical report and intervention guidelines. *Preventive Medicine, 19,* 198–212.

Orleans, C. T., Schoenbach, V. J., Wagner, E. H., Quade, D., Salmon, M. A., Pearson, D. C., Fiedler, J., Porter, C. Q., & Kaplan, B. H. (1991). Self-help quit smoking interventions: Effects of self-help materials, social support instructions, and telephone counseling. *Journal of Consulting and Clinical Psychology, 52,* 439–448.

Orleans, C. T., & Slade, J. (1993). *Nicotine addiction: Principles and management.* New York: Oxford University Press.

Prochaska, J. O., & DiClemente, C. C. (1983). Stages and processes of self-change of smoking: Toward an integrative model of change. *Journal of Consulting and Clinical Psychology, 51,* 390–395.

Prochaska, J. O., DiClemente, C. C., Velicer, W. F., & Rossi, J. S. (1993). Standardized, individualized, interactive, and personalized self-help programs for smoking cessation. *Health Psychology, 12,* 399–405.

Prochaska, J. O., Redding, C. A., & Evers, K. E. (1997). The transtheoretical model and stages of change. In K. Glanz, F. M. Lewis, & B. K. Rimer (Eds.), *Health behavior and health education* (2nd ed., pp. 60–84). San Francisco: Jossey-Bass.

Project MATCH Research Group. (1997). Matching alcoholism treatments to client heterogeneity: Project MATCH posttreatment drinking outcomes. *Journal of Studies on Alcohol, 58,* 7–29.

Ramirez, A. G., & Gallion, K. J. (1993). Nicotine dependence among blacks and Hispanics. In C. T. Orleans & J. Slade (Eds.), *Nicotine addiction: Principles and management* (pp. 350–364). New York: Oxford University Press.

Rimer, B. K., Orleans, C. T., Fleisher, L., Cristinzio, S., Resch, N., Telepchak, J., & Keintz, M. K. (1994). Does tailoring matter? The impact of a tailored guide on ratings and short-term smoking-related outcomes for older smokers. *Health Education Research, 2,* 69–84.

Schwartz, J. L. (1985). *Review and evaluation of smoking cessation methods: The United States and Canada, 1978–1985.* Bethesda: National Institutes of Health.

Shiffman, S. (1993). Smoking cessation treatment: Any progress? *Journal of Consulting and Clinical Psychology, 61,* 718–722.

Silagy, C., Mant, D., Fowler, G., & Lodge, M. (1994). Meta-analysis on efficacy of nicotine replacement therapies in smoking cessation. *Lancet, 343,* 139–142.

Smoking Cessation Clinical Practice Guideline Panel and Staff. (1996). The Agency for Health Care Policy and Research *Smoking Cessation Clinical Practice Guideline. Journal of the American Medical Association, 275,* 1270–1280.

Spoth, R. (1992). Simulating smokers' acceptance of modifications in a cessation program. *Public Health Reports, 107,* 81.

Strecher, V. J., Kreuter, M., DenBoer, D. J., Kobrin, S., Hospers, H. J., & Skinner, C. S. (1994). The effects of computer-tailored smoking cessation messages in family practice settings. *Journal of Family Practice, 39,* 262–270.

Strecher, V. J., & Rosenstock, I. M. (1997). The health belief model. In K. Glanz, F. M. Lewis, & B. K. Rimer (Eds.), *Health behavior and health education: Theory research and practice* (2nd ed., pp. 41–59). San Francisco: Jossey-Bass.

Sutton, S. (1996). Can "stages of change" provide guidance in the treatment of addictions? A critical examination of Prochaska and DiClemente's model. In G. Edwards & C. Dare (Eds.), *Psychotherapy, psychological treatments and the addictions* (pp. 189–205). Cambridge, UK: Cambridge University Press.

Taylor, C. B., Houston-Miller, N., Killen, J., & DeBusk, R. F. (1990). Smoking cessation after acute myocardial infarction: Effects of a nurse-managed intervention. *Annals of Internal Medicine, 113,* 118–123.

U.S. Department of Health and Human Services. (1988). *The health consequences of smoking. Nicotine addiction: A report of the Surgeon General.* Rockville, MD: U.S. Department of Health and Human Services, Public Health Service, Office on Smoking and Health.

U.S. Department of Health and Human Services. (1990). *The health benefits of smoking cessation: A report of the Surgeon General* (Publication No. (CDC) 90-8416). Washington, DC: U.S. Department of Health and Human Services, U.S. Government Printing Office.

U.S. Department of Health and Human Services, Public Health Service. (1989). *Reducing the health consequences of smoking: 25 years of progress* (DHHS Publication No. (CDC) 89-8411). A report of the Surgeon General. Centers for Disease Control, Center for Disease Prevention and Health Promotion, Office of Smoking and Health.

Velicer, W., Fava, J. L., Prochaska, J. O., Abrams, D. B., Emmons, K. M., & Pierce, J. P. (1995). Distribution of smokers by stage in three representative samples. *Preventive Medicine, 24,* 401–411.

Velicer, W. F., Prochaska, J. O., Bellis, J. M., DiClemente, C. C., Rossi, J. S., Fava, J. L., & Steiger, J. H. (1993). An expert system intervention for smoking cessation. *Addictive Behaviors, 18,* 269–290.

Velicer, W. F., Prochaska, J. O., Rossi, J. S., & Snow, M. G. (1992). Assessing outcome in smoking cessation studies. *Psychological Bulletin, 111*, 23–41.

Windsor, R. A., Cutter, G., Morris, J., Windsor, R. A., Cutter, G., Morris, J., Reese, Y., Manzella, B., Bartlett, E. E., Samelson, C., & Spanos, D. (1985). The effectiveness of smoking cessation methods for smokers in public health maternity clinics: A randomized trial. *American Journal of Public Health, 75*, 1389–1392.

# 12

# Stepped Care for Alcohol Problems: An Efficient Method for Planning and Delivering Clinical Services

## MARK B. SOBELL
## LINDA C. SOBELL

Compared to many health and mental health problems, knowledge about effective treatments for alcohol problems is modest and incomplete. Despite this state of affairs, health care professionals still must make decisions about what types of services should be used, with whom, and when. Although rarely used in the alcohol abuse field, there are principles that can help determine rational treatment decisions at the individual- as well as health-care-systems level. This approach has been termed "stepped care" (Sobell & Sobell, 1993b).

Stepped care is not new. The practice of medicine, in fact, is governed by such an approach. For example, physicians begin by evaluating a person's presenting problems, and then, based on the evaluation, an individualized treatment plan is developed. The treatment selected is expected to be the least intensive and yet have a good chance of a successful outcome. For example, if a person had an angina attack, the recommended intervention would not be immediate bypass surgery. Similarly, if a person is diagnosed with mild hypertension, an early intervention involves changes in diet and exercise, with medication prescribed if the problem persists or worsens. For individuals with very high blood pressure, a more intensive intervention might be the first step. The underlying principle, however, would still be to use the least intensive intervention that is judged as having a reasonable chance of success. Failure to respond to treatment would necessitate further assessment and more intensive or alternative treatment. Finally, whatever interventions are recommended, they should have a solid empirical base, or at least be consistent with current standards of practice.

In summary, the provision of health care services is based on three principles:

1. Assessment and treatment should be individualized. Different types and intensities of assessments and treatments should be used depending upon the presenting problem and other client characteristics.
2. The recommended treatment should be the one that is least intensive but likely to resolve the problem. More intensive treatments are reserved for more extreme problems.
3. Recommended treatments should be consistent with the contemporary research literature.

## THE STEPPED-CARE APPROACH

This chapter describes how the use of a stepped-care approach can improve clinical service delivery for alcohol problems. This approach is shown in Figure 12.1. The term stepped care refers to the way different intervention decisions are linked together, and to the guidelines used in making clinical decisions.

The stepped-care guidelines in Figure 12.1 are similar to those that apply to the provision of other health care. Considering the individual's history and presenting symptoms, current living situation, resources, and attitudes, the intervention should have a reasonable probability of a positive outcome. The judgment of a positive outcome should have a basis in the research literature as well as contemporary standards of care. As noted in Figure 12.1, this is where the concept of matching is important.

In the treatment of alcohol problems, client–treatment matching is receiving increasing attention (Mattson, 1993). At a general level, matching is straightforward. For example, a brief cognitive-behavioral outpatient treatment would not be viewed as appropriate for a cognitively impaired, homeless alcohol abuser. At the level of specific client–treatment matching, the process is less clear, however, as demonstrated by the recent results from Project MATCH (Allen et al., 1997). Project MATCH was a multicenter, randomized clinical trial that compared the effectiveness of three different manualized treatments: 12-step-based, cognitive-behavioral, and motivational enhancement. Development of the latter two ap-

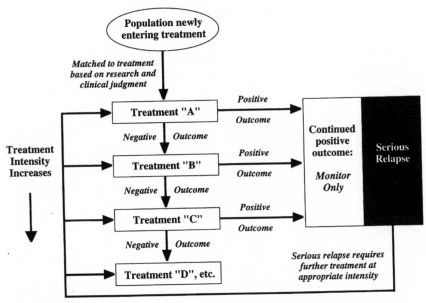

**FIGURE 12.1.** A stepped-care approach to the delivery of health care services. Adapted with permission of the authors from Sobell and Sobell (1993b).

proaches was based on research, whereas the former derived from popular but relatively unevaluated methods.

The main finding of Project MATCH was that the approaches did not differ significantly in treatment effectiveness (Allen et al., 1997). The approaches did differ, however, in terms of resource requirements and how much they imposed upon clients' lives. The motivational enhancement treatment involved 4 sessions, whereas the other two treatments involved 12 sessions each. Although there was no evidence that one treatment should be preferred over another, from a public health standpoint, the differences between treatments were great. For a more expensive treatment to be preferred over a less expensive treatment, the more expensive treatment should produce a much better outcome. It is not enough to produce a similar outcome to a less expensive treatment, as more cases can be treated with the same funds using the less expensive treatment.

A similar example to Project MATCH involves our recently completed randomized clinical trial that evaluated the effectiveness of guided self-change, a brief cognitive-behavioral motivational intervention for alcohol and drug abusers, delivered in either an individual or group format (Sobell

& Sobell, 1995; Sobell, Sobell, Brown, & Cleland, 1995). Guided self-change treatment was inspired by several lines of research that developed in the early 1980s.

One line of research that was relevant to the development of guided self-change treatment was research on natural recoveries from alcohol and other drug problems. It was becoming clear that many people had overcome substance use disorders without the assistance of formal help or treatment (Sobell, Sobell, & Toneatto, 1992). Recognition of this phenomenon necessitated a rethinking of how behavior change comes about, since, prior to that time, substance use had often been viewed as an inappropriate coping or problem-solving response. Use of the inappropriate response likewise was thought to reflect skills deficits. Yet naturally recovered individuals had overcome these deficiencies, if these were in fact their reasons for substance use in the first place.

A second important influence at the time was a report from Great Britain that male alcohol abusers who were treated by just one session of counseling/advice, had an outcome no different than that of men randomly assigned to receive the standard package of care, including even inpatient care if deemed necessary (Edwards et al., 1977). The key question, again, was how did people manage to do so well without professional help.

The third line of work that was important was Prochaska and DiClemente's work on stages of change, and in particular their separation of the phenomenon of deciding to change (motivation) and acting to bring change about (Prochaska & DiClemente, 1986). If in some cases the barrier to change was not a lack of skill but a lack of desire, that could explain how people could change on their own or as a result of a minimal intervention.

Finally, there was accumulating evidence that a large proportion of the total population of persons with alcohol problems had problems of low to moderate severity rather than being chronic alcoholics. Severity of dependence also was coming to be viewed as an important individual-difference variable because the British trial of treatment versus advice had reported an interaction such that less dependent individuals did better with brief rather than intensive treatment, and vice versa for those more severely dependent (Orford, Oppenheimer, & Edwards, 1976). Although that finding was reevaluated nearly 20 years later (Edwards & Taylor, 1994) and severity of dependence was found not to interact with treatment type, the earlier report spurred a large amount of research on brief treatments for the less severely dependent.

Guided self-change (GSC) was one of those treatments developed specifically for problem drinkers. An additional factor influencing GSC was Bandura's cognitive social learning theory (Bandura, 1986). Its contributions were important because it suggested that choice was an important factor in determining motivation, particularly choice of goal (Sobell, Sobell, Bogardis, Leo, & Skinner, 1992).

The major procedures involved in GSC treatment are described elsewhere (Sobell & Sobell, 1993a). Briefly they include goal self-selection, self-monitoring, brief readings and homework assignments, personalized feedback, and motivational interviewing by the therapist throughout. Recent versions of the treatment also incorporated decisional balance exercises developed by Janis and Mann (1977) to help clients evaluate the sources of their motivation. The emphasis throughout the treatment is on helping the individual to evaluate his or her drinking, become committed to change, and take actions to institute change.

In our recent study of the effectiveness of GSC (Sobell & Sobell, 1995; Sobell et al., 1995), the treatment was extended to drug abusers. Goals were self-selected, but it was recommended that drug abusing clients attempt to become abstinent. The study's main aim was to evaluate the effectiveness of the treatment delivered in a group as compared to individual format. Participants were 232 alcohol abusers and 55 drug abusers who had voluntarily sought treatment at the Addiction Research Foundation in Toronto. For clients in the group therapy condition the procedures were the same as in individual therapy, but topics were discussed in a round-robin fashion with the therapists responsible for promoting the use of group process and participation by all members (Sobell et al., 1995). As in Project MATCH, although there was marked improvement from pretreatment to follow-up, the major finding was that there were no significant differences in outcome between conditions for both alcohol and drug abusers. However, the group format was considerably more cost-effective, achieving a cost savings of 42% over the cost of providing individual treatment.

A final issue in matching decisions is client attitudes. It makes little sense to refer clients to treatments that they believe are inappropriate, and where the referrals are likely to result in those individuals dropping out of treatment. Client–treatment matching decisions, therefore, involve consideration of the feasibility as well as the efficacy of interventions.

Clinical judgment, as used in Figure 12.1, refers to a clinician's consideration of all features of a case in light of the scientific knowledge base guiding intervention decisions. An important distinction, however, is that clinical judgment should not be confused with a clinician's beliefs. In the alcohol field, clinicians sometimes have unquestioning devotion to a single type of intervention, seeing that approach as the treatment of choice for all clients (Miller & Hester, 1986). Such an approach is not consistent with "clinical judgment" as used here.

Finally, the relative cost of the available options should also be considered. Although this guideline primarily affects public services, it has increasing relevance for private services as insurers pursue cost containment. From a public health standpoint, funding is a major concern, because a limited amount of funding must be apportioned to achieve an equitable distribution of services. Today, as never before, the cost of treatment is an important consideration in the choice of interventions.

Until recently, the alcohol treatment field has not offered services consistent with a stepped-care approach. The field also has been deficient in developing and evaluating an array of services for the diversity of problems identified in epidemiological studies (Institute of Medicine, 1990).

The remainder of this chapter is devoted to discussions of how a stepped-care approach can be used by clinicians at the level of individual case management and by managers and health care policymakers at the level of health care systems planning. Other issues relevant to the role of stepped care in the treatment of alcohol problems are also discussed.

## APPLYING STEPPED CARE TO INDIVIDUAL TREATMENT PLANNING

Stepped care is relevant to both assessment and treatment planning. Research has shown that a large number of people have alcohol problems of low severity, and that such individuals often respond well to brief interventions (Bien, Miller, & Tonigan, 1993; Sobell & Sobell, 1993b). This, combined with the current emphasis on health care cost containment, suggests that, in many cases, a comprehensive assessment is not necessary. In fact, many studies of brief treatments of problem drinkers have been conducted in general medical settings and have involved very minimal assessment (e.g., Chick, Ritson, Connaughton, Stewart, & Chick, 1988).

With respect to nonintensive (i.e., brief) interventions, a concern is sometimes raised about individuals who do not respond well to such treatment. This concern is addressed by stepped care because it is a dynamic, performance-based procedure. If an individual does poorly in treatment, the stepped-care model suggests additional treatment planning, beginning with further assessment. At each level of care, the decision about what to do next is based on the individual's case characteristics, what has been learned from the failure to respond to treatment, and what clinical judgment and research suggest as the most appropriate next level of care. Neither assessment nor treatment are conceived of as single entities, but as processes that can be repeatedly enacted based upon treatment outcome. The performance-based aspect of the stepped-care model is one of its greatest strengths, as it results in the most intensive and, typically, the most expensive interventions being reserved for more severe cases or where less intensive interventions have failed.

An example of a performance-based stepped-care approach is a study currently being conducted by Breslin and his colleagues (Breslin, Sobell, Sobell, Cunningham, & Kwan, 1995). Results from a previous study found that problem drinkers who continued to have some heavy drinking days during the early course of a GSC treatment were likely to have poorer treatment outcomes than problem drinkers who reduced their heavy drinking early in treatment, even when pretreatment drinking levels were statistically controlled. In the Breslin et al. study, at the time of clients' third treatment session, those who continued to manifest heavy drinking early in treatment were randomly assigned to two groups. In one group, clients received a fifth session of treatment that involved additional motivational enhancement procedures, including a reevaluation of the basis for their motivation and the provision of personalized reminder cards that they could use when they found themselves in high-risk situations. In the control group, the fifth session involved a continuation of procedures used in the fourth session. The hypothesis that the enhanced motivational session will result in better treatment outcomes is currently being evaluated. This study illustrates how decisions about the need for additional care can be based on clients' early responses to treatment (i.e., performance-based).

Another important issue relating to a stepped-care model, and one that has assumed importance in the alcohol field, is the use of motivational interventions (see Chapter 4, this volume; Miller & Rollnick, 1991; Prochaska & DiClemente, 1986). If an individual is not committed to changing his or her behavior, then the intervention should address the individual's motivation before focusing on behavior change procedures. For example, it is not unusual for persons who have alcohol problems that are not severe to be extremely ambivalent about how important it is to change. They may have suffered few if any consequences of their drinking; thus, the trade-off is between the "risk" posed by continued heavy drinking episodes and the positive rewards also associated with the drinking. Until the individual has resolved this conflict and become committed to change, it makes little sense to have a clinical agenda that involves taking strong actions to change.

Two final issues regarding the application of a stepped-care approach to individual treatment planning concern (1) whether such an approach should be evaluated by research, and (2) whether the treatments that should be involved in a stepped-care model and the criteria used to move from one treatment to another should be specified.

The alcohol field needs a stepped-care approach, because most clients are still offered only one treatment, regardless of their histories or problem severity (Miller & Hester, 1986). Whereas other fields of health care have required that intensive approaches be justified and limited to the most severe cases, in the alcohol field, intensive approaches have become the standard approach, with less intensive treatments being viewed as in need of justification. However, the question of whether less intensive treatments can be effective for some proportion of clients has already been answered by numerous research studies (see Chapter 9, this volume, and reviews by Anderson & Scott, 1992; Bien et al., 1993; Kahan, Wilson, & Becker, 1995; Saunders & Foulds, 1992). In light of the evidence supporting brief interventions for low-dependence alcohol abusers, to assign such individuals to intensive treatment (e.g., 28-day inpatient program) would be unconscionable. Clearly, there is sufficient evidence for using a steppedcare approach with problem drinkers. In medicine, for example, it would not be seen as reasonable to conduct a study where bypass surgery was performed on all individuals who experienced an angina attack when it is known that less intensive treatment is sufficient in most cases.

With regard to specifying treatments that compose the ideal steppedcare approach, such an endeavor would also have little value. Considering stepped care to be a set of principles or rules has two advantages. First, it considers that individual differences should always be taken into account when making treatment decisions. Second, there are advantages to considering the stepped-care approach as a heuristic in a field where new knowledge is rapidly accruing and where the nature of the treatment system is similarly changing. Today's most appropriate treatment may be tomorrow's memory. Also, the setting and available resources place obvious constraints on treatment options. For example, if the treatment of choice is not locally available, it may be necessary to use an alternative treatment. Considering stepped care as a set of principles allows the field to keep up with changes in knowledge and to work within the existing service system.

The following example illustrates how the procedure can be applied. Consider someone who requests treatment and is evaluated as a problem drinker. Although a brief, self-change treatment is likely to be the treatment of choice (Sobell & Sobell, 1993b), that does not guarantee effectiveness. The outcome needs to be determined empirically, and further treatment decisions need to be performance-based. If the outcome is positive, then no further intervention is needed. If the outcome is negative, then further intervention is warranted and might involve a greater amount of the same treatment (e.g., additional sessions or additional procedures of the same sort) or an alternative intervention. If the client continued to show little or no progress, then more intensive interventions could be considered, or motivational issues could be reexamined. Other factors might also be relevant. For example, if research shows that clients' beliefs about what treatments are likely to be effective for them contribute to positive outcomes, then assessing and matching treatment orientation to clients' beliefs would be an important consideration in treatment selection (Cunningham, Sobell, & Sobell, 1996; Orford & Keddie, 1986). The heart of the stepped-care method is that reasonable procedures are sequentially invoked. Such an approach has benefits for individuals in terms of not intruding unnecessarily into their lifestyle, as well as benefits for the health care system by using costly resources only when necessary.

The value of allowing clients choice in treatment has been the subject of speculation but has seldom been explicitly tested. In areas other than substance abuse, the literature on the role of choice in therapy is sparse and inconsistent (Van Dyck & Spinhoven, 1997). In alcohol treatment, the issue of choice has focused on goal choice. Two studies have explicitly tested goal choice (Booth, Dale, & Ansari, 1984; Orford & Keddie, 1986) and found some support for the concept, but the designs have been confounded by self-selection; that is, subjects who had a strong preference for a particular goal were assigned to their preferred goal, and only those who did not express a strong preference were randomized to goals. A strong test of the importance of goal choice would require having subjects with a strong goal preference randomly assigned to either their preferred goal or to a nonpreferred goal. It also is known that problem drinkers prefer to select their own goal (Sobell et al., 1992). Of course, at a more general level choice is an integral feature of most treatments, beginning with an individual choosing to seek treatment and complying with treatment recommendations.

## APPLYING STEPPED CARE FOR HEALTH SYSTEMS PLANNING

To the extent that it is possible to estimate treatment needs (e.g., how many people may require brief interventions), the stepped-care approach can also guide health systems planning. As cost containment continues, the need for an efficient health care system is critical. Using a stepped-care approach is one way that health care managers will be able to lower costs. It is important, however, to distinguish between stepped care and managed care. Because managed care emphasizes cost savings, some researchers have questioned whether managed care accords much priority to producing positive outcomes for clients (Appelbaum, 1993). The paramount priority for stepped care, however, is efficiently achieving a positive treatment outcome.

A practical example of how stepped care can contribute to health care planning is that, until recently, residential, 28-day inpatient programs were the rule rather than the exception for treatment of alcohol problems in the United States (McCaul & Furst, 1994). These programs have continued despite an accumulation of epidemiological data showing that there is an imbalance between treatment needs and the types of services available (Sobell & Sobell, 1993b). In particular, there is a deficiency of treatment resources for individuals who have low-severity alcohol problems. As the alcohol field continues to evolve, it is clear that there needs to be a shift to increase the availability of outpatient treatments, particularly short-term interventions (Institute of Medicine, 1990). Other factors to be considered include whether services already exist or need to be established. One way of conserving resources is to encourage existing programs to change the services they offer. For example, if an area had an excess of residential programs and few outpatient programs, some residential programs could be encouraged to offer outpatient services, with the goal of phasing out their residential services over time.

The role of a stepped-care approach in planning such changes in the health care system would be to suggest the overall plan for the types and amounts of services necessary, as well as to identify where linkages among different agencies might result in more efficient services. From the standpoint of efficiency, there is no reason why any one facility needs to provide a comprehensive range of services, and there are benefits to agencies linking different services together. Thus, as economic pressures mount, greater linkages between facilities can be expected. Because stepped care is a rational approach to service delivery that emphasizes efficiency without sacrificing quality of care, it is also applicable to government health care (e.g., national health insurance) and to other systems of care (e.g., health maintenance organizations).

A concern sometimes expressed about stepped care is that a client might inadvertently be assigned to an approach that is not sufficiently intensive or that may even result in deterioration. This concern is not limited to the alcohol field but applies to all health care. It reflects our incomplete knowledge about client–treatment matching. The value of a stepped-care approach is that monitoring of progress is a key procedure. Thus, instead of assuming that a square peg will fit into a round hole, given sufficient time and motivation, the stepped-care approach emphasizes identifying poor fits and taking actions aimed at improved outcomes.

Finally, from a community planning standpoint, stepped care is not restricted to treatment services. For example, self-help organizations and methods to facilitate recoveries from alcohol problems without treatment are relevant. From the standpoint of minimizing intrusiveness and resource requirements, attempts at self-change should be encouraged when appropriate, complemented by advice on when to seek professional services, join a self-help group, or both. For example, we are presently conducting a controlled trial with persons in the community who are concerned that they may have a drinking problem are offered an opportunity to receive materials by mail that will allow them to evaluate their drinking and encourage them to attempt self-change. A randomly assigned control group receives educational materials. In accordance with a stepped-care approach, persons who attempt but do not succeed at self-change will be offered referral to an appropriate treatment program (Sobell et al., 1996).

Last, it must be acknowledged that stepped-care principles are likely to run counter to the views of many therapists in the alcohol field who have come to believe that one particular approach is appropriate for all cases. The stepped-care approach, therefore, is more likely to be adopted by service providers who are not ideologically wedded to a particular approach, and by policy planners and health care managers for whom the preservation of ideology is secondary to providing effective and efficient treatment.

## SUMMARY

The stepped-care model provides rational guidelines for selecting services for an individual, as well as for planning community health care services. The model is consistent with how professionals have provided services for other health problems. Economic pressures and the need to deliver effective and efficient services can be expected to favor the use of a stepped-care approach. The ultimate benefactors from such a change will be individuals with alcohol problems.

## ACKNOWLEDGMENT

The preparation of this chapter was supported in part by Grant No. 2 RO1 AA08593-04A1 from the National Institute on Alcohol Abuse and Alcoholism.

## REFERENCES

Allen, J. P., Mattson, M. E., Miller, W. R., Tonigan, J. S., Connors, G. J., Rychtarik, R. G., Randall, C. L., Anton, R. F., Kadden, R. M., Litt, M., Cooney, N. L., DiClemente, C. C., Carbonari, J., Zweben, A., Longabaugh, R. H., Stout, R. L., Donovan, D., Babor, T. F., DelBoca, F. K., Rounsaville, B. J., Carroll, K. M., Wirtz, P. W., Bailey, S., Brady, K., Cisler, R., Hester, R. K., Kivlahan, D. R., Nirenberg, T. D., Pate, L. A., Sturgis, E., Muenz, L., Cushman, P., Finney, J., Hingson, R., Klett, J., & Townsend, M. (1997). Matching alcoholism treatments to client heterogeneity: Project MATCH posttreatment drinking outcomes. *Journal of Studies on Alcohol, 58*, 7–29.

Anderson, P., & Scott, E. (1992). The effect of general practitioners' advice to heavy drinking men. *British Journal of Addiction, 87*, 891–900.

Applebaum, P. S. (1993). Legal liability and managed care. *American Psychologist, 48,* 251–257.

Bandura, A. (1986). *Social foundations of thought and action: A social cognitive theory.* Englewood Cliffs, NJ: Prentice-Hall.

Bien, T. H., Miller, W. R., & Tonigan, J. S. (1993). Brief interventions for alcohol problems: A review. *Addiction, 88,* 315–336.

Booth, P. G., Dale, B., & Ansari, J. (1984). Problem drinkers' goal choice and treatment outcome: A preliminary study. *Addictive Behaviors, 9,* 357–364.

Breslin, F. C., Sobell, L. C., Sobell, M. B., Cunningham, J. C., & Kwan, E. (1995, November). *Prognostic markers for a stepped care approach: The utility of within treatment drinking variables.* Poster presented at the 29th Annual Meeting of the Association for Advancement of Behavior Therapy, Washington, DC.

Chick, J., Ritson, B., Connaughton, J., Stewart, A., & Chick, J. (1988). Advice versus extended treatment for alcoholism: A controlled study. *British Journal of Addiction, 83,* 159–170.

Cunningham, J. A., Sobell, L. S., & Sobell, M. B. (1996). Are disease and other conceptions of alcohol abuse related to beliefs about outcome and recovery? *Journal of Applied Social Psychology, 26,* 773–780.

Edwards, G., Orford, J., Egert, S., Guthrie, S., Hawker, A., Hensman, C., Mitcheson, M., Oppenheimer, E., & Taylor, C. (1977). Alcoholism: A controlled trial of "treatment" and "advice." *Journal of Studies on Alcohol, 38,* 1004–1031.

Edwards, G., & Taylor, C. (1994). A test of the matching hypothesis: Alcohol dependence, intensity of treatment, and 12-month outcome. *Addiction, 89,* 553–561.

Institute of Medicine. (1990). *Broadening the base of treatment for alcohol problems.* Washington, DC: National Academy Press.

Janis, I. L., & Mann, L. (1977). *Decision-making: A psychological analysis of conflict, choice, and commitment.* New York: Free Press.

Kahan, M., Wilson, L., & Becker, L. (1995). Effectiveness of physician-based interventions with problem drinkers: A review. *Canadian Medical Association Journal, 152,* 851–859.

Mattson, M. E. (1993). Project MATCH: Rationale and methods for a multisite clinical trial matching patients to alcoholism treatment. *Alcoholism: Clinical and Experimental Research, 17,* 1130–1145.

McCaul, M. E., & Furst, J. (1994). Alcoholism treatment in the United States. *Alcohol Health and Research World, 18,* 253–260.

Miller, W. R., & Hester, R. K. (1986). The effectiveness of alcoholism treatment: What research reveals. In W. R. Miller & N. Heather (Eds.), *Treating addictive behaviors: Processes of change* (pp. 121–174). New York: Plenum.

Miller, W. R., & Rollnick, S. (1991). *Motivational interviewing: Preparing people to change addictive behavior.* New York: Guilford Press.

Orford, J., & Keddie, A. (1986). Abstinence or controlled drinking in clinical practice: A test of the dependence and persuasion hypotheses. *British Journal of Addiction, 81,* 495–504.

Orford, J., Oppenheimer, E., & Edwards, G. (1976). Abstinence or control: The outcome for excessive drinkers two years after consultation. *Behaviour Research and Therapy, 14,* 409–418.

Prochaska, J. O., & DiClemente, C. C. (1986). Toward a comprehensive model of change. In W. R. Miller & N. Heather (Eds.), *Treating addictive behaviors: Process of change* (pp. 3–27). New York: Plenum.

Saunders, J. B., & Foulds, K. (1992). Brief and early intervention: Experience from studies of harmful drinking. *Australian and New Zealand Journal of Medicine, 22,* 224–230.

Sobell, L. C., Cunningham, J. C., Sobell, M. B., Agrawal, S., Gavin, D. R., Leo, G. I., & Singh, K. N. (1996). Fostering self-change among problem drinkers: A proactive community intervention. *Addictive Behaviors, 21,* 817–833.

Sobell, L. C., Sobell, M. B., Brown, J., & Cleland, P. A. (1995, November). *A randomized trial comparing group versus individual guided self-change treatment for alcohol and drug abusers.* Poster presented at the 29th Annual Meeting of the Association for Advancement of Behavior Therapy, Washington, DC.

Sobell, L. C., Sobell, M. B., & Toneatto, T. (1992). Recovery from alcohol problems without treatment. In N. Heather, W. R. Miller, & J. Greeley (Eds.), *Self-control and the addictive behaviours* (pp. 198–242). New York: Maxwell Macmillan.

Sobell, M. B., & Sobell, L. C. (1993a). *Problem drinkers: Guided self-change treatment.* New York: Guilford Press.

Sobell, M. B., & Sobell, L. C. (1993b). Treatment for problem drinkers: A public health priority. In J. S. Baer, G. A. Marlatt, & R. J. McMahon (Eds.), *Addictive behaviors across the lifespan: Prevention, treatment, and policy issues* (pp. 138–157). Beverly Hills, CA: Sage.

Sobell, M. B., & Sobell, L. C. (1995, July). *Group versus individual guided self-change treatment for problem drinkers.* Paper presented at the World Congress on Behavioural and Cognitive Therapies, Copenhagen, Denmark.

Sobell, M. B., Sobell, L. C., Bogardis, J., Leo, G. I., & Skinner, W. (1992). Problem drinkers' perceptions of whether treatment goals should be self-selected or therapist-selected. *Behavior Therapy, 23,* 43–52.

Van Dyck, R., & Spinhoven, P. (1997). Does preference for type of treatment matter? *Behavior Modification, 21,* 172–186.

# 13

## Evaluation of Substance Abuse Treatment Programs in the Era of Managed Care: The Role of Cost–Benefit Analysis

RENÉ P. McELDOWNEY
JOHN G. HEILMAN

Weighing the costs incurred against the benefits received from a program or production process is standard practice in many sections of the economy, but it is by no means universal. The substance abuse (SA) field has been particularly slow to embrace this concept, in part because the benefits received from SA treatment and interdiction programs are too individualistic and complex to be measured by standard costing techniques. This perception is changing, however, as the economic impact of SA on the health care system and the broader economy is increasingly recognized. The high costs associated with SA and the U.S. government's largely failed War on Drugs have caused many within the public and private sectors to take another look at how treatment and interdiction resources are allocated. Economic and related considerations that have promoted this reevaluation include the following:

• SA has widespread, negative economic consequences. In 1990, the U.S. economy lost over $238 billion because of SA-associated costs related to lost economic productivity, crime, medical care, and SA treatment (Robert Wood Johnson Foundation, 1994). Alcohol abuse was most costly ($99 billion), followed by smoking ($72 billion) and illicit drug abuse ($67 billion).

- The number of illicit drug users has declined since 1985, but federal spending to reduce the drug problem has increased 400% since 1986 (Leen, 1998). In 1994, for example, the drug control budget was over $12.5 billion (Robert Wood Johnson Foundation, 1993). Most expenditures were aimed at reducing the drug supply through interdiction efforts and increased criminal penalties for drug trafficking and possession. Less than 20% of the budget was specifically earmarked for SA treatment, and treatment availability remains inadequate in many urban areas with high concentrations of substance abusers (Nadelman, 1998).
- Drug demand reduction strategies such as treatment appear to be more cost-effective in reducing drug use compared to interdiction and other drug supply reduction strategies commonly used in the U.S. War on Drugs (Rand Drug Research Policy Center, 1995).
- Within the health care arena, cost–offset studies have demonstrated that SA treatment tends to more than to pay for itself by reducing utilization of other medical services, which otherwise is higher among substance abusers compared to nonabusers (Fuller, 1995; Holder, 1987; Holder & Blose, 1992). Untreated substance abusers access the health care system up to 10 times more often than do nonabusers, and their families receive medical care at a rate up to five times more often than do families of nonabusers (Sax, Dougherty, Esty, & Fine, 1983).
- Compared to inpatient treatments for substance abuse, similar or better outcomes have been achieved by several less intensive, lower cost outpatient treatments (Holder, Longabaugh, Miller, & Rubonis, 1991; see Chapters 8–12, this volume).

Evaluating the economic dimension of various approaches to reducing SA is consistent with more general trends in health care and other areas of public policy. In an era of escalating health care costs and cries for smaller government, economic analysis of spending practices will increasingly determine which programs will be funded and the amount of funding they will receive (Holder, Longabaugh, Miller, & Rubonis, 1991). To compete effectively with other policy and budgetary priorities, health care, including SA treatment programs, must demonstrate both clinical efficacy (improved patient functioning) and economic utility (positive net economic return) (Holder et al., 1991). This chapter addresses this issue by discussing the evaluation of SA treatment programs in the current era of managed health care. As managed health care organizations have become the dominant players in the medical services industry, major shifts in emphasis have taken place in the conceptualization and evaluation of health services, including SA services. Although these changes are matters of tendency and degree, they nevertheless carry profound implications for the future of SA policies and services. The present chapter explores these implications.

Specifically, the conceptual underpinnings of SA services have shifted from an emphasis on medical treatment aimed at curing a disease through lifelong abstinence to an emphasis on psychological and social services aimed at improving a substance abuser's functional status, even if complete and permanent abstinence is not achieved. Furthermore, evaluation of these services is expanding beyond effectiveness studies to include efficiency studies. For purposes of this chapter, the notion of *effectiveness* emphasizes the impact of treatment on medical and behavioral outcomes. The notion of *efficiency* emphasizes the relationship of such results to the costs incurred to achieve them (i.e., cost–benefit and cost-effectiveness analyses that relate costs to outputs and outcomes). It is important to note that while cost–benefit analysis requires that outcomes and resources be measured in the same units, cost-effectiveness analysis does not (Yates, 1994). This chapter focuses on the implications of cost–benefit analysis for the development of SA policy and programs and the consequences for some of the major stakeholders in this arena. The chapter does not detail procedures for conducting a cost–benefit analysis of a specific treatment program. This information is available in Yates (1994, 1995), who discusses methods and justifications for incorporating cost variables into clinical research.

Our discussion has four objectives. One is to provide an introduction to evaluation in general and to cost–benefit analysis in particular. A second objective is to show how and why cost–benefit analysis will likely play a central role in the evaluation of health services and SA services. A related objective is to describe the Health Plan Employer Data and Information Set, or HEDIS system. The fourth objective is to suggest the implications of the HEDIS system for the future development of SA services.

To achieve these objectives, the chapter is organized into three parts. The first part provides a history of program evaluation. It is not specific to SA services but lays a necessary foundation for applications to the SA field. Applications to the evaluation of health services and current issues in the field then are discussed, including the use of the HEDIS system of collecting and analyzing program performance data. The final section integrates material from preceding sections to suggest some conclusions about the scope and limitations of cost–benefit analysis as a growing force in the field of SA programs and policies.

## PROGRAM EVALUATION
## AND COST–BENEFIT ANALYSIS

This section raises issues that relate to the conduct and use of program evaluation, including how the field has developed and how different types of evaluation activity relate to the policy process. The concepts of cost–benefit analysis and program theories and paradigms are discussed.

## The Growth and Transformation
## of Program Evaluation

Program evaluation did not exist as an organized field of professional activity in the 1960s, when government-sponsored social programs burgeoned during the Johnson administration, but those initiatives almost certainly propelled the field's development. Less than three decades later, the profession was robustly present, and evaluation has become a firmly established component of the public policy process (Rossi & Freeman, 1993). At the same time that program evaluation was becoming institutionalized in the policy process, it underwent a transformation with respect to its scope, underpinning assumptions, and research methods.

With respect to changes in scope, two pioneers in the field, Peter Rossi and Howard Freeman (1993), noted:

> Social programs and the evaluation activities that have accompanied them emerged from the transfer of responsibility for the nation's social and environmental conditions. . . . [B]efore World War I, the furnishing of human services was seen primarily as the obligation of individuals and voluntary associations. . . . Human services grew at a rapid pace with the advent of the Great Depression, and, of course, so did government in general during the period surrounding World War II. (pp. 16–17)

These events, combined with a broad range of related social forces and developments, including increasing deficits, the evident ineffectiveness of some large-scale social programs, the consumer movement, and calls for the limitation and reinvention of government, all contributed to an enlargement of the role and scope of evaluation activities in the mid- to late 1960s that continues today. For instance, a powerful confirmation of the place of evaluation in public policy appears in the passage by Congress of the 1993 Government Performance and Results Act. It mandates most federal agencies to submit strategic plans to Congress, along with plans for evaluation, and deems these "functions and activities . . . to be inherently Governmental functions" (S. 20, 103 Congress, 1st session, section 306e).

The same forces that contributed to the growth of evaluation also contributed to a fundamental change in the assumptions underlying evaluation and to a differentiation of the roles that evaluation plays in the policy process. Prior to the mid-1960s, evaluation research was viewed as an "application of social research techniques to the study of large-scale human service programs" (Rossi & Freeman, 1993, p. 14) and relied heavily on experimental designs as set forth by Campbell and Stanley (see Suchman, 1967, pp. 91–114). The reliance on experimental design reflected "the emphasis of evaluation [through the 1960s] on assessing the gains achieved in social and human conditions from social programs" (Rossi & Freeman, 1993, p. 22). During the 1970s and 1980s, however, evaluation activities were broadened to address not only program impact but also program design, implementation, and cost-effectiveness. Findings of limited effectiveness and serious questions about the benefits-to-costs ratios of federal initiatives indicated "the importance of undertaking program evaluation both before putting programs into place on a permanent and widespread basis and whenever modifications are made to them" (Rossi & Freeman, 1993, p. 22).

These developments led not only to a differentiation of evaluation questions and research methods, but also to increased attention to notions of program theories and paradigms. Both terms refer to sets of assumptions that link program activities to desired outcomes. The next two sections develop these points.

## Evaluation and the Policy Process

The experience of the late 1960s indicated that when programs failed to have their intended effect, the causes could potentially be traced to several points within the policy process. The practice of evaluation grew to include questions and methods appropriate to each stage of the policy process. Many different evaluation questions arise as the policy process plays out, and no single evaluation procedure can answer equally well all of the resulting questions.

The policy process generally includes phases or activities that form a cycle. The phases tend to overlap (see Dunn, 1988, p. 721) but can be treated as distinct for purposes of discussion. In settings that are reasonably well structured, the policy cycle typically begins when a problem is identified and finds a place on the political agenda. Alternative solutions, possibly including inaction, are proposed. Some solutions are considered, possibly through rational analysis. A solution is selected, and implementation takes place. The effectiveness of the policy is then evaluated in a manner that may or may not be systematic, and that may or may not take into account the benefits obtained in relation to the costs incurred. The program continues, is terminated, or is redesigned.

It is important to note that the manner in which evaluation results affect program status is heavily dependent on the style of decision making of policymakers or program managers. Appendix A summarizes different frameworks for decision making (Dye, 1984). Although detailed discussion of these models is beyond the scope of this chapter, the overarching point is that the translation of evaluation findings into policy outcomes is far from automatic. It is shaped and constrained by the values and processes that govern the decision in question. This point is returned to at the close of the chapter.

As summarized in Table 13.1, specific evaluation activities tend to be more applicable to certain phases of the policy cycle than to others. Definitions of the different evaluation activities are given in Appendix B.

In addition to drawing distinctions between different types of evaluation procedures, a distinction also is often made between two general uses of evaluation study results. *Summative* evaluation is concerned with deciding "whether programs should be started, continued, or chosen from among two or more alternatives" (Posavac & Carey, 1989, p. 12), whereas *formative* evaluation provides feedback that assists individual program design and implementation (Yates, 1994). Thus, summative evaluation is concerned with the impact of evaluation on the overall allocation of resources among different types of programs, whereas formative evaluation is concerned with fine-tuning and improving an individual program (cf. Yates, 1994, 1995). The distinction between specific programs and general policy also comes into play when dealing with program theories and paradigms, which are considered next.

## Program Theories and Paradigms

Ideally, policies are formulated and programs are designed and implemented on the basis of assumptions about how program activities will lead to desired improvements. At the level of individual programs, this set of assumptions is often referred to as a *program theory* or model, which may be implicit or explicit, and consists of "assumed causal relationships among

**TABLE 13.1. Evaluation Activities and the Policy Process**

| Stages of the policy process | Evaluation activities and issues |
| --- | --- |
| Problem identification | Needs assessment (what, where, how much) |
| Identify alternative solutions | Develop and specify policy options |
| Choice of a solution[a] | Policy analysis |
| Policy implementation | Monitoring |
| Impact assessment | Naturalistic methods, experimental methods, *ex post* cost–benefit analysis |
| Policy redesign | Draw on results of all of the above |

[a]See models of decision making in Appendix A.

resource inputs, and outcomes or outputs" (Rossi & Freeman, 1993, p. 58). Understanding a program's theory in detail is a key initial step in evaluating the program, because it will have wide-ranging effects on the goals, characteristics, operations, and outcomes of the program. Articulating the theory and its specific manifestations in terms of program processes and outcomes is basic to the evaluation process. See Suchman (1967, pp. 52–56) and Patton (1986, pp. 150–174) for discussions of how this is conducted.

When the issue is not evaluation of a particular program in a particular setting, but rather evaluation of competing approaches to programming, then more general theories or *paradigms* that underlie the different approaches to programming also can be articulated. In order to understand the implications of cost–benefit analysis, it is important to keep the different paradigms in mind. In the field of mental health (MH) and SA services, two distinct sets of organizing assumptions, or paradigms, have commonly guided the design of specific programs, namely, the physical disease paradigm and the mental health paradigm. Table 13.2 sets forth some of the differences between these two familiar paradigms, which re-

### TABLE 13.2. Physical Disease and Mental Health Paradigms

| Point of comparison | Physical disease | Mental health |
| --- | --- | --- |
| Conceptual approach | Treat biological causes | Treat social, psychological, and environmental causes |
| Locus of treatment | Inpatient, medical | Outpatient, in social setting |
| Treatment regimen | Established protocols | Emergent, based on facts of individual case |
| Staffing approach | Homogeneous | Heterogeneous |
| Salient staff skills | Technical competence | Humanistic characteristics such as empathy |
| Admission process | Brief history, bodily exam, detoxification | Detailed history, explore pattern of substance abuse and its consequences; detoxification, if needed, is only the first step |
| Focus of treatment | Patient as biological unit | Social system of which patient is a part |
| Treatment goal | Abstinence as cure | Mitigation of dysfunctional patterns; restoration of satisfactory functioning |
| Follow-up care | Limited after discharge | Goal is continued stability and maintenance of positive change |
| Economic cost | Relatively expensive | Relatively inexpensive |

flect alternative approaches to MH/SA treatment. The important point is that they lead to decidedly different questions throughout the evaluation process.

## Cost–Benefit Analysis

Cost–benefit analysis involves relating costs of services to outputs or outcomes such as the amount of services delivered or the impact of services on the recipients. Cost per unit of service delivered provides a measure of program efficiency; cost per unit of beneficial impact provides a measure of program effectiveness. Some variation exists in the meaning assigned to the terms "cost–benefit" and "cost-defectiveness." For some writers (e.g., Yates, 1995), the central issue is whether program outcomes can be measured in the same units as the resources, such as money, that go into the program. If they can, then the process is cost–benefit analysis; if not, the process is cost-effectiveness analysis. Others (e.g., Holder et al., 1991) have viewed the effectiveness question as asking whether treatment recipients are better off after they have initiated treatment, and the benefit question as asking whether society is better off after those in need have initiated treatment. In either case, the measures permit direct comparisons of different treatment programs.

The analysis of costs is standard practice in many fields and is essential for program management and accountability. Ideally, the analysis of costs should be broken down into different categories, such as "variable versus fixed, incremental versus sunk, recurring versus nonrecurring, and hidden versus obvious" (Posavac & Carey, 1989, p. 194), though these distinctions are absent in the emerging SA cost-analysis literature. High costs may lead to program discontinuation, no matter how many positive effects can otherwise be demonstrated. For instance, Mitlying (1975/1976) reported on the costs per hour of services delivered through a publicly funded alcohol treatment program. At $60 per hour of treatment, the program was seen as prohibitively expensive and was discontinued.

Another important issue in cost–benefit analysis is choosing the perspective from which costs and benefits are to be determined. Rossi and Freeman (1993) identified three different "accounting perspectives" from which costs and benefits can be estimated, including the perspective of (1) individual program participants or targets, (2) program sponsors, and (3) communal aggregates or society. If programs are to be compared, then the perspective from which costs and benefits are determined should be consistent across programs.

For example, from the standpoint of individual participants in a SA treatment program, costs may be limited to their own financial contribution, the time spent in receiving services, and the opportunities forgone through the investment of their time and money (Yates, 1980). The benefits would be the results that they personally experience (e.g., improved functioning and better health). From the sponsor's perspective, the relevant costs and benefits are those that accrue to the funding organization. Suppose that employees who participate in a company-sponsored treatment program for alcohol problems show reduced rates of absenteeism from work. The gain in productivity would be a benefit from the perspective of the sponsoring company, but not necessarily from the perspective of the individual worker. Finally, Rossi and Freeman (1993) observed that

> the communal perspective takes the point of view of the community or society as a whole, usually in terms of total income . . . [and] implies that special efforts are being made to account for secondary or indirect project effects—that is, effects on groups not directly involved with the intervention. Moreover, in the current literature, communal cost–benefit analysis has been expanded to include equity considerations, or the distributional effects of programs among different subgroups. (p. 378)

As cost–benefit analysis has gained ascendancy in the assessment of health and MH/SA services, so has the communal perspective, referring to costs and benefits for society at large. In order for these developments to be consistent with some degree of rationality in policymaking, it needs to be shown that societal costs and benefits of health-related programs can be measured and related to each other with reasonable validity and reliability. In the SA field, several recent contributions suggest that this goal is being accomplished. The cost of treating alcoholics is addressed in Goodman, Holder, Nishiura, and Hankin (1992) and in Holder and Blose (1992). Holder (1987) also dealt with the general health care cost savings that may be associated with alcoholism treatment, and Holder et al. (1991) provided a well-researched framework for relating the costs of treatment to the benefits derived by the patient recipients. As summarized by Holder and Blose (1992, p. 293), "Taken as a whole this body of research has established the potential of alcoholism treatment to stimulate a reduction in the total cost of health care."

## EVALUATION OF MENTAL HEALTH AND SUBSTANCE ABUSE PROGRAMS

MH/SA services are under increasing pressure to demonstrate efficient use of funds, high standards of care, and effective outcomes. Recent changes in funding resources, national politics, and employer attitudes have given rise to the popularity of performance measures. These factors and the various institutions and societal developments that influence them are discussed next.

## Focus of MH/SA Evaluation Efforts, 1970s–1990s

From a policy and program evaluation standpoint, the emphasis during the 1970s was on the amount of monies devoted to a particular system or program, and health and social programs, including MH/SA programs, became preoccupied with, and judged by, the level of inputs allotted to them. The rationale was that increased inputs would automatically yield higher quality outputs, and inputs were primarily defined in terms of financial resources, levels of staffing, and the procurement of new technologies (Harrison & Sheldon, 1994). During the 1980s, the focus of health and social programs began gradually to shift due to growing concerns about rising health care costs and mounting national debt. New policies were explicitly designed to encourage cost containment and to facilitate more efficient use of financial resources. This shift in governmental policy began to have far-reaching effects in how MH/SA programs were operated, evaluated, and financed, and it increased concern with overall service delivery systems, rather than with the amount of inputs or levels of funding for individual programs. Quality of service was increasingly equated with adherence to established clinical protocols (preestablished written treatment procedures) and required an appropriate orchestration of interdisciplinary teams of service providers. MH/SA interdisciplinary teams variously included subdoctoral counselors, social workers, psychologists, psychiatric nurses, and psychiatrists. The interdisciplinary team focus coincided with a trend in medicine toward considering the whole person rather than just the "biological patient."

To its credit, this systems approach produced some much needed efficiencies and better use of financial resources (Harrison & Sheldon, 1994). But it did not achieve significant long-term reductions in health care inflation. By the early 1990s, the situation had become so dire that health care policymakers actively sought new avenues to control health care costs and to evaluate system performance, and government and employers became increasingly interested in the value and efficiency of the health care system as a whole (Frater & Sheldon, 1993). The traditional U.S. fee-for-service (FFS) system and its perverse incentives that encouraged expensive, acute intervention at the expense of cost-saving preventive care (Holder et al., 1991) have been increasingly scrutinized and modified, either through explicit policy changes (e.g., in insurance coverage) or through the effects of market competition, primarily among managed care (MC) organizations.

The rising costs of FFS health care have caused many government officials and private businesses to consider MC. Whereas FFS medicine pays only when a patient visits a health care provider, MC ties financial remuneration to keeping patients healthy and seeks to avoid costly treatments and procedures. The shift toward MC is likely due to several converging factors (Harrison & Sheldon, 1994). First is the persistence of economists in arguing for the instrumentalist view of health care and its overall value to society. Second is the rising influence of health care consumerism, both at the individual and health-care-purchaser level (Seligman, 1995). Third is the increased media coverage of rising health care costs and health policy debates. And, finally, national demographics are changing. As the average age of Americans rises, more demands are being put on the health care system, which is financially and structurally ill-equipped to meet the often chronic health care needs of an aging population (Harrison & Sheldon, 1994).

## Frameworks for MH/SA Service Delivery and Evaluation

All of these developments have prompted concern with the effects of health care interventions on patients' health status (Frater & Sheldon, 1993). However, unlike many other areas of evaluation research, the desired outcome of MH/SA services can be difficult to define or measure and depend on the accounting perspective taken. Patients, mental health care professionals, and community officials often have differing opinions on what constitutes a positive outcome (Jenkins, 1990). For example, some stakeholders value only complete abstinence from addictive substances, while others regard reduced substance abuse or reduced substance-related problems as acceptable outcomes. These differing viewpoints make the systematic evaluation of MH/SA services problematic. Similarly, the practice of psychology, psychiatry, and other relevant disciplines is theoretically and professionally heterogeneous, and this heterogeneity inevitably spills over into the organization of services and the practice patterns of mental health professionals. This heterogeneity also makes establishing evaluation criteria and procedures difficult, as does the apparent greater variability in accepted practice standards for many MH/SA disorders compared to many medical diagnostic and treatment procedures.

Another issue is that quality indicators usually used in evaluating medical outcomes (e.g., eradication of disease and attainment of normal function levels) do not generalize easily to the evaluations of MH/SA services (Turner, 1989). If mental illness is a disease like other medical conditions, then the traditional medical model approach should apply, but "if it is more a personality disturbance based on dysfunctional learned repertoires, or inadequate adjustment to societal living, then the medical model is harder to apply" (Turner, 1989, p. 79). For example, one of the main factors used to evaluate medical quality is the technical competency of a physician. But in treating MH/SA problems, therapist warmth and empathy, which form the basis of the therapeutic alliance, are at least as important as questions of technical proficiency (Harrison & Sheldon, 1994). Furthermore, MH/SA treatments may include the whole family, not just the individual patient, and valued outcomes may involve such subjective measures as self-worth and emotional state. These difficulties are further compounded by the complexities of the multidisciplinary team approach and the increasing importance of external agencies and networks, such as social service counselors, teachers, and probation officers, who operate outside the usual system of health care delivery.

## Economic Factors in MH/SA Service Evaluation: The HEDIS System

Once regarded as trendy and experimental, MC is now seen by many as a major approach to controlling health care costs (Holder & Blose, 1992; Kongstvedt, 1996). This is true for both the private health care industry and federal and state governments in the case of Medicare and Medicaid programs for the elderly and poor, respectively. Over half of the nation's state governments are either actively considering using MC as a way of delivering Medicaid care or are currently doing so. And many predict that Medicare MC will be the way of the future as Congress attempts to deal with an increasing elderly population in an era of balanced budgets and a fiscally troubled Medicare Trust Fund (Nelson, 1996).

In the private sector, rising health care costs also have persuaded corporate America to adopt managed health care plans. During the past two decades, nearly all of the nation's Fortune 500 companies have experienced substantial increases in the cost of providing medical and MH/SA coverage for their workers, sometimes ranging from 15% to 20% per year. In reaction to these spiraling costs, over 50% of employer-sponsored health care plans now utilize some sort of MC plan (Jensen, Morrisey, Gaffney, & Liston, 1997). This has caused a major shift in how health care is both purchased and delivered.

Because MC relies on centralized data collection and recordkeeping, cost-conscience purchasers of health care can now obtain information on individual health plans and can compare their coverage and performance against other health insurers and MC plans (Cahill, 1994). One of the more popular systems for evaluating medical and mental health coverage is the employer-based cost–benefit analysis system known as HEDIS (Health Employer Data and Information Set). Developed by the nation's largest MC accrediting agency, the National Committee for Quality Assurance (NCQA), HEDIS is an integrated system that measures a variety of factors normally associated with quality health care. HEDIS began in 1989 with the support of four large private employers and a major health maintenance organization. Its objectives were as follows:

- To systematize the measurement process, using standardized definitions and specific methodologies for deriving performance measures.
- To enable employers to evaluate and follow trends in health plan performance and to compare performance across plans.
- To develop a common set of reporting standards that will address the needs of multiple stakeholders, including suppliers, purchasers, and consumers of health care.
- To address the needs of purchasers to track the "value" their health care dollar is purchasing and to hold a health plan "accountable" for its performance.

The NCQA/HEDIS group adopted performance measures based on a defined set of health care services and targeted for assessment and improvement five domains, including (1) quality of care, (2) access to care and patient satisfaction, (3) membership and utilization, (4) finances, and (5) descriptive information on health plan management and activities. Determining what to measure in each area depended on two factors: the ability of a health plan to collect a specific measure and the relevance of the data to the purchaser community. Thus, for example, the area of quality of care has been further broken down into the following subfields: (1) preventive services, (2) prenatal care, (3) acute and chronic illness, and (4) mental health, including SA services. For MH/SA services, the HEDIS system concentrates on the following parameters: (1) inpatient discharges, (2) percent of plan members who receive ambulatory services, (3) percent who receive follow-up care, and (4) readmittance rates.

The interpretation and use of these measures has been variable; the results can be ambiguous, and on occasion, the same data have produced different decisions about the utility of a plan or its features. For example, little argument exists about the value of childhood immunizations, but other HEDIS measures, such as those outlined for MH/SA evaluation, tend to be more imprecise and, therefore, open to varying interpretation. The only HEDIS factor for SA services that seems to have consensus regarding its utility in evaluation plans is readmittance rates. Programs with lower readmission rates are regarded as being more effective, but readmission rates obviously can be influenced by factors other than treatment effectiveness, including program readmission criteria, client characteristics (e.g., problem severity, economic resources), and program aftercare provisions.

It is cause for concern that the best HEDIS measure of SA program effectiveness (readmission rates) is one that is exceedingly crude in relation to the advances in measuring SA treatment outcomes that have occurred over the past two decades (see Donovan & Marlatt, 1988; Litten & Allen, 1992). The refined set of measures now available to assess key dimensions of SA disorders, including substance use, related psychosocial problems, and dependence levels, are conspicuously absent in HEDIS. The gap between the scientific literature on SA treatment outcomes and the cost-driven assessment schemes developed within the MC industry urgently needs to be addressed. Incorporation of cost-related indices into these existing scientific measurement schemes is likely to produce a superior assessment foundation for conducting cost–benefit analysis of MH/SA services (Yates, 1995).

While admittedly still evolving, the HEDIS system has become a widely adopted tool in the assessment of health service quality and value. Government officials have enlisted the expertise of its developers to help generate a similar system for the assessment of Medicaid and Medicare utilization. Even though many of its measures are rudimentary, the HEDIS system is quickly becoming the evaluation method of choice. A more positive contribution of HEDIS and related systems is the promotion of more systematic evaluation of health and mental health services. This will continue to change the organization and climate of health care systems in favor of evaluation activities as government and private purchasers demand greater accountability for the services they purchase. Clearly, the age of cost-irrelevant health care has ended, and cost–benefit analysis will increasingly influence health care decision making.

## The Importance of MH/SA Service Evaluation

As noted earlier, substance-related problems exact huge costs in terms of lost productivity, social problems, and health care expenses (Merrill, 1993; National Institute on Drug Abuse, 1991). State and local governments are perhaps under the most pressure to address SA problems, for these governments are responsible for providing MH/SA services for most of the nation's poor and disabled. This has put a tremendous strain on their budgets, which must balance competing health care interests with ever-declining tax revenues and federal funding cutbacks. As the demand for MH/SA services grows and funding becomes more scarce, it is only logical that the use of cost–benefit evaluation methods such as HEDIS will increase.

The precepts of specialized managed MH/SA care are based on the philosophy that early intervention, adequate follow-up, and outpatient care are effective alternatives to expensive hospitalization and restrictive treatment (Kongstvedt, 1996). Most experts consider the avoidance of costly inpatient treatment as one of the most cost-effective ways to control MH/SA expenditures (Holder & Blose, 1992). One study (Nelson, 1996) found that the average inpatient costs per day for SA services were approximately $267, compared to only $86 per day for outpatient clinical care. Thus, one of the principal indicators used in evaluating MH/SA treatment from the perspective of MC is the number of days of inpatient care. Most MC plans have strict referral guidelines and use various utilization review methods to reduce expensive hospital-based treatment.

Preliminary results indicate that managed outpatient treatment can be just as effective as inpatient care (Miller & Hester, 1986) and can be delivered at much lower costs (Holder et al., 1991; Nelson, 1996). However, when access to inpatient treatment is restricted in MC plans, outpatient treatment utilization does not always increase (e.g., Ma & McGuire, 1998), as would be expected if care were being appropriately shifted from an inpatient to an outpatient setting. Such findings raise legitimate concerns about whether MC plans can maintain, much less increase, access to MH/SA treatment for the population in need (Mechanic, Schlesinger, & McAlpine, 1995).

Another example comes from a Medicaid pilot project in Massachusetts (Nelson, 1996). Starting in 1992, the Medicaid agency initiated a pilot program to determine if health care costs could be reduced by enrolling MH/SA patients in managed behavioral health care. The goal was to restrain costs while maintaining quality of care by (1) controlling inpatient admissions, (2) monitoring utilization, and (3) contracting with lower cost, nonphysician mental health professionals. A 1994 evaluation of the program showed that the number of service users increased slightly from 21.3% to 22.3%, while the 30-day recidivism rate dropped from 19.5% to 18.9%, and overall expenditures decreased by 22%, or $46 million. Such positive results make managed mental health care an attractive proposition for state officials (Nelson, 1996). This enthusiasm should be tempered, however, by the negative effects of MC on costs, access, or both that have been observed in some states (e.g., Chang et al., 1998).

There also are legitimate concerns about the ability of a uniform medical model system of evaluation like HEDIS to evaluate MH/SA services adequately. This evaluation system tends to emphasize features of care that are most quantifiable and easily measured, rather than those that may relate most directly to positive outcomes. The evaluation and measurement of MH/SA outcomes within systems like HEDIS are not well developed. The MH/SA field thus has an opportunity and responsibility to shape the future of evaluation of its services.

## CONCLUSIONS

MH/SA evaluation has undergone over a decade of unprecedented change. Political and fiscal pressures continue to shape society's conceptions of health and government, and current trends in SA policy reflect the nation's limited financial resources, rising health care demands, and increased calls for public accountability. Cost–benefit analysis is at the center of this debate, as the various factions and stakeholders seek a verifiable mechanism to hold down costs without diminishing the quality and level of care.

As programs and procedures are increasingly scrutinized in terms of dollars expended and benefits received, the winners and losers will depend in large part on the evaluation system being used, and it will be the system used (e.g., HEDIS), rather than the various players involved, that will increasingly drive MH/SA treatment. Indications are that some of the winners are likely to include employer purchasers of health care and individual consumers of care. As treatment shifts from costly institutional settings to outpatient services, costs are likely to drop, and for many persons with MH/SA problems, less restrictive outpatient treatment is a viable alternative to inpatient care. Another likely employer benefit is the potential for increased worker productivity and decreased absenteeism. By holding the providers of health care accountable, the HEDIS system also encourages intervention at earlier stages, rather than at the more costly, later stages of problem development.

In theory, a cost–benefit approach to MH/SA services should increase the availability of care, although this has not always occurred within MC plans (Mechanic et al., 1995). Whereas traditional SA treatment programs often required lengthy institutional confinement, the cost-driven shift to outpatient care should remove a significant barrier to receiving care, namely, the time required for treatment participation. This shift also should make MH/SA services more affordable, thus increasing their accessibility to more affected people. Although reductions in the monetary and time costs of treatment will remove impediments to utilization, these changes will not assure that those in need of services will use them because of the stigma associated with MH/SA problems and their treatment (see Chapter 1, this volume).

Greater inclusion of MH/SA treatment coverage in MC health plans alongside coverage of physical health problems should help decrease this stigma. However, some fear that greater coverage of MH/SA treatment will increase demand and costs beyond a level that reflects genuine need because the demand for MH/SA services appears to be more elastic than the demand for medical care (e.g., Manning et al., 1987). This concern has perpetuated the long-standing trend for health plans to provide less generous coverage for MH/SA disorders than for physical health problems, a disparity that has recently been addressed in new federal mental health "parity" regulations (Frank, Koyanagi, & McGuire, 1997). The effects of the regulations remain uncertain, but they are not likely to close the gap in coverage between MH/SA and medical care because they allow for several exemptions.

Thus, providers of MH/SA services are likely to experience mixed results. As HEDIS or other cost–benefit measures become commonplace, many institutional treatment programs are likely to go out of business or to have to refocus their care. This is particularly true for the for-profit inpatient programs, which reportedly have high recidivism rates. Another likely consequence is that third-party payers will attempt to set reimbursement rates for services at the level acceptable to the lowest competent provider. In the MH/SA area, this typically is at the level of subdoctoral counselors or therapists. Doctoral level professionals will need to differentiate their more specialized services and to demonstrate their effectiveness in a cost–benefit framework in order to justify higher reimbursement rates.

Perhaps the largest benefactor of the cost–benefit approach to MH/SA service evaluation in terms of dollars will be the federal government. With an increased emphasis on early follow-up and outpatient care, the HEDIS system is projected to be a powerful tool in the overall effort to trim governmental health care costs. HEDIS provides government officials a means to hold providers accountable for treatment results. Programs that do a poor job can be identified and dropped from approved provider lists.

But the question of effectiveness still remains. For all of its possibilities, HEDIS and other cost–benefit evaluation systems tend to be rather crude and to focus on what is easily measurable, rather than on the more central elements of successful behavior change. Of necessity, these systems must rely on simple and easy-to-obtain measures to avoid being impracticably expensive and complex, but simple measures are frequently so rudimentary as to be meaningless or easily misconstrued. As Lebow and Newman (1987) asserted, what are needed are simple measures that are not simple-minded. In this regard, the SA field enjoys an advantage in that an array of clinically feasible measures of key outcomes are available in the clinical research literature (Donovan & Marlatt, 1988; Litten & Allen, 1992). The challenge will be in integrating them with the cost indices now so highly prized by MC companies and health care purchasers. Growing concerns about balancing the quality and cost of care, along with patient (i.e., consumer) activism due to problems with MC, will almost certainly create opportunities to revise evaluation schemes and their attendant measures.

Capitalizing on these opportunities requires an understanding of how the health care industry conducts program evaluation and uses the resulting data, which differs in significant ways from the conventional clinical research process, and which grew out of a tradition that has its roots in business and management, more so than in science. An optimal evaluation approach will likely be an interdisciplinary process, drawing from health economics, the program evaluation and policy expertise of the social sciences, and the treatment outcome clinical literature, while also considering the needs and perspectives of other stakeholders, including the purchasers, suppliers, and consumers of health care.

## APPENDIX A: MODELS OF POLICY CHOICE

A model is a simplified picture of the real world focused through a key "lens" that makes problems easier to analyze by drawing attention to a limited issue. No one model completely describes, explains, or fits all cases. Some models are especially well suited to describing economic choices, others are well suited to describing policy choices, and still others can be applied in both realms. In all cases, the model of choice that is operative will influence the policy outcome. This overview draws on material from Dye (1984) and Allison (1971).

- *Rational–comprehensive choice.* Costs and benefits of all plausible options are known and compared, and the option that yields the greatest net benefit is selected. A common criterion for determining the greatest net benefit is efficiency (i.e., the ratio of benefits to costs is positive and higher than the ratio for any other option).
- *Incrementalism.* Choices are made that continue past patterns of activity with only small (incremental) changes. The incrementalist view suggests that the rational–comprehensive model is unrealistic. Decision makers have limited resources, including time and information, and prefer to stay with arrangements that are known and that may have large sunk costs in them.
- *Pluralism (group theory).* The pluralist theory focuses on the competition of different group interests that is a common feature of social existence. Choices represent the outcome, or equilibrium, achieved by competing group interests.
- *Elite theory.* Decisions are influenced by the social elite—the few who are in the top strata of society in terms of economic power, political power, prestige, or all three dimensions.
- *Organizational process.* In cases where organizations are the setting in which decisions are made, outcomes often can be explained through reference to organizational structures (departments, committees, ad hoc groups, and procedural rules, including meeting schedules and rules of order). The notion of "standard operating procedures" plays an important role in this approach.
- *Bureaucratic politics.* Again, where bureaucratic organizations form the setting for decision making, outcomes may be explained by the preferences of bureaucratic actors to protect their organizational interests and to expand their bud-

gets, staffs, and responsibilities. Often, bargains struck among bureaucratic and political interests explain outcomes effectively.

## APPENDIX B: OVERVIEW OF EVALUATION ACTIVITIES

### Needs Assessment

The assessment of needs provides a definition of the problem to be addressed by stating not only what the problem is but also where and how widely it occurs. For a recent review of nine different models for assessing alcohol and other drug-related service needs, see DeWit and Rush (1996).

### Identifying Alternative Solutions

The specification of policy alternatives involves proposing strategies for addressing the problem and indicating whom the targets of the strategies will be. "Do nothing" serves as one option.

### Choice among Solutions

Once alternative policies or courses of action have been proposed, a process of selection among them takes place. It involves both the evaluation of alternatives and the authoritative choice among them. The methods of policy analysis (see Stokey & Zeckhauser, 1978, p. 584; Weimer & Vining, 1991, p. 584) offer formally structured and systematic ways of evaluating alternatives; the process of decision making often reflects less than the comprehensive rationality embodied in many methods of policy analysis. For an overview of some ways in which policy decisions are made, see Allison (1971), Dye (1984), and Appendix A.

### Monitoring

Once a choice is made and a policy is implemented, monitoring activities provide management with information concerning the extent to which activities envisioned in the policy are actually being carried out, how many resources are being invested in these activities, the extent to which services are reaching members of the target population, and the process by which those who provide services are dealing with their clients.

### Impact Assessment

Issues of program impact, meaning the extent to which the intended effect of program services occurs among recipients and the extent to which observed outcomes are attributable to the services, are often studied through experimental or quasi-experimental methods (Babbie, 1989). It is important to note that qualitative or "naturalistic" research methods are increasingly advocated as supplements or alternatives to experimental assessments of program impact (Erlandson, Harris, Skipper, & Allen, 1993).

## Cost–Benefit Analysis

The analysis of benefits and costs addresses the relationship between the resources invested in program activities and the extent to which the effects are attributable to program activities. If outcomes are difficult to observe or to quantify, then outputs, meaning levels of programmatic activity, may be related to costs. A large literature deals with issues that arise under the headings of cost–benefit analysis and cost-effectiveness analysis (see Yates, 1980, 1994, 1995).

## ACKNOWLEDGMENT

We thank Brian Yates for commenting on a draft of the chapter and James Murphy for assisting with library research.

## REFERENCES

Allison, G. T. (1971). *Essence of decision: Explaining the Cuban missile crisis.* Boston: Little, Brown.

Babbie, E. R. (1989). *The practice of social research.* Belmont, CA: Wadsworth.

Cahill, K. (1994, November). Group therapy. *CFO: The Magazine for Senior Financial Executives*, pp. 71–80.

Chang, C. F., Kiser, L. J., Bailey, J. E., Martins, M., Gibson, W. C., Schaberg, K. A., Mirvis, D. M., & Applegate, W.B. (1998). Tennessee's failed managed care program for mental health and substance abuse service. *Journal of the American Medical Association, 279*, 864–869.

DeWit, D. J., & Rush, B. (1996). Assessing the need for substance abuse services: A critical review of needs assessment models. *Evaluation and Program Planning, 19*(1), 41–64.

Donovan, D. M., & Marlatt, G. A. (Eds.). (1988). *Assessment of addictive behaviors.* New York: Guilford Press.

Dunn, W. N. (1988). Methods of the second type: Coping with the wilderness of conventional policy analysis. *Policy Studies Review, 7,* 720–737.

Dye, T. R. (1984). *Understanding public policy* (5th ed.). Englewood Cliffs, NJ: Prentice-Hall.

Erlandson, D. A., Harris, E. L., Skipper, B. L., & Allen, S. D. (1993). *Doing naturalistic inquiry: A guide to methods.* Newbury Park, CA: Sage.

Frank, R. G., Koyanagi, C., & McGuire, T. G. (1997). The politics and economics of mental health "parity" laws. *Health Affairs, 16,* 108–119.

Frater, A., & Sheldon, T. A. (1993). The outcomes movement in the USA and UK. In M. F. Drummond & A. K. Maynard (Eds.), *Purchasing and providing cost effective health care.* Edinburgh: Churchill Livingstone.

Fuller, M. G. (1995). More is less: Increasing access as a strategy for managing health care costs. *Psychiatric Services, 46,* 1015–1017.

Goodman, A. C., Holder, H. D., Nishiura, N., & Hankin, J. R. (1992). An analysis of short-term alcoholism treatment cost functions. *Medical Care, 30,* 795–809.

Harrison, S., & Sheldon T. (1994). Psychiatric services for elderly people: Evaluating system performance. *International Journal of Geriatric Psychiatry, 9,* 259–272.

Health Employer Data and Information Set. (1993). *HEDIS 2.0 handbook.* Washington, DC: National Committee for Quality Assurance.

Holder, H. D. (1987). Alcoholism treatment and potential health care cost saving. *Medical Care, 25,* 52–71.

Holder, H. D., & Blose J. (1992). The reduction of health care costs associated with alcoholism treatment: A 14-year longitudinal study. *Journal of Studies on Alcohol, 53,* 293–302.

Holder, H., Longabaugh, R., Miller, W. R., & Rubonis, A. V. (1991). The cost effectiveness of treatment for alcoholism: A first approximation. *Journal of Studies on Alcohol, 60,* 517–540.

Jenkins, R. (1990). Towards a system of outcome indicators for mental health care. *British Journal of Psychiatry, 157,* 500–514.

Jensen, G. A., Morrisey, M. A., Gaffney, S., & Liston, D. (1997). The new dominance of managed care: Insurance trends in the 1990s. *Health Affairs, 16,* 125–136.

Kongstvedt, P. R. (Ed.). (1996). *The managed health care handbook* (3rd ed.). Gaithersburg, MD: Aspen.

Lebow, J., & Newman, F. L. (1987). The utilization of simple measures in mental health program evaluation. *Evaluation Program Planning, 10,* 189–190.

Leen, J. (1998, January 12). A Shot in the Dark on Drug Use? *Washington Post Weekly, 15,* 32–33.

Litten, R., & Allen, J. (Eds.). (1992). *Measuring alcohol consumption.* Totawa, NJ: Humana Press.

Ma, C. A., & McGuire, T. G. (1998). Costs and incentives in a behavioral carve out. *Health Affairs, 17,* 5–69.

Manning, W. G., Newhouse, J. P., Duan, N., Keeler, E. B., Leibowitz, A., & Marquis, M. S. (1987). Health insurance and the demand for managed care: Evidence from a randomized experiment. *American Economic Review, 77,* 251–277.

Mechanic, D., Schlesinger, M., & McAlpine, D. D. (1995). Management of mental health and substance abuse services: State of the art and early results. *Milbank Quarterly, 73,* 19–55.

Merrill, J. (1993). *The cost of substance abuse to America's health care system: Report 1. Medical and hospital costs.* New York: Columbia University Press.

Miller, W. R., & Hester, R. K. (1986). The effectiveness of alcoholism treatment: What research reveals. In W. R. Miller & N. Heather (Eds.), *Treating addictive behaviors: Processes of change* (pp. 121–174). New York: Plenum Press.

Mitlying, J. (1975/76). Managing the use of staff time: A key to cost control. *Alcohol Health and Research World, Winter,* 7–10.

Nadelman, E. A. (1998). Commonsense drug policy. *Foreign Affairs, 77,* 111–126.

National Institute on Drug Abuse (1991). *See how drug abuse takes the profit out of business.* Rockville, MD: U.S. Department of Health and Human Services.

Nelson, H. (1996). *Treating drug abusers effectively: Researchers talk with policy makers.* New York: Milbank Memorial Fund Publication.

Nigro, F. A., & Nigro, L. G. (1989). *Modern public administration* (7th ed.). New York: Harper & Row.

Osborne, D., & Gaebler, T. (1993). *Reinventing government: How the entrepreneurial spirit is transforming the public sector.* New York: Plume.

Patton, M. Q. (1986). *Utilization-focused evaluation* (2nd ed.). Beverly Hills, CA: Sage.

Posavac, E. J., & Carey, R. G. (1989). *Program evaluation: Methods and case studies* (4th ed). Englewood Cliffs, NJ: Prentice-Hall.

Pressman, J. L., & Wildavsky, A. (1973). *Implementation: How great expectations in Washington are dashed in Oakland; or, why it's amazing that federal programs work at all, this being a saga of the economic development administration as told by two sympathetic observers who seek to build morals on a foundation of ruined hopes.* Berkeley: University of California Press.

RAND Drug Research Policy Center. (1995). *Projecting future cocaine use and evaluating control strategies* (Research Brief No. 6002). Santa Monica: Rand Corporation.

Robert Wood Johnson Foundation. (1994). *Costs of drug addiction: Report 14.* Princeton, NJ: Princeton University Press.

Rossi, P. H., & Freeman, H. E. (1993). *Evaluation: A systematic approach* (5th ed). Newbury Park, CA: Sage.

Rundall, T. G. (1994). The integration of public health and medicine. *Frontiers of Health Services Management, 10,* 3–22.

Sax, L., Dougherty, D., Esty, K., & Fine, M. (1983). *The effectiveness and cost of alcoholism treatment* (Health Technology Case Study No. 22). Washington, DC: Office of Technology Assessment.

Seligman, M. E. P. (1995). The effectiveness of psychotherapy: The Consumer Reports study. *American Psychologist, 50,* 965–974.

Stokey, E., & Zeckhauser, R. (1978). *Primer for policy analysis.* New York: Norton.

Suchman, E. A. (1967). *Evaluative research.* New York: Russell Sage Foundation.

Turner, W., III. (1989). Quality comparisons in medical/surgical and psychiatric settings. *Administrative Policy in Mental Health, 17,* 79–90.

Weimer, D. L., & Vining, A. R. (1991). *Policy analysis: Concepts and practice.* Englewood Cliffs, NJ: Prentice-Hall.

Yates, B. T. (1980). *Improving effectiveness and reducing costs in mental health.* Springfield, IL: Charles C Thomas.

Yates, B. T. (1994). Toward the incorporation of costs, cost-effectiveness analysis, and cost–benefit analysis into clinical research. *Journal of Consulting and Clinical Psychology, 62,* 729–736.

Yates, B. T. (1995). Cost-effectiveness analysis, cost–benefit analysis, and beyond: Evolving models for the scientist–manager–practitioner. *Clinical Psychology: Science and Practice, 2,* 385–398.

# Author Index

# Subject Index

379